LIBRARY/NEW ENGLAND INST. OF TECHNOLOGY

SO-EIJ-501

HV 1454.2 .U6 B37 2003

Batavia, Andrew I.

Independent living

NEW ENGLAND INSTITUTE
OF TECHNOLOGY
LIBRARY

NEW ENGLAND INSTITUTE
OF TECHNOLOGY
LIBRARY

Independent Living

Independent Living

A Viable Option for Long-Term Care

Andrew I. Batavia

NEW ENGLAND INSTITUTE
OF TECHNOLOGY
LIBRARY

ABI Professional Publications
Clearwater, Florida

l-04   # 53164048

Published by
ABI Professional Publications
P.O. Box 17446
Clearwater, FL 33762

Copyright 2003
Andrew I. Batavia

ISBN 1-886236-34-8

NEW ENGLAND INSTITUTE
OF TECHNOLOGY
LIBRARY

Manufactured in the United States of America. All rights reserved, which include the rights to reproduce this book or any portion thereof in any form whatsoever, except as provided by U.S. Copyright Law. For information contact ABI Professional Publications.

Dedicated to my wife,
Cheryl Nicholson Batavia,
whose partnership and support
have contributed enormously
to my quality of life.

Acknowledgments

This book was supported by a Mary Switzer Distinguished Research Fellowship from the National Institute on Disability and Rehabilitation Research (NIDRR), U.S. Department of Education. I am grateful to my NIDRR project officer, Ellen Blasiotti, for her ongoing support. I also want to thank my publisher, Art Brown, whose valuable suggestions assisted me in keeping on course. My able personal assistant of three years, James Cadigan, helped me in keeping track of the stacks of books, articles and papers in my office. Several superb researchers and scholars reviewed versions of the manuscript or provided me valuable information, including Gerben DeJong, Pamela Doty, Marshall Kapp, and Margaret Nosek. They contributed substantially to the academic rigor of the book, providing many interesting insights and suggestions. Of course, any errors that may be contained within are my responsibility alone.

I also want to thank my brother, Mitchell Batavia, Ph.D., who is a member of the faculty of New York University, for the excellent technical assistance he provided in helping me develop the figures in this book. His contribution was invaluable. Also essential for other reasons was the contribution of my children, Joe and Katey, without whom this book would have been finished much sooner, but also without whom it would have had far less meaning to me. As I have already indicated, it was only through the autonomy I was able to maintain through receiving assistance under the independent living model that I have been able to raise these beautiful children, the most fulfilling thing I have ever done in my life. As always,

I greatly appreciate the strong support of my entire family, including my parents Renee and Gabriel, Donna, Mitch, Genia, David, T.J., Ellen and Clifford.

This book is dedicated first and foremost to my wife Cheryl, who has been a wonderful friend, partner and the best personal assistant I have ever had. It is also dedicated to the many other individuals who have provided me personal assistance services over the years. Without their assistance, I could not have achieved what I have achieved, in part because I could never have gotten out of bed. There are millions of people with similar needs in the United States and throughout the world. In a real sense, this book is dedicated to them too. They struggle on a daily basis to ensure that their basic needs are met, and they deserve a full range of options for their long-term care. I hope this book contributes in a significant way to our understanding of these options, and to thereby increase the long-term care options available.

A.I.B.

Contents

Preface

I first started thinking about the topic of this book in 1973, although I did not think of it as long-term care at that time. In that year, at the age of 16, my spinal cord was severed in an automobile injury that rendered me paralyzed from below my shoulders and unable to use my legs, arms or hands.

At Rusk Institute of Rehabilitative Medicine in Manhattan, where I spent much of a year being rehabilitated after my broken neck was stabilized, I learned many things about adapting to my physical condition. One important set of lessons concerned how to hire and employ a personal assistant to help me in getting bathed, dressed and everything else I could no longer do independently. To me, this was not a long-term care issue; long-term care was for old people in nursing homes, not someone who just a few months earlier had run a marathon. I thought of my new need for personal assistance as a basic survival issue. If I could not achieve an affordable means by which to meet my basic needs, I would not be able to work, have my own home, and raise a family—goals I had always taken for granted.

Coincidentally, just about when I was flying through a windshield from the backseat of a stranger's car and being patched together again by some of this country's best health care providers in my home state of New York, something important was happening across the country. I was not then aware that these happenings would profoundly affect my life. A new social movement was being established primarily by working-age people with disabilities who wanted to live productive lives in their homes and chosen communities. This "independent living movement" would challenge the paternalistic way our society has always perceived and treated people with disabilities. It would alter the expectations of people with disabilities about what they could do with their lives. Although I regret that I was not around early enough to have been among the founders of this movement, I was among its early recruits and strong proponents.

Almost precisely two years after my injury, I found myself living over 3000 miles from home in one of the most unusual cities in the country: Berkeley, California. In addition to being the site of well-publicized demonstrations against the Vietnam War and other causes a few years earlier, Berkeley was the birthplace of the independent living movement. Partly through the efforts of its disability rights advocates, the University of California at Berkeley was one of only three college campuses in the country in 1975 that was being recommended to highly-motivated students with major disabilities. Consequently, once I was accepted, there was really no question that I would be attending this great university. The bigger question was whether and how I was going to survive my first year on my own in this distant and very strange land with no friends or relatives around to help in emergencies.

Berkeley in the 1970s had the highest concentration of people with disabilities living independently anywhere in the United States and possibly the world. Consequently, there were more people who required personal assistance services than any other community in the country. Those users of personal assistance services who had established themselves earlier generally had their pick of the best personal assistants in the community. Those of us who were recent arrivals had a much more limited choice. Consequently, many of the individuals who responded to my employment ads were people who were then referred to as "street people," largely vagabonds and other holdovers from the 1960s, many of whose brains had not fully recovered from that turbulent period.

In Berkeley, a person with a major disability would typically hire several different individuals for a specified number of hours at a time. I hired a weekday morning assistant, a weekday evening assistant, a weekend morning assistant and a weekend evening assistant. Each of these individuals would have to be trained by me, and paid by me on the basis of number of hours worked. Consequently, at the age of 18, while a freshman at one of the most challenging universities in the country, I had a payroll that was larger than some of the small businesses in the city. Because the work force was highly mobile, I was constantly in the process of searching for and training new assistants. At any point in time, it was not unusual for me to have in my employ one or two itinerant musicians, artists, members of Eastern religions or communes, and many self-proclaimed hippies.

I can recall very vividly one evening when I was in bed, my morning assistant – an extremely quiet and reserved individual – came bursting into my dormitory room loudly talking nonstop nonsense. He proceeded to open my window wide and throw his prized $500 guitar out the window into a tree, fortunately missing all innocent bystanders. He then departed my room leaving both the window and hall door wide open, and progressed outside to finish the job on his guitar by smashing it several times against the aforementioned tree, fortunately not in view of any environmentalists or music lovers.

After my dormitory mates closed my window and covered my exposed body, we debated the likelihood that my assistant, who had previously proven to be among my most dependable assistants, would show up the following morning. At 8:00 a.m., he entered my room as always without uttering a word, put on the Bob Dylan album as always, and began to bathe me. After a little while, riddled with curiosity, I asked him "Mike, what happened last night?" He quietly replied, "Bad trip, man," which was all I ever learned about the previous evening. He continued to work for me until the end of the academic year without another incident.

On one weekend, another personal assistant was scheduled to meet me at 11:30 p.m. in my dormitory room to assist my getting to bed. The great claim to fame of this individual, who was of the bisexual persuasion, was that he had attended over 100 consecutive weekend showings of the movie cult classic, *Rocky Horror Picture Show*, with its homosexual themes and an audience that participates by dressing up as the film's characters. On this particular Saturday evening, he was going to his show and I was going on a date with an attractive young lady whom I was set upon impressing. It turned out that I did leave a strong impression on her. Upon returning from our date, she opened my room door for me, and waiting in my waterbed was my dedicated assistant dressed in fishnet stockings and a wig. This required a certain amount of explanation.

In retrospect, I am somewhat amazed that I survived my freshman year of college, and that I did so with high grades. One could not imagine an environment less conducive to study, with strangers constantly wandering in and out of my life and the necessity to manage the equivalent of a small business enterprise without the possibility of profits. Even more important than the formal education I received that year was the informal education. Through the process of recruiting, interviewing, training, supervising and on a couple of occasions, firing personal assistants, I developed instincts about people and insights about the process that would benefit me for the rest of my life. After Berkeley, I had little doubt that I would be able to survive virtually anything, and that I could handle the many challenges that I would face in ensuing years.

After my freshman year at Berkeley, I transferred to the University of California, Riverside, and later attended Harvard Law School for my Juris Doctor degree and then Stanford University Medical School for my Master's degree. At each of these places, I refined the model under which I received personal assistance services. I tended to hire students who were in need of the income and who were much more stable than the workers I hired at Berkeley. Consequently, I did not need to hire as many individuals, and they stayed with me much longer, reducing the arduous task of training. I got better and better at managing the work relationship, which is a complex relationship in part because it often results in friendship, and the friendship can never take precedence over the work requirements.

Over the 29 years since my injury, I estimate that I have employed about 50 personal assistants. They have stayed with me from a few weeks to several years. Some have since become doctors, teachers and other professionals, and have taken their experience working with me to their professional endeavors. Most bring back warm memories; a few have disappeared from memory over time; some remain good friends; five attended my wedding as honored guests; and one has since become my wife of the past ten years.

With the assistance of these individuals, I have been able to maintain a sufficient level of independence to live in my own homes and maintain an active and challenging career, including jobs in the White House, the U.S. Senate, the Justice Department, the Department of Health and Human Services, an independent federal agency, a research center, a top consulting firm, a major law firm, and now at Florida International University, a Carnegie I research university. Five years ago, my wife and I adopted the two most wonderful children from Siberia. None of this would have been possible if my only choice was to receive my "long-term care" in a nursing home or other institution.

PURPOSE OF THE BOOK

The primary purpose of this book is to examine very closely the "independent living model" of care under which I and thousands of other mostly young and working-age people with disabilities are receiving our long-term care. This model also is increasingly being used by older people with disabilities. The independent living model will be compared with the more traditional models of long-term care under which the vast majority of Americans requiring extensive assistance receive their care – the "informal support model" and the "medical model." A fundamental premise of this book is that the independent living model has not received the attention it deserves from the mass media, the public and policymakers at all levels.

To the best of my knowledge, this book presents the first comprehensive comparison of all the major models of long-term care. In analyzing the various models, I attempt to be as objective as possible in pointing out the strengths and weaknesses of each model, and I hope others will do so as well in reviewing the analysis. Although I personally favor the independent living model for myself, as one person with a disability who strongly values personal autonomy, I definitely would not recommend it for everyone. It should be clear from my description of the model in this preface that it can have some major shortcomings and that management skills are key to success. As discussed in the book, such management skills may be provided by the consumer of services or by a surrogate if the consumer does not have the capacity to exercise such skills.

An enormous literature is available on issues of long-term care, including institutional care, home and community-based care, and personal assistance services. Hundreds of books and thousands of journal articles have been devoted to this topic; however, most of these publications are written from the perspective of providers or advocates for elderly people. Therefore, most of the long-term care literature does not address or reflect the independent living values of working-age people with disabilities or many older people with disabilities. Most of this literature focuses on the medical model of long-term care. Only in the last decade has there been a significant number of articles that address the independent living model.

The empirical work on long-term care and personal assistance services has had limited success in enhancing understanding so as to make long-term care services available to consumers in a manner that satisfies their needs, including the need for autonomy and independence. The current literature is highly fragmented and relatively inaccessible, except for that on the elderly. It is grounded in a theoretical framework that is not adequately known or understood by most policymakers or the public. This book attempts to consolidate our knowledge and understanding about this essential issue for all Americans.

This book hopefully will be considered important for several reasons at several levels and to several audiences.

- First, knowledge of the independent living model is important for consumers of long-term care and their families, and for individuals who wish to serve as personal assistants under the independent living model.
- Second, health care providers need to be familiar with the long-term care options for their patients, including options under the independent living model.
- Third, the synthesis of the research will provide government officials with knowledge about the independent living model and a basis for comparing it with the medical and informal support models; this will allow them to better understand the implications of their long-term care policies and develop policies consistent with the needs and desires of consumers.
- Finally, this book is intended to inform other key long-term care policymakers in the private sector, including insurance executives, officials of accrediting agencies, and foundation executives who address long-term care issues.

The greatest challenge of writing this book was to make it comprehensible, meaningful and useful to four very diverse groups: consumers and their families and personal assistants; health care providers; government officials; and private sector officials who address long-term care. The risks of writing to several different groups with different levels of sophistication, vocabularies, perspectives and interests are obvious. Yet, ignoring any of these groups, which will need to communicate with each other on an informed basis in addressing our long-term care policy, would have been more problematic.

The inherent challenge of writing this book was to do so in a manner that will make it accessible to the educated consumer, while avoiding undue jargon, acronyms and technical material. Separate technical sections and extensive endnotes are included to meet the needs of the more sophisticated analyst and to provide primary sources of information. The general public is encouraged to ignore this explanatory material, which is unnecessary for a general understanding of the subject matter. Those readers who are more knowledgeable of these issues and find the level of discourse somewhat pedantic will hopefully bear with me, recognizing the challenge of reaching a diverse readership, including many people who have never examined long-term care or personal assistance services.

Some may view this book with some skepticism, particularly some professional providers of long-term care. They may feel threatened by a work that considers seriously a model of care that does not use trained health care workers and in which they would play no major role. I ask that they recognize I am not proposing the independent living model as an alternative to the other models of long-term care, but rather as one option from which consumers may choose. There will be an enormous demand for long-term care over the coming decades, as the large baby boom population ages and becomes more disabled. No single model or set of providers will be able to accommodate this demand alone. All three models and variations of each model will be essential to meet this growing need for quality long-term care.

ORGANIZATION OF THE BOOK

The first half of this book (chapters 1 through 7) is arranged in a manner to allow the reader to assess the three models of long-term care independently. The second half (chapters 8 through 13) considers the various issues that must be addressed in implementing the independent living model. There is a small amount of overlap in the content of some of the chapters to allow readers to treat each chapter independently if they wish. For example, the reader who is already familiar with the independent living movement and related social movements that affect long-term care may wish to peruse or skip over that chapter. Generally, it is preferable to read this book sequentially in that the chapters are ordered in a logical sequence to offer a comprehensive understanding of the issues.

Chapter 1 provides an overview of the long-term care issue.

Chapter 2 provides an assessment of the long-term care population from several different perspectives. The objective is to provide a general picture of who needs long-term care services, who receives such services currently, how such services are received, and how these parameters are likely to change over time. Only by understanding this population can we develop an understanding of the models and services of long-term care that meet their needs.

Chapter 3 offers a brief history and philosophy of the independent living movement. As indicated, this book is written from an independent living perspective. Those who contend that the book is biased are, in a sense, correct, although this does not take away from the validity of the analysis or its potential importance. Every analysis is written from some perspective, but the values and assumptions of the analysis are not always stated explicitly. Many analyses of long-term care that have been conducted implicitly adopted the perspectives and values of medical model providers. What is unique about this book is that it explicitly adopts the values of the independent living movement. Once critics understand these values, they are free to criticize them, the criteria based on them, and the conclusions of the analysis.

Chapter 4 considers the two key related concepts of consumer direction and consumer choice, distinguishing them and discussing their evolution and application to different populations of people with disabilities who require long-term care.

Chapter 5 examines in depth the three models of long-term care—the informal support model, the medical model and the independent living model. These models are considered both theoretically and in their practical implementation.

Chapter 6 then discusses the various sub-models of the independent living model. Specifically, it examines different state programs, the Cash and Counseling Demonstration and Evaluation, and support from intermediary service organizations.

Chapter 7 defines and applies six specific criteria for assessing models of long-term care: affordability; quality, accountability; autonomy; security and manageability. In applying the criteria to each model systematically, the strengths and weaknesses of each model are identified, analyzed and presented graphically.

Chapter 8 looks at financing options that are available to expand access to personal assistance services under the independent living model. In doing so, it briefly summarizes the current mechanisms of financing such services.

Chapter 9 considers workforce issues, such as whether the number of potential personnel to serve as nurses aides under the medical model and as personal assistants under the independent living model will be adequate to meet the needs of the rapidly growing long-term care consumer population. This chapter also examines public policies that affect the current and potential workforce.

Chapter 10 considers options for ensuring quality under the independent living model. Mechanisms based upon structure, process and outcome are examined with respect to compatibility with this model.

Chapter 11 examines how personal assistance services fit into the broader health care system, including the relationship of such services to acute care services provided by managed care organizations.

Chapter 12 discusses the ways in which variations of the independent living model have been implemented in other countries, such as the Netherlands, Austria, France and Germany.

Chapter 13 draws general conclusions from the overall analysis of the comparison of the three broad models of long-term care, and the specific issues concerning implementation of the independent living model. It concludes that the independent living model should be one of the options available to consumers. This model is increasingly likely to be included as an option for long-term care over time.

Andrew I. Batavia
Florida International University
January 2003

IN REMEMBRANCE
Andrew I. Batavia
1957–2003

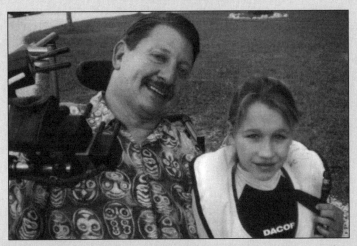

The true measure of any man's legacy is how many lives he has touched. And the legacy of Drew Batavia is far reaching. While working in the Office of the United States Attorney General, Drew helped usher in a new era of independence and opportunity by crafting portions of *The Americans with Disabilities Act of 1990*. Afterward, he fought to ensure that this landmark piece of legislation reached its fullest potential as executive director of the National Council on Disability and later as a member of Senator John McCain's staff. Throughout his life Drew continued to fight for everyone's right to equal opportunity and in 1997 became a teacher and mentor for the next generation of leaders by joining the faculty at Florida International University. Drew Batavia touched countless lives.

I am proud to have counted Drew a friend and colleague. When we founded National Rehabilitation Hospital in 1986, he joined our team to help create a research center whose mission was to empower people with disabilities. Today, the NRH Center for Health & Disability Research is one of the leading policy research centers in Washington. Indeed, we owe a great debt to the legacy of Drew Batavia.

—Edward A. Eckenhoff
   President and Chief Executive Officer
   National Rehabilitation Hospital
   Washington, D.C.

One of the central choices of our time, in health and in other areas, is finding the proper balance between individual (personal) and collective (social) responsibility. If too much weight is given to the former, we come close to recreating the "jungle"—with all the freedom and all the insecurity that the jungle implies. On the other hand, emphasizing social responsibility can increase security, but it may be the security of the "zoo" purchased at the expense of freedom.

Victor R. Fuchs, Ph.D.
Who Shall Live? 1973

1

The Jungle vs. the Zoo

One seldom hears anyone say, "I can't wait to live in a nursing home." Nursing facilities conjure up images of large numbers of elderly people waiting to die in a highly institutionalized setting, with care provided in an impersonal and regimented manner. While the best nursing homes may provide an excellent quality of care and recreational activities, few individuals would choose to live for the remainder of their lives in such facilities if they had the option to receive comparable services and opportunities in their homes and communities. This book considers an option that has not been adequately examined by the public for people of all ages with virtually any type of disability to obtain their long-term care and assistance while living "independently" at home.[1]

THE NATURE OF LONG-TERM CARE

Traditionally, people with disabilities who have been able to receive long-term care in their homes and communities received such services from family members and friends who were not compensated financially, or from health care workers through nursing homes and home health agencies. Yet living at home itself does not guarantee that individuals will receive their care according to their preferences. One of the most prominent experts on long-term care has said, "One's own home can be as restrictive as a nursing home, if an individual is homebound and is not getting the services that would facilitate some independence."[2]

1

Despite dissatisfaction with the limited options available, until recently our nation's long-term care policy has focused almost exclusively on providing institutional care and other medically oriented care. This policy has been in effect because policymakers have concentrated primarily on the sickest members of the frail elderly population, many of whom have major cognitive problems and limited decisional capacity. Due to their extensive need for medical services, it is not surprising that determinations have been made to provide their care in health care facilities or at their homes by health care personnel.

However, the majority of people who need long-term care do not require constant medical attention. They need help in conducting basic life activities, which could potentially be provided by any capable person willing and able to provide such assistance and to some extent by assistive technology (e.g., wheelchairs, environmental control systems, communication devices, adapted tools and utensils, and automatic door openers). The goal is to assist consumers in doing what they would otherwise be able to do for themselves, if not for their functional limitations.

Moreover, there is nothing inherent in the nature of long-term care that requires such services to be provided by health care professionals. Long-term care has been defined as: "assistance given over a sustained period of time to people who are experiencing long-term inabilities or difficulties in functioning because of a disability."[3] This definition does not focus on medical assistance, and the vast majority of long-term care services can be and are provided by people who are not health care professionals.[4]

Compared with other types of health care, long-term care is unique in the extent to which it pervades every aspect of the recipient's life. In a very real sense, long-term care becomes the context in which all other aspects of life are affected. As Kane and her colleagues pointed out in *The Heart of Long-term Care*:

> Long-term care is not an extension of acute care—it is distinctive in its very nature. Because long-term care continues for prolonged periods, it becomes enmeshed in the very fabric of people's lives. Unlike the situation with acute care, where lifestyles may be temporarily disrupted in pursuit of tangible gains in health (for example, by an admission to the hospital), the predominant strategy in long-term care emphasizes integration of treatment and

living. The point is not to ignore or undervalue health care for those getting long-term care, but to incorporate health care into the context of daily life. Ironically, this principle is most dramatically violated in the most visible embodiment of long-term care, the nursing home.[5]

LONG-TERM CARE SERVICES

Although there are many ways to conceptualize and categorize long-term care services, one straightforward and instructive approach is to divide them into three components: personal assistance services; medical and health care services; and other support services.

Personal Assistance Services

While many analysts would begin by describing medical and other health care services for long-term care consumers, the essence of long-term care is the provision of non-medical personal assistance services that help people with disabilities with functions they are not able to perform without assistance, or that they can perform only with great effort. Such life functions are often referred to as "the activities of daily living" (ADLs) and "the instrumental activities of daily living" (IADLs).[6]

ADLs include basic self-help functions, such as bathing, dressing, eating, using the toilet, and transferring in and out of beds and chairs. IADLs include other tasks necessary for independent living in the community, such as cooking, cleaning, shopping, doing laundry, using a telephone, reading mail, following instructions, and paying bills. An individual's ability to conduct both ADLs and IADLs, or to have them conducted on the individual's behalf, is essential for the individual to function as independently as possible.

In this book, "personal assistance services" are defined as any services provided to assist people with substantial disabilities with the ADLs and/or IADLs. Such services are necessary for people who have limitations in their abilities to conduct such activities independently without assistance. Due to their non-medical nature, these services can be provided by virtually anyone willing and able to provide them. There is no reason to believe that people trained under the health care system will provide these personal assistance services better than those without such training.

Medical and Health Care Services

The general public perception is that the vast majority of long-term care services are medical in nature, because of the disproportionate press coverage of long-term care services provided in institutions such as nursing homes. In fact, most hours of human interaction in these facilities entail the provision of personal assistance services. It is true that long-term care consumers, like all people, have medical needs. Due to their chronic conditions and disabilities, some of these individuals require extensive medical assistance. On average, people with disabilities have greater health care needs than people without disabilities; however, such averages may obscure the fact that some people with disabilities and long-term care needs require less than average medical care, depending in part on their particular disabilities and medical conditions.[7] Enormous variation exists in medical need, demand and use within the disability population.

Even for those long-term care consumers with substantial medical problems, the need for non-medical personal assistance services typically demands substantially more hours of intervention than the need for medical services. Those services that are truly medical in nature must be performed by health care professionals. The clearest example is any type of surgical intervention. Surgery obviously requires extensive medical training, in part because it is potentially harmful or even lethal; the public must be protected against unqualified individuals conducting surgical procedures. The same is not true of most non-invasive procedures.

Many services that health care professionals might characterize as medical or health care services are actually in a gray area between medical and personal assistance services. *See* Figure 1. Many of these services, such as the insertion of urinary catheters, enemas, and suppositories and the application of dressings, have been labeled medical in nature. However, these services really do not require extensive medical training and generally do not pose a substantial risk of harm; virtually anyone of average intellect can be trained to perform these services competently and safely. After all, the nursing home aides and home health aides who regularly perform these functions are just average individuals with relatively little training.

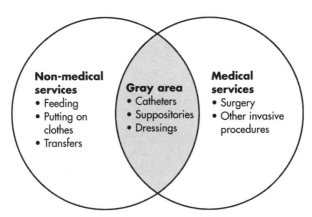

Figure 1: **Non-Medical vs. Medical Long-Term Care Services**

There is an ongoing debate over which types of services should be provided by health care professionals and which may be performed by anyone.[8] For example, bathing and dressing the consumer are not health care procedures, and may be performed by anyone willing and able to do so. Of course, even these non-medical services can pose certain risks of harm under certain circumstances. For example, some individuals with disabilities have very fragile bones (e.g., from osteoporosis) or painful hypersensitivity (e.g., from arthritis or decubitus ulcers), and they must be bathed and dressed very carefully to avoid harm. However, the general point remains valid, that anyone of average intellect and physical capability can learn to conduct such functions competently and safely without health care training and credentialing.

Some procedures that may appear to require some health care training, such as the application of an external catheter needed by a person with urinary incontinence or the insertion of a suppository for bowel evacuation, should not be considered medical procedures; they really do not require the training and expertise of a health care professional. Even some procedures that are more invasive or technical, such as the insertion of an internal urinary catheter or the changing of a wound dressing, can be taught easily to non-health care workers. Such procedures are performed competently many thousands of times every day throughout the country by family members and personal assistants with no health care training.

This debate over who may perform certain procedures considers whether state Nurse Practice Acts prohibit non-health-care professionals from performing these functions. Appendix A provides an

A Note on Terminology

There is no consensus on what to call people who receive long-term care services. The term "patient" is deeply rooted in the medical model of care, and implies that the individual receiving care is a passive recipient of care prescribed by health care professionals. In this book, the term "consumer" or "recipient" is used to characterize the individual who receives long-term care. These terms are more neutral than other terms, in that they are not biased on the basis of residency versus non-residency, program status, or long-term care model. The term "patient" is only used when referring to an individual who is in the process of receiving actual medical services. This terminology has important implications, because the concept of "patient" is associated with the "sick role" in which such individuals are excused from normal societal expectations such as work, a notion rejected by independent living advocates.

The term "medical model" may mean different things to different people. In this book, medical model is used very specifically to refer to long-term care directed and provided under the supervision of health care professionals. Although the term is often used by disability rights advocates in a derogatory fashion due to the control that is allegedly exercised over consumers, that connotation should not be inferred by readers.

In this book, the often-used term "home and community-based services" (HCBS) is used very broadly to include all services provided in the consumer's home or community, including home care under the medical model and personal assistance services under the independent living model. The term "home care" is used exclusively to refer to services provided in the consumer's home by health care professionals and para-professionals under the medical model. The term "personal assistance services" refers exclusively to human services provided under the independent living model to assist people with disabilities in the activities of daily living and the instrumental activities of daily living in any setting according to the direction of the consumer.

Even the term "care" is objectionable to many independent living advocates, who regard the term as a paternalistic sentiment of the medical model. They prefer the term "assistance," which is more neutral with respect to models of care and less paternalistic. They also reject "home-based care," stressing that such services are often needed in work, school and other settings, as well as the home. However, the general public is accustomed to referring to long-term care services as care. Throughout the book, both terms "care" and "assistance" are used generically and synonymously to describe the same services; "care" is typically used in describing services under the medical model and "assistance" is typically used in describing services provided under the independent living model.

The terms "informal care" and "formal care" are used frequently in the long-term care literature. Informal care should be interpreted as unpaid care, as implied by the informal support model. Formal care should be interpreted as paid care. Formal care can be provided under either the medical model or the independent living model.

Finally, terms relating to consumer control of services tend to be used very loosely and inconsistently in the health care literature. In this book, the terms "consumer direction," "consumer control," and "consumer autonomy" are used synonymously to refer to the self-determination of consumers over when, how and by whom their long-term care services are provided. The term "consumer-directed personal assistance services," as used in this book, refers exclusively to services provided under the independent living model.

It is hoped that the conventions used in this book, which entail more narrow and precise definitions of terms than often used in the field, will be adopted for discourse on long-term care generally. For the debate on long-term care to advance, it will be necessary to apply a clear and consistent nomenclature. A glossary is provided to achieve this objective.

extensive discussion of this issue. Independent living advocates argue strongly that the consumer should be able to decide who can perform such functions, because consumers should be allowed to control their own bodies; the consumers would perform the functions themselves if they could.[9] People with paraplegia can catheterize themselves using their arm and hand function, so why shouldn't people with quadriplegia be allowed to hire assistants to conduct the same procedure under their supervision simply because they do not have adequate arm and hand function?

Other Support Services

Other than personal assistance services and medical/health care services, long-term care entails a variety of other support services, including case management, social work, home modifications, assistive technologies, psychosocial rehabilitation and other specialized products and services. Although these support services are not the focus of this book, it is important to recognize that they are often essential to the optimal functioning of consumers. Moreover, some of these services can serve as partial substitutes for personal assistance services; the amount of personal assistance services needed may be reduced as a result of the availability of such other support services.

The prime example of support services serving as a partial substitute for personal assistance is assistive technology. For example, a home modification involving the installation of an automatic door opener can result in less need for personal assistants to be available to the consumer. Although such a door opener may cost over a thousand dollars, it could save tens of thousands of dollars in personal assistance over a period of years. Another example is a wheelchair cushion that allows consumers to sit in their wheelchairs for longer periods of time, thereby allowing them to be on their own for longer periods without having their assistants available. Still another example concerns the use of service animals such as dogs trained to assist people who are blind, deaf or paralyzed.

Although the benefits of support services, assistive technology and service animals can be dramatic, they should not be viewed unrealistically as full substitutes for personal assistance services. A person with substantial disabilities will require a certain level of services that can only be provided by another human being. The support services should be regarded as an important component of the package of services needed by consumers of long-term care, the most central of which is typically personal assistance services.

MODELS OF LONG-TERM CARE

When Americans think about long-term care, they visualize care under what has been referred to as "the medical model." Under the medical model of long-term care, individuals trained as health care workers, supervised by physicians and nurses, provide services to the consumer, who is considered a "patient."[10] The broad array of different types of medical model providers, which are heavily regulated, includes nursing homes, home health agencies, adult day care centers, and assisted living facilities, as well as individual practitioners. The public has focused primarily on the medical model as a result of constant press coverage of nursing homes, home health agencies and other health care providers of long-term care. Indeed, the concept of the long-term care institution as *the* provider of long-term care in this country is so ingrained that most Americans would say that they are not familiar with other models of long-term care; however, the medical model is not even the most prevalent model of long-term care in this country.

The dominant model of long-term care is, and has always been, the "informal support model." Under this model, the family members and friends of the individual needing care provide assistance that is not compensated financially. The obvious advantage of this model to the consumer and other potential payors (e.g., state and federal government) is that it is affordable, in that uncompensated assistance does not entail direct financial costs for them. The disadvantage is that it often imposes large physical and emotional costs on the family members and friends providing care, and it sometimes results in unhealthy relationships of dependency.

A third model of long-term care that is largely unknown to the public, and even to much of the health care industry, is the "independent living model," often referred to as "consumer-directed personal assistance services."[11] This model involves the provision of compensated personal assistance services to the consumer—the person who requires the long-term care services—by an individual who is not a health care worker. The provider under this model is called a "personal assistant,"[12] and is recruited, hired, trained, managed, and

if necessary, fired by the consumer.[13] The consumer, or a surrogate acting on behalf of the consumer, typically places an advertisement for a
personal assistant in a local newspaper, and then proceeds to hire
such an individual from among the respondents to the ad. The consumer or surrogate, rather than a health care provider, then supervises the personal assistant. In stark contrast with the medical model, the
consumer controls the services provided under the independent living
model.[14]

Under the independent living model, the personal assistant "is,
above all, someone chosen by the consumer to meet his or her *individualized* needs."[15] The model has been described as follows:

> There is no single set of services that fits every individual
> with a disability. Flexibility is a hallmark of consumer-direct-
> ed personal assistance programs: the [assistant] performs
> whatever personal assistance services are needed to allow
> the consumer to live at home, go to school or go to work just
> as an able-bodied person might. No one consumer is like any
> other: each has individual service needs and specific prefer-
> ences regarding the type of caregiver and the type of care to
> be received, including needs and preferences that are related
> to the maintenance of health and physical condition.[16]

Independent living should not be confused with assisted living,
although there are some similarities.[17] Like the independent living
model, assisted living allows the consumer to live in a residential
"home" setting.[18] However, a distinguishing characteristic of assisted
living is that the resident "belongs" to the assisted living facility,
which arranges for the availability of assistance for all residents. The
assisted living workers may be health care workers hired and supervised by the facility; therefore, assisted living may be conceptualized
as a variation of the medical model of long-term care. Even if assisted
living facilities were to hire individuals who are not health care workers, to the extent permissible in their states, assisted living cannot really be considered a variation of the independent living model unless
the rules of the facility permit the resident to act as the supervisor of
the assistant.

COMPARING MODELS OF LONG-TERM CARE

Figure 2 presents the relationship among the three general models
of long-term care: the informal support model, the medical model and

A Note on Values and Criteria

Saying that the goal of this book is to assess the three models as objectively as possible is not to suggest that the analysis is value-free. Any assessment of long-term care options, or of any other societal options for that matter, depends largely on the values of the assessor. Whether the values are considered explicitly or implicitly, any non-arbitrary assessment must rely on values. Ideally, to enhance the rationality, validity and reliability of the assessment, the assessor's values should be applied consistently in the form of well-defined criteria. Each model should then be evaluated according to each criterion.

This book is written from an independent living perspective. This perspective is justified because many, and probably most, Americans wish to live as independently as possible under any and all circumstances. They wish to live in this manner even if they will someday become too disabled to be able to care for themselves without assistance. Independent living does not necessarily mean that the consumer must achieve goals alone. For those consumers who cannot fulfill a need without assistance, or who can satisfy the need only with great effort and difficulty, independence means locating the assistance necessary and ensuring that it is provided in a manner consistent with the consumer's desires. The focus is on consumer control, not independent function. In analyzing long-term care options, the fundamental value or goal that will be applied is that people should be able to obtain affordable long-term care in a manner that allows them to control their lives.

The values inherent in this book's analysis are applied through the following operational criteria: accountability, affordability, autonomy, manageability, security and quality. These criteria are defined and applied in analyzing the three models in Chapter 7. In this book, these criteria are not weighted. Much more must be known about how consumers value and prioritize criteria before they can be weighted accurately. If the readers value some of the criteria more than others, they are free to weigh those sections of the analysis more heavily. If readers disagree with some or all of the criteria, they are welcome to criticize the criteria applied and to substitute their own criteria. Whether one agrees or disagrees with the analysis is less important than that the analysis makes transparent the values being applied and assesses each model explicitly according to these values.

the independent living model. It considers differences in several key characteristics: who provides direction; whether there is a plan of care; whether there is nurse supervision; who provides care and assistance; what training is required; who receives payment; who ensures accountability; what is the role of the recipient of services; and what type of benefit is provided. The models may be summarized generally as follows:

- Under the informal support model, the family provides direction, there is no nurse supervision or formal training, there is no payment and little accountability, and recipients serve in the role of dependents;
- Under the medical model, providers direct services, nurses supervise aides who have health care training, providers receive payment and are held accountable, and the recipients are considered patients; and

- Under the independent living model, recipients of services train and provide direction to their assistants, pay their assistants, and ensure accountability in the role of self-directed consumers.

This theoretical framework is not the only way in which to conceptualize long-term care.[19] For example, critics of this framework might argue that the distinction between institutional and non-institutional care is more important than distinctions between who is providing the services. Certainly, whether care is provided in an institutional setting is a key issue, and is captured in the framework to the extent that institutional care is provided almost exclusively by health care workers under the medical model. Non-institutional care is provided under all three models. The reason for the emphasis on who is providing care (i.e., health care workers vs. other workers) and under what circumstances (i.e., professional supervision vs. consumer direction) is that these considerations have major implications for consumer control and independence.

Most people receiving long-term care do not receive it exclusively under one single model. For example, most people who receive care primarily under the medical or independent living model still receive at least some supplemental assistance from uncompensated family members and friends when their primary provider of services is not available, or simply to assist the primary provider. Many people who receive their care primarily under the informal support model may occasionally receive formal support services from health care professionals or personal assistants. Others may receive care under two of the models approximately in equal parts. Still, considering the three models in their pure forms is valuable to derive insight into the situations of those who receive services under them exclusively or primarily, and to infer about services under a hybrid, mixed model.[20]

To those who have never heard of the independent living model of consumer-directed personal assistance services, and who conceive of long-term care as inherently medical in nature, the very idea of the independent living model is probably very radical and possibly threatening. It may conjure up images of people with no health care training practicing medicine without a license. This is not an accurate portrayal of the independent living model. Unfortunately, this is sometimes the image conveyed by some medical model providers of long-term care, whose financial interests may be threatened by widespread adoption of the independent living model.

As discussed above, long-term care may be divided into several

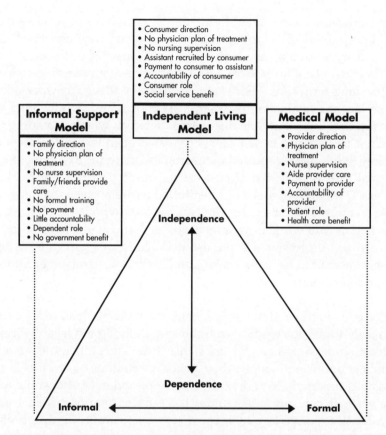

Figure 2: **Three Models of Long-Term Care for Persons
with Disabilities**

Note: This figure was adopted from figures entitled "Continuum of Attendant Care Programs" in DeJong And Wenker 1983 and "Toward a national Personal Assistance Program" in Batavia, DeJong, and McKnew 1991.

components, most of which involve personal assistance of a non-medical nature, but some of which may require medical expertise. Under the independent living model, personal assistants do not do anything that must be done by health care professionals and that consumers would not do for themselves if not for their disabilities. When the consumer has a medical problem, the individual addresses the problem by going to the appropriate health care provider, such as a primary care physician or a specialist.

Some dismiss the independent living model as an unviable policy option, claiming that policymakers will never accept a model of care in which the consumer controls services provided with government or private insurance funds. They argue that such an approach lacks accountability. They may be surprised that programs of consumer-directed personal assistance services already exist in most of the states and several countries, and mechanisms of consumer account-ability are built into these systems.[21] The limited availability of the independent living model is more a result of political opposition by vested interests than legitimate policy concerns about security and accountability.

THE JUNGLE AND THE ZOO

Perhaps the most fundamental policy issue addressed by this book is how much freedom versus how much security we as a society demand for our recipients of long-term care. In this regard, Professor Fuchs' analogy to the jungle and the zoo, quoted at the beginning of this book, seems particularly applicable to the circumstances of long-term care.[22] As he suggests, there are inherent tradeoffs between free-dom and security in all areas of public policy. Such tradeoffs are par-ticularly apparent in the general field of health care. Nowhere are they more stark than in the area of long-term care.[23]

Overprotective long-term care policy carries the risk of restricting the freedom of long-term care consumers, creating the security of the zoo. This analogy, though intended to raise consciousness about the relevant tradeoffs between freedom and security, hits close to home in some instances. Many nursing homes and other institutional settings resemble zoos in a manner that is disturbing to many. They have vis-iting hours; meal times, bathing and other activities typically are scheduled inflexibly according to the schedules of the "keepers;" res-idents are provided everything they need based on the determina-tions of the staff and regulatory/accrediting agencies; and residents who cause problems may receive consequences for their actions (e.g., physical or chemical restraints).[24]

Yet, equally disturbing is the opposite scenario—the freedom and insecurity of the jungle—in which those consumers who are vulnera-ble have no protections and may fall prey to predators and other haz-ards to their health and well-being. There are dangers associated with living in the community, particularly in certain low income neighbor-hoods that may be the only affordable locations for many consumers. There is certainly no shortage of potential risks, including abusive and

A Note on Key Studies

Certain studies have been particularly important in this area, and are discussed and referenced throughout this book. For purposes of brevity, they will be abbreviated as follows: the 1984 study by the World Institute on Disability (the 1984 WID study);[i] 1988 World Institute on Disability study (the 1988 WID study);[ii] the Commonwealth Commission survey of Medicaid personal care service consumers aged 65 and older in Michigan, Maryland and Texas (the Commonwealth study);[iii] the Cash and Counseling Demonstration and Evaluation (Cash and Counseling Study);[iv] the study of the California In-home Services Program (the California Study);[v] the MEDSTAT study of fiscal intermediary service organizations (MEDSTAT Study),[vi] and the Report of the National Blue Ribbon Panel on Personal Assistance Services.[vii]

[i] Litvak, S., Zukas, H. and Heumann, J.E. 1987. Attending to America: Personal Assistance for Independent Living. A Survey of Attendant Services in the United States for People of All Ages with Disabilities. Berkeley, CA: World Institute on Disability.
[ii] Litvak, S. and Kennedy, J. 1991. Policy Issues Affecting the Medicaid Personal Care Services Optional Benefit. Oakland, CA: World Institute on Disability.
[iii] Commonwealth Commission on Elderly People Living Alone. 1991. The Importance of Choice in Medicaid Home Care Programs: Maryland, Michigan, and Texas. New York: Commonwealth Fund.
[iv] Simon-Rusinowitz, L., Mahoney, K., Desmond, S.M., et al. 1997. "Determining Consumer Preferences for a Cash Option (AQ1): Arkansas Survey Results." Health Care Financing Review, 19(2): 73-96; Simon-Rusinowitz, L., et al. 1998. Telephone Survey Technical Report: Consumer Preferences for a Cash Option Versus Traditional Services in New Jersey. Baltimore, MD: University of Maryland Center on Aging.
[v] Benjamin, A.E. and Matthias, R. 2000. "Comparing Consumer-Directed and Agency-Directed Models: California's In-Home Supportive Services Program." Generations, 24(3): 85-87; Benjamin, A.E., Matthias, R. and Franke, T.M. 2000. "Comparing Consumer-Directed and Agency Models for Providing Supportive Services at Home." Health Services Research 2000 Apr; 35 (1 Pt 2): 351-66; Benjamin, A.E., Matthias, R. and Franke, T.M. 1998. Comparing Consumer-Directed and Agency Models for providing supportive services at home. Final Report under HHS Contract #100-94-0022. Los Angeles, CA: School of Public Welfare, University of California, Los Angeles.
[vi] Flanagan, S.A. and Green, P.S. 1997. Consumer-Directed Personal Assistance Services: Key Operational Issues for State CD-PAS Programs Using Fiscal Intermediary Service Organizations. Cambridge, MA: MEDSTAT, Inc.
[vii] Dautel, P.J. and Frieden, L. 1999. Consumer Choice and Control: PersonalAttendant Services and Supports in America (Report of the National Blue Ribbon Panel on Personal Assistance Services). Houston, TX: Independent Living and Research Utilization Program, available on the Internet at www.ilru.org.

negligent caregivers, incompetent providers, and thieves and con artists. The traditional paternalism of medical model providers is justified under certain circumstances, particularly when consumers have diminished mental capacities and limited ability to protect themselves.

There may be no area of health care policy in which the tradeoff between freedom and security is as prominent, or has greater implications for the life of the recipient of services, than long-term care. Figure 3 presents the theoretical freedom-security continuum of long-term

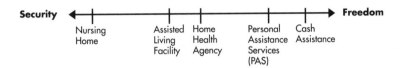

Figure 3: **The Jungle vs. The Zoo: The Freedom-Security Continuum of Long-term Care**

care, illustrating the range of choices from the most secure, least free (i.e., institutional care) to the most free, least secure (e.g., personal assistance services using cash payments to personal assistants who consumers do not know well prior to hiring them). This graphic depiction of the tradeoff between freedom and security identifies basic tendencies in different types of long-term care providers and settings.

Of course, there is nothing deterministic about this set of relationships. It is theoretically possible to find a nursing home that offers as much freedom as a particular personal assistance relationship at a consumer's home. Conversely, it is possible to find a highly restrictive personal assistance relationship that is as limiting as any nursing home. As a general rule, however, this continuum fairly characterizes the levels of freedom and security related to the different providers and settings of long-term care, and the general tradeoffs between them.

Despite these tradeoffs, freedom and security have not received equal consideration in long-term care. Long-term care policymakers traditionally have focused so extensively on providing adequate security that issues of freedom often have been neglected.[25] In recent years, as the principles of patient autonomy and self-determination have become more and more ingrained in our health care system, there has been a lot of rhetoric concerning patient rights to control their care in the nursing home. Although this is clearly a step in the right direction, there are real limitations as to how much control an individual can exercise in any institutional setting.

At the risk of extending the jungle-zoo analogy beyond its welcome, there has been a strong movement over the past two decades in zoology to eliminate bars and allow the animals to live in a setting resembling their natural habitat; yet, in the final analysis, the animals are not able to roam wherever they wish, or do whatever they want to do whenever they want to do it. To a lesser degree, the same is true concerning human long-term care institutions. Residential institutions, by their very nature, are not compatible with substantial freedom. While we are willing to accept such restrictions for other animals, few of us would willingly accept them for ourselves.

2

Long-Term Care Consumers

The first question policymakers typically ask when considering a long-term care program is: how much will it cost? Implicit in that question is another question: how many consumers will be served? Answering these difficult questions depends upon an understanding of the need, demand, and use of long-term care services, including the unmet demand for personal assistance services under the independent living model. We must develop an understanding of who is the consumer, what services the consumer needs, and where the consumer needs to receive such services. This chapter examines these issues in attempting to provide insight about the consumers of long-term care.

THE CHALLENGE OF COUNTING CONSUMERS

The key question of how many individuals require long-term care services is not as simple as it may seem. Several related questions must be answered initially, some of which cannot be answered fully because of data limitations. First, how many people require assistance in conducting basic life activities? Second, how many of these people require such a significant amount of assistance as to be deemed as requiring long-term care services? Third, how many of these consumers are already receiving such services on an uncompensated basis from family members and friends? Fourth, how are these numbers likely to change over time as a result of demographic and other factors?

Estimates of the number of people who require personal assistance and other long-term care services vary based upon different definitions of these terms and different assumptions concerning these parameters. For example, many different definitions of disability have been devised for different purposes, each of which yields a different number of estimated people with disabilities. Estimates also vary based upon the survey instruments and research methodologies used, and the year in which the survey was administered. For these reasons, some of the numbers below may appear inconsistent with each other. Although there is no consensus on precise numbers of the population of people with disabilities and the various components of that population, we have a good sense of the general ranges of these parameters.

Level of disability and the need for personal assistance are typically assessed by an individual's ability to conduct certain basic life activities, the "activities of daily living" (ADLs) and "instrumental activities of daily living" (IADLs) discussed in Chapter 1.[1] The U.S. Department of Commerce estimated in 1997 that about 20% of Americans (almost 60 million people) have limitations in at least one of these basic life activities; however, this does not mean that 60 million Americans require long-term care.[2] Although we are interested in the number of individuals who require some assistance on a daily basis, our primary concern is in understanding the number of people who require a sufficient intensity of care and assistance as to require long-term care in a nursing home or some alternate setting.

Altogether, the Commerce Department estimates that about 9 million people of all ages require personal assistance services to carry out daily activities.[3] The Urban Institute recently estimated a somewhat higher number, based on about 9 million adults currently receiving long-term care services and another half million children who require such services.[4] Still others have contended that access to personal assistance services is a key lifestyle issue for over 10 million people with disabilities in this country.[5] Whatever is the most accurate number of people who require personal assistance and other long-term care, this number will grow substantially over time, as the population ages and becomes more disabled and chronically ill. About 7.3 million people—over 80% of all individuals who receive long-term care or assistance—receive such services in community settings.[6]

Of course, access to long-term care affects far more individuals than those who are direct consumers of such care. It also affects family members, friends and any other individuals providing personal assistance services under the informal support model. The number of individuals who require long-term care and are already receiving such care from family members and friends under the informal support model is not clear, because no records are required under this model. The Commerce Department estimated that approximately 80% of the estimated 9 million people who require personal assistance—over 7 million people—receive such assistance from relatives under the informal support model.[7] Although it is not clear how many of the remaining 20% receive their care under the medical model or the independent living model, it is clear that the medical model dominates; it appears that only 2-5% of long-term care in this country currently is provided under the independent living model, although this estimate is speculative. *See* Figure 4.

The model of long-term care that is most appropriate for a particular consumer depends upon the individual's needs, desires, capabilities, and willingness to accept responsibility for controlling one's care. No single model of care is best for everyone; therefore, before examining the different models of care, it is important to understand

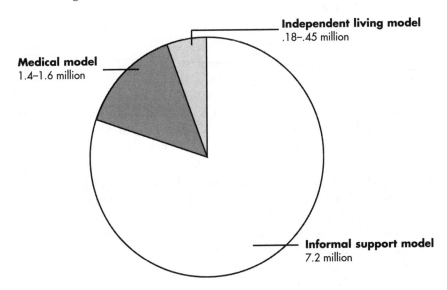

Figure 4: **Long-term care consumers receiving assistance under the three models of long-term care: the informal support model, the medical model, and the independent living model**

the long-term care population and its specific characteristics. This examination reveals an extremely diverse population with basically one characteristic in common: substantial functional limitations and the consequent need for long-term assistance.

A DIVERSE DISABILITY POPULATION

Several characteristics of long-term care consumers may affect the choice of a model of care. These include age, impairment, disability and cultural background.

Age

Age is one of the best predictors of the need for long-term care. The older one gets, the more likely it becomes that he or she will develop functional limitations reducing the capacity for self-care and therefore creating the need for personal assistance and other long-term care.[8] However, there is a general misconception that the vast majority of elderly people require long-term care, and that the vast majority of long-term care consumers are elderly. Altogether, only about 16% of people over age 65 require assistance with their ADLs and/or IADLs.[9] However, this proportion ranges substantially, from about 9% of those ages 65-69 to over 50% for those over age 85.[10]

The skewed perception that the long-term care population is almost exclusively elderly is based in part on the further misconception that nursing homes care for the vast majority of long-term care consumers. In fact, while 91% of nursing home residents are age 65 and older,[11] and the average age of a nursing home resident is 81,[12] nursing homes care for only about 20% of all long-term care consumers. The vast majority of consumers, about 80%, receive their care and assistance while living in the community. Altogether, the long-term care population consists of about 55% of consumers age 65 or older and 45% of consumers under that age. See Figure 5. Of the estimated 7.3 million adults receiving long-term care services in the community, 3.9 million (53%) are age 65 or older, and 3.4 million (47%) are ages 18 to 64. See Figure 6.

The need and demand for long-term care are expected to increase dramatically over the next few decades. As the baby boom population ages into retirement, a growing percentage of the population will be elderly. The number of individuals age 65 and above is expected to

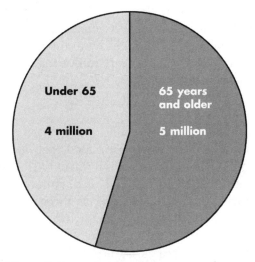

Figure 5: **Long-term care consumer by age**

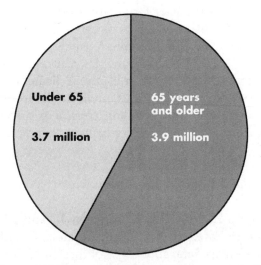

Figure 6: **Adults receiving long-term care in the community by age**

double over the next 35 years, from 35.5 million in 2000 to 70 million in 2035.[13] The number of older adults who have at least two limitations in ADLs will grow by a third over the next 25 years.[14] Many of these individuals will require long-term care services. Home-based long-term care is expected to grow at a much more rapid rate than institutional care.[15] Between 1992 and 1996, the number of people receiving home health care under the medical model doubled from 1.2 million to 2.4 million.[16] Although the numbers are much smaller, the rate of growth of home-based care under the independent living model appears to be even greater.

Children Requiring Long-Term Care

The Department of Commerce estimated that about 12% of children between ages 6 and 14 have disabilities.[17] The Urban Institute similarly estimates that slightly over 12% of children between ages 5 and 17 have difficulty conducting one or more activities, but only 0.9% of these 51 million children have difficulty with self-care.[18] Therefore, approximately 1% of the population under age 18 requires at least some long-term care assistance.[19] The majority of these are children with mental retardation and other developmental disabilities.[20] Approximately 64% of them live in the community.[21]

Although meeting the long-term care needs of children with disabilities is an important topic, this book focuses primarily on meeting the needs of adults who require long-term care. It should be noted, though, that the same general principles that apply to adults also apply to children. Children with substantial disabilities who are too young or otherwise emotionally and intellectually immature to claim decisional capacity may still maintain consumer direction and consumer choice through the use of surrogate decision-makers.[22] *See* Appendix B.

Working-Age Adults Requiring Long-Term Care

Approximately 2.7% of people between 18 and 64 years of age require long-term care, totaling approximately 5 million people.[23] Based on 1990 Census data, about 86% of these individuals live in the community, primarily in private residences.[24] A much smaller percentage lives in some type of institutional setting, such as nursing homes (181,000 individuals), special intermediate care facilities for mental retardation (118,000 individuals), other facilities for mental retardation (109,000 individuals), and facilities for the mentally ill (144,000 individuals).[25] Among the 3.4 million adults of ages 18 to 64 who receive long-term care in the community, about 71% receive assistance from unpaid caregivers only; 6% receive care from paid caregivers only and another 6% receive assistance from both paid and unpaid caregivers.[26] Therefore, the informal support model clearly predominates among the working-age disabled population.

Older People Requiring Long-Term Care

People over 65 years of age comprise the single largest age group of long-term care consumers; however, only about 22% of this population, 7.3 million seniors, requires long-term care.[27] Due in part to the large absolute number of these individuals who reside in nursing homes, about 1.4 million in 1994,[28] and their high visibility through press reports, there is a general misconception that most of these individuals live in nursing homes. Among the 18.6 million people of ages 65 -74, only 1% live in nursing homes and 7% receive long-term assistance in the community. Among the 10.9 million of ages 75 through 84, only 5% reside in nursing homes, and 15% receive assistance in the community. Finally, among the 3.6 million of age 85 and older, 23% reside in nursing homes and 29% receive assistance in the community.[29] Therefore, only among "the oldest of the old" (ages 85 +) do a majority of individuals receive long-term care (52%); fewer than half of these individuals receive their care in nursing homes.[30]

Among the population of people 65 years old and older, 28% of their personal health expenditures are for long-term care; 21% of such expenditures are for nursing home care and 7% are for home- and community-based care.[31] Therefore, about 75% of the expenditures for their long-term care are for institutional care provided under the medical model. This substantial percentage suggests the strong bias in favor of institutional care in this country for the elderly population. Considering that only about 25% of all long-term care is provided in institutions, the percentage also suggests the disproportionate costs associated with institutional care.[32] Although the high cost of institutional care may be justified to some extent by the extent of its residents' disabilities and co-morbidities, and the comprehensive scope of its services, these factors alone cannot account for the discrepancy in costs.

The ability of elderly people living in their own homes to remain in the community is affected by many factors such as finances, health, family support, a sense of identity, and a feeling of independence.[33] One study estimates that about two-thirds of elderly long-term care users who live in the community use no formal long-term care services and receive all their care without providing compensation under the informal support model.[34] According to another analysis, among the 3.9 million adults of ages 65 and older who receive long-term care in the community, about 57% receive assistance from unpaid caregivers only; 7% receive care from paid caregivers only, and another 36% receive assistance from both paid and unpaid caregivers.[35] These findings demonstrate the strong prevalence of the informal support model among the older population. Those who receive formal support in the community pay primarily out of pocket; out-of-pocket spending accounts for 42% of their long-term care expenditures.[36]

Some have asserted that an "elderly mystique" has created a presumption against giving elderly people autonomy and consumer direction in their long-term care.[37] According to Cohen:

> ... the elderly with disabilities (those elderly receiving or in need of long-term care) are the victims of low goal formulation and underestimated potentials for self-realization and full participation as family members; neighbors; church, synagogue and club members; community residents; citizens; and friends. ... It is suggested that the elderly themselves have bought into an elderly mystique which holds that the potentials for growth, development, and continuing engagement virtually disappear when disabled. The energy of formal and informal providers is directed toward maintaining activities of daily living and keeping the elderly person out of a nursing home. This results in a perception of little or no choice by the elderly themselves, and hence diminished exercise of autonomy.[38]

While such an elderly mystique may in fact exist, it is a cultural phenomenon that is not inherent in older people. Many such individuals do not adopt this self-fulfilling prophecy of permanent dependence. Moreover, to the extent that such a mystique exists, it is likely to diminish over time, particularly as the baby boom generation becomes elderly. Irrespective of age, the majority of consumers indicate that they want to be able to control their long-term care.[39]

Comparing Older and Younger Consumers

Whether or not an elderly mystique exists, there appear to be differences between younger and older people with disabilities as to specifically how they arrange and receive their long-term care services. Like younger people with disabilities, the vast majority of older people strongly prefer to receive their personal assistance and other long-term care at home.[40] Support for consumer-directed care under the independent living model is stronger among the younger disabled population, which is more familiar with this model than the older population; however, such support is still considerable among older individuals with disabilities.[41]

One study of differences in service experience and outcomes between recipients over and under age 65 who direct their own services in California's Medicaid program concluded:

> Findings indicate that although younger recipients embrace self-direction more enthusiastically than older ones, age differences are small on a majority of service outcomes. On average, older users embrace this [independent living] model and manage within it much like younger users. Some differences emerge between the young-old (65-74) and old-old (75+), but these are neither consistent nor determinative. . . . Old age is far from an inevitable barrier to self-direction. As with other age groups, there are opportunities and obstacles to be addressed as this newer approach to home care is disseminated.[42]

These conclusions are consistent with data from other countries as well, as discussed in Chapter 12. In the Netherlands, the average age of consumers who receive services under the independent living model is 57.5 years compared with an average age of 71 years for consumers who receive services under the medical model.[43] Similarly, in Germany's consumer-directed program, younger consumers were more likely to choose a cash payment under the independent living model.[44] However, in both countries, significant numbers of elderly people are receiving their long-term care services under the independent living model.

Impairment

Consumers of long-term care have a broad array of different chronic conditions and illnesses. Among elderly consumers, the most common chronic conditions resulting in the need for long-term care are arthritis, coronary heart disease, visual impairments, stroke and respiratory conditions. Among working-age consumers, long-term care services are needed most frequently by people with back problems, mental retardation, mental illness, coronary heart disease and respiratory conditions. Among children, the most common conditions leading to the need for long-term care are mental retardation, other developmental disabilities (e.g., cerebral palsy, spina bifida), mental illnesses, and respiratory conditions.

Other less prevalent conditions that may result in a level of disability necessitating long-term care occur to greater or lesser extent in all three age groups, such as multiple sclerosis, muscular dystrophy, amyotrophic lateral sclerosis (ALS, known as Lou Gehrig's disease), post-polio syndrome, spinal cord injury resulting in paraplegia or quadriplegia, and acquired immunodeficiency syndrome (AIDS). In aggregate, individuals with these conditions constitute a significant and rapidly growing population of people who require, or may eventually require, long-term care services.

All of the above conditions may affect whether one requires long-term care. However, this does not necessarily mean that individuals with such conditions require care in a nursing home or even under the medical model of long-term care. Again, whether a consumer's impairment is associated with a debilitating level of morbidity, disability, cognitive loss, and reduced physical energy may affect the individual's desire and ability to take on the responsibilities of managing care under the independent living model. Social factors also have a profound impact on whether a person with a specific impairment is able to live independently.[45]

Disability

A disability is a substantial functional limitation (i.e., a limitation in a major life activity). People who require long-term care have disabilities, by definition. If they were not disabled in some significant way, they would be able to conduct their activities, including self-care, without assistance and, therefore, would not require long-term care services. However, simply because one has a chronic condition or illness does not necessarily mean the individual has a disability. Moreover, simply because one has a disability does not necessarily mean that the individual requires long-term care. Such care is typically required only by people with very substantial disabilities, although people with minor disabilities may require a relatively small amount of assistance on occasion.

This book is concerned almost entirely with disabilities requiring very substantial or full-time personal assistance services. The Department of Commerce estimated that about 20% of Americans have disabilities. These Americans are defined as having difficulty performing certain functions (seeing, hearing, talking, walking, climbing stairs, and lifting and carrying), having difficulty performing activities of daily living, or having difficulty with certain social roles (doing school work for children, working at a job or working around the house for adults).[46] About 10% of Americans have "severe disabilities," defined as being unable to perform one or more of the above activities.[47] About one-third of these people with severe disabilities—about 9 million people—require personal assistance services.[48]

About 25% of all adults who receive long-term care in the community receive assistance with three to six ADLs, suggesting a substantial level of disability.[49] *See* Figure 7. These data suggest that 75% of these adults of all ages have limitations in only one or two ADLs, and are receiving long-term care services in the community to address the limitations associated with mild to moderate disabilities. Presumably, a relatively small amount of assistance provided under the informal support model will suffice for most of these individuals, to the extent that they have family members or friends willing and able to provide uncompensated care.

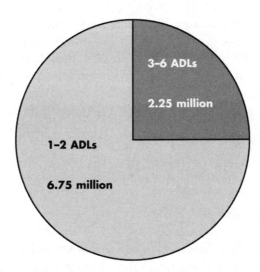

Figure 7: **Long-term care consumers by level of disability**

Cognitive Function

One type of disability that deserves particular attention is diminished cognitive function. This disability may result from a variety of impairments, such as Alzheimer's disease and brain injury. Senile dementia, which is a general term that encompasses a wide range of disorders involving irreversible and increasing memory loss sometimes accompanied by personality changes and disturbing behavior, is a growing source of nursing home patients. It has been estimated that between two and four million Americans have experienced diminished cognitive function related to dementia.

People with dementia or other mental problems often do not have the cognitive capacity to direct their lives on a consistent basis. Of all long-term care consumers, they are probably most in need of care under the medical model. To the extent that the independent living model is applicable to them would depend largely on the availability of a surrogate, such as a family member, who is willing and able to manage a personal assistance relationship, including hiring, training, monitoring, and possibly firing personal assistants present. These issues pertaining to decisional capacity are addressed in Appendix B.

Gender

Women are more likely to have functional impairments than men. Women with disabilities are also more likely than men with disabilities to be institutionalized. One of the findings of the Framingham Study of people who have had strokes was that older women, whether or not they are married, with moderate to severe residual impairment and little formal education, were at highest risk of institutionalization.[50] Although marriage protects men from institutionalization, it does not necessarily protect women, in part because women have longer life expectancies than men and tend to outlive their husbands.[51] Many women, who comprise the majority of nursing home patients, have nobody able and willing to take care of them.

Race and Ethnicity

African-Americans are more likely to have functional impairments than Caucasians. For example, in the 55 to 64 age bracket, some 35% of blacks have severe disabilities compared with 20% of whites, not of

Hispanic origin, and 28% of people of Hispanic origin (who may be of any race).[52] Such high disability rates are also associated with the lower incomes of people in these groups, and their greater exposure to environmental conditions that may result in disability. Predictably, these groups with high disability rates also have high rates of need for long-term care services.

Cultural Background

Closely related to race and ethnicity is cultural background. One's belief system is likely to affect whether one is willing to seek paid long-term care services, as well as selection of the model of preference for receiving such services. Among the most important determinants of belief system are racial and ethnic background through culture. Some have alleged that certain groups, such as African-Americans, have a strong cultural tradition of taking care of their own, which explains in part why they use the informal support model extensively. Others have dispelled this notion as a myth, concluding that the poorer economic circumstances of many African-Americans explain their use of the medical model.

In providing long-term care services under any model, one needs to be sensitive to cultural issues. One prime example relates to the native American community.[53] Under traditional tribal belief systems, the immediate family is expected to take care of family members who are sick or disabled.[54] In recent times, this expectation has been modified somewhat. Now, the belief is that the community has this responsibility, particularly when the immediate family does not have the caregiving capacity.[55] The American Indian Choices project at the University of Montana has assisted local tribes in establishing a planning process for organizing and providing long-term care services in a manner compatible with their cultural beliefs.[56]

Some have asserted that our national culture has served as an impediment to the expansion of consumer-directed long-term care.[57] Professor Zola argued that the integration of people with disabilities into the mainstream of American life has been hampered by certain American values, such as "an overreliance on technologic solutions to personal and social problems, and our continuing reluctance to fully admit patient-consumers as partners in their own rehabilitation."[58] Paternalism is a cultural characteristic that can have a substantial impact on public policy, particularly affecting people with disabilities.

Income and Resources

One's financial circumstances are likely to affect the way in which the individual receives needed long-term care. People with major disabilities who are from families with very substantial financial resources are able to pay for services under the medical model or the independent living model without being subject to enormous stress. Those from families with very low incomes and resources may be eligible for Medicaid. Depending upon the state in which the individual lives, he or she may have several long-term care options, including the independent living model in some states, or only the option to live in a nursing home.

Those individuals who are not eligible for Medicaid, possibly because their income and resources are slightly above the state's eligibility levels or because their disability is slightly less limiting than required for disability eligibility, have fewer options than those under Medicaid. The only option for those not eligible for Medicaid may be to receive care from uncompensated family members or friends under the informal support model, if such family members or friends are available and willing to help. Otherwise, they may have to spend down their resources in an effort to become eligible for Medicaid. Some people who are not able to receive support, primarily those with mental disabilities, become homeless.

Private Long-term Care Insurance

One financial resource that deserves specific attention is long-term care insurance coverage. Although such coverage is still very rare, access to a good long-term care plan can provide access to long-term care services. Depending upon the specific coverage package of a plan, funds may be available for consumer-directed personal assistance services. Some plans pay a cash benefit to the consumer who may purchase such services under the independent living model.

One recent study of community-dwelling long-term care insurance claimants and their informal caregivers found that the typical private health insurance package covered a maximum of $80 per day for a period of approximately four years.[59] Their private insurance policies paid for all the costs of care for 70% of respondents.[60] On average, the monthly private insurance benefit was $1,527, compared with an average public insurance home care benefit of $450 under Medicaid waiver programs.[61] Private insurance claimants received 59 hours of care per week, on average, compared with 45 hours per week for those without insurance.[62] Their private insurance paid for an average of 36 hours of care per week, constituting about 60% of their care.

Approximately 60% of respondents received their care from home health aides under the medical model; the remainder received care from other types of providers.[63] About 23% rely totally on formal services; therefore, all their caregivers are compensated. The remaining 77% received at least some of their care under the informal support model compared with 90% for those without insurance.[64] About 60% of respondents would have to reduce their level of formal care if they did not have their private policy, and many indicated that they would have to increase their level of informal care.[65] Approximately half indicated that without insurance, they would require institutional alternatives such as nursing homes and assisted living facilities.[66] Interestingly, about two-thirds of informal caregivers surveyed indicated that they have not reduced their level of care, suggesting that formal care is not a substitute for informal care.[67]

Some 86% of claimants indicated that they were satisfied with their insurance policy, and those with a disability policy design (i.e., cash benefits) were most satisfied.[68] About 75% indicated that they had no difficulty understanding their coverage, and 70% found it easy to file a claim under their policy.[69] About 90% of respondents who filed with their companies had no disagreements or had all disagreements resolve to their satisfactions.[70] Some 75% believed they had enough coverage, while 25% wished they had purchased more extensive coverage.[71] A large majority of claimants indicated that their needs were being met. Those who indicated their needs were unmet or undermet said that this was related to service availability, scheduling, continuity and coordination of caregivers, and quality of caregivers.

THE SETTINGS OF LONG-TERM CARE

Another way of getting an understanding of long-term care in this country is by examining where it is provided. As indicated above, the variety of long-term care settings includes nursing homes, other large institutions such as intermediate care facilities for the mentally retarded, smaller community-based residential facilities such as assisted living facilities, and the consumer's home.

The most prominent institutional setting for long-term care is the nursing home, which provides a broad array of services exclusively under the medical model. In 1997, there were 1.6 million residents living in the approximately 17,000 nursing homes in this country.[72] In the same year, the average private pay rate per day rate at nursing homes was $125 per day, and the average annual cost was about $50,000.[73]

The assisted living facility is another institutional setting that has been growing in popularity in recent years. In 1998, about half a million consumers lived in the approximately 11,500 assisted living facilities.[74] The major advantage of assisted living from the perspective of many consumers is that it allows them to reside in a setting that resembles a traditional home, and to have access to assistance as needed. Many consumers who reside in assisted living facilities probably do not know that they could achieve the same objectives through the independent living model.

Moreover, assisted living facilities typically reject individuals who require skilled nursing care.[75] Therefore, a consumer could become comfortable at an assisted living facility, only to have to leave when health or functional status deteriorates. Only 24% of residents at assisted living facilities require assistance in three or more ADLs, compared with 83% of residents in nursing homes; 34% of assisted living facility residents have cognitive impairments compared with 71% of nursing home residents.[76]

The most prominent community-based setting for long-term care is the consumer's home. Care is provided at the home setting under all three major models of long-term care. Under the informal support model, care is provided by family members and friends free of charge. Of course, from a broad economic perspective, such care is not really free because it is provided at the cost of time, effort, body strain and injury, and foregone opportunities to receive income from alternative efforts. There is no completely objective way in which to estimate such costs. Estimates would vary depending in part on the individual's earning capacity in the job market.

Under the medical model, home-based care is provided by home health aides under the supervision of physicians and nurses at home health agencies. In 1997, the average charge for a skilled nursing visit by a registered nurse employed by a Medicare-certified home health agency was $88 per visit; the average charge for a visit by a home health aide was $58, often for only a few hours.[77] A comparison between the costs of home health services under the medical model and personal assistance services under the independent living model in California reveals that the independent living model had a unit cost of about one-third of the medical model with no difference in safety or unmet needs.[78]

LONG-TERM CARE SERVICES NEEDED BY CONSUMERS

A broad array of services is needed by people with disabilities. As presented in Table 1, these services may be divided into those that require the work of a health care professional and those that do not. For example, the diagnosis of disease and prescription of medications obviously must be done by a professional physician. However, assisting the consumer in complying with medical instructions, including taking prescribed medications, does not require the skills of a trained health care professional or paraprofessional. Most consumers conduct the functions on their own, or would do so on their own if not for their disabilities. Consumers should be and generally are able to delegate these functions to whomever they wish, professional or not. Whether non-professional providers are legally prohibited from performing such functions in some states, and whether such prohibitions are actually enforced, as discussed in Appendix B, is largely a function of the political power of health care professionals in those states.

The issue of which services non-professional providers are competent to provide has obvious implications for selecting the optimal model of long-term care for any particular consumer. Each consumer must be considered as a unique individual in assessing the best model of care. A consumer who requires all or most of the services that must be provided by health care professionals, possibly because the individual has multiple co-morbidities (i.e., several concurrent diseases) and secondary complications (e.g., bedsores, infections), may be more inclined to receive services under the medical model. Consumers who require relatively few services that must be provided by professionals may be more attracted to the independent living model.

This set of generalizations is not to suggest that some consumers will not, or even should not, choose the exact opposite model as that predicted. Many consumers with several co-morbidities and complications will still choose the independent living model because of the control it offers. Such decisions could not be considered irrational, as long as consumers recognize that they will need to seek out the services of health care professionals to meet the needs that cannot be met by the personal assistant. Conversely, relatively healthy consumers who are not particularly concerned about control or costs may choose the medical model for its relative convenience.

Table 1: Services that Require Professional vs. Non-Professional Skills

Professional	Non-Professional[1]
skilled nursing	personal assistance
residential care	chore services (shopping, cooking, etc.)
diagnosis/medical care/medical supervision	implementing medical instructions
prescribing medication	administering medication
physical therapy	implementing exercises/range of motion
speech therapy	implementing therapy instructions
family/caregiver education and training	implementing care plan
family/caregiver counseling	disability/disease support groups
professional counseling	peer counseling
legal services	[no related service]
financial/benefits counseling	[no related service]
mental health services	implementing mental health plan
vision care	[no related service]
audiology	[no related service]
dental care	implementing dental plan
nutrition counseling	implenting nutritional plan
hospice care	implementing hospice plan
professional transportation	personal transportation
recreational therapy	recreational assistance
telephone reassurance	telephone reassurance
professional respite care	personal respite care
professional companion	personal companion
emergency care/response system	personal emergency response system

[1]All services that can be provided by non-professionals can, of course, also be provided by health care professionals, but typically at a much greater financial cost and not necessarily a higher quality of service.

SUMMARY

Altogether, almost 10 million Americans require long-term care services. Contrary to some popular belief, the vast majority of these individuals receive care in their homes and communities, primarily under the informal support model. This is true for elderly people as well as younger people who require long-term care, though a somewhat larger percentage of older people live in nursing homes and other institutions. The individual's home is by far the preferred setting for long-term care services. An increasing number of such services are being provided in the home under all three models of long-term care.

3

A Brief History of the Independent Living Movement

The long-term care landscape has been shaped by many societal forces. One of the most powerful is the independent living movement—a social movement of, by, and for people with disabilities who have sought to eliminate the social, environmental and other barriers preventing them from living independently in their homes and communities.[1] Independent living advocates demand policies that eliminate barriers to independent living. The beginning of the movement is best identified as the early 1970s, although it had important direct precursors as early as the 1950s.[2] This chapter considers the historical and social context in which the independent living movement was established and has evolved to influence long-term care.

RELATED SOCIAL MOVEMENTS

Before discussing the independent living movement and its relevance to long-term care, we must understand four related social movements that have also affected it: the broader civil rights movement, the consumer rights movement, the de-institutionalization movement, and the normalization movement.

The Civil Rights Movement

The civil rights movement in this country has had a profound impact on the thinking of all disenfranchised groups, including people with disabilities.[3] Such individuals have been inspired by the

movement's successes in identifying sources of prejudice and discrimination and opposing such attitudes and behaviors through a
variety of efforts; these have included demonstrations, sit-ins, litiga-
tion and lobbying for legislation. The manifestation of the civil rights
movement in the disability community has been labeled the "disability rights movement," in which people with disabilities first sought
civil rights, such as the right to vote, and later sought benefit rights,
such as the right to income and medical assistance benefits.[4]

Some might argue that the disability rights movement and the
independent living movement are really two terms for the same ongoing social movement, or that the independent living movement is just
the most recent stage of the broader disability rights movement.
Others would contend that they are two separate social movements
conceptually and politically, and that they are distinguished by the
independent living movement's focus since the 1970s on the ability to
live in one's own home. Although this is in part a debate over seman-
tics, it illustrates the important point that the struggle by people with
disabilities to control their lives dates back over a century, well before
what we now refer to as the independent living movement.[5]

Over time, the disability rights movement has altered the general
belief in our society that people with disabilities are vulnerable,
exploitable, and incapable of personal autonomy. Until recently, the
paternalism that has dominated our nation's approach to disability
was largely accepted by most people with disabilities, who allowed
others to control their lives. Such control has often been detrimental
to people with disabilities. After decades of political struggle by disability rights advocates, Congress enacted with overwhelming support, and President George H.W. Bush signed, the Americans with
Disabilities Act of 1990 (the ADA).[6] The enactment of this landmark
civil rights legislation demonstrated a national consensus that competent adults with disabilities can and should exercise control of their
lives in the mainstream of our society.[7]

Our society has recognized several important rights for people
with disabilities, including the right to be free of involuntary steril-
ization,[8] to marry, and to raise a child.[9] People with disabilities also
have the right to a free and appropriate education under the
Individuals with Disabilities Education Act (IDEA),[10] and the right
to access public services, public transportation, privately-owned
places of public accommodation and places of employment under
the ADA.[11]

The Consumer Rights Movement

Like the disability rights movement, the consumer rights movement of the 1960s was largely about autonomy and control.[12] For the first time, the well-established warning, "Let the buyer beware," was challenged by advocates who maintained that consumers have rights that may be protected in a court of law. The movement was personified publicly by attorney Ralph Nader and his "Nader's Raiders." An army of public interest attorneys and consumer rights advocates fought corporate invulnerability on many fronts, including federal and state legislatures and courts. The result was a variety of federal and state consumer protection laws and court decisions protecting the rights of consumers.

The consumer rights movement made substantial contributions to the independent living movement in terms of philosophy and consistent terminology.[13] The independent living movement was based on a similar distrust of the sellers and providers of services for people with disabilities, particularly physicians and other health care professionals.[14] Independent living advocates adopted the term "consumer" to refer to the recipient of personal assistance and other independent living services. A consumer is a person whose demands must be satisfied; i.e.,"The customer is always right." This concept represented a stark departure from the traditional treatment of people with disabilities as "patients." A patient is traditionally a passive recipient of services and is supposed to follow doctor's orders. Thus, this change in language reflected a fundamental change in the way in which people with disabilities saw themselves and expected other people to treat them.

People with disabilities were offended that, no matter where they lived or whether they were currently receiving medical services, they were always placed in the role of the dependent, subservient patient. In recognizing the implicit contribution of the consumer rights movement, an early history of the independent living movement concludes that the underpinnings of the movement were "revolutionary":

> Among them was a rejection of the medical model. If anything needed to 'Get better,' it was American society; if anyone should be in charge, it was not the doctor. People with disabilities, said the Berkeley group [that founded the independent living movement], were consumers, not patients. Like all consumers, they needed to select rather than settle.[15]

Due to the negative experiences of the early independent living advocates being patronized by their physicians and the medical profession generally, the particular style of self-help consumerism they adopted focused primarily on issues of demedicalization of disability. This rejection of paternalism and any manifestation of the medical model in long-term care and other areas became a fundamental principle of the independent living movement.[16] Replaced with a demand for consumer involvement and consumer control of organizations and services under the independent living model for people with disabilities, this fundamental principle remains central today. This principle is evident in the ongoing commitment of independent living advocates to the de-institutionalization of people with disabilities.[17]

The De-institutionalization Movement

The United States has a long and mostly shameful history of institutionalizing people whom our society wanted to hide from the public's view, including people with physical or mental disabilities who lacked resources.[18] From the Colonial period, our society has operated or financed institutions housing "the unfortunate," including poor people with disabilities.[19] Until the 1930s, however, these social policies focused primarily on addressing indigence through poor relief; the long-term care needs of frail elderly people or others with disabilities was largely an afterthought.[20] People with disabilities who had family members willing to take care of them or financial resources to pay for such services received their care at home. In this sense, the informal support model and the independent living model, although they did not have names at the time, were really the first models of long-term care in our country.

The home has always been, and remains today, the place of choice to receive long-term care in this country. By receiving care at home, the individual with a significant disability could receive individualized attention and was not exposed to the rampant disease and harsh conditions of the public institution. What we are now calling the independent living model or consumer-directed personal assistance services was not a major social innovation early in our history; it was merely common sense. If disabled people with resources had nobody to take care of them, they hired domestic servants to assist them with their needs. Those without resources who had nobody to take care of them had no option but to rely upon the benevolence of a society that has never been overly concerned about poor people, relying upon a variety of institutions that have evolved over the generations.[21]

In the Colonial period, the social response to poverty was primarily a system of locally-based "outdoor" (i.e., non-institutional) relief, in which poor people received assistance and had reciprocal community obligations consistent with their functional capabilities.[22] Some large towns and cities established almshouses, but these early institutions were dominant only between 1820 and 1865. A new belief that poverty was primarily the result of moral turpitude created an institutional response to reform and punish poor people, as well as keep them away from "respectable" people.[23] The horrible conditions of the almshouses were also intended to encourage people to work at any wage and for families to care for their family members in need.[24]

As an alternative to the almshouses, the private home for the aged arose in the early 19th century for "worthy" women of "appropriate caste and nativity."[25] These community-based residences designed to provide humane long-term care and assistance developed in a few communities throughout the country.[26] However, the vast majority of people with long-term care needs, who did not have resources or family members willing to help, received whatever little assistance they got in the almshouse and similar institutional settings.

By the middle of the 19th century, there were some efforts at institutional reform. Dorothy Dix and other reformers, in responding to almshouse conditions such as placing people with mental retardation or mental illnesses "in cages, closets, cellars, stalls and pens," demanded that the states take over these local institutions.[27] Consequently, the states got into the business of building and running large specialized institutions for people who previously were served in the almshouses. Systematically, the reformers attempted to transfer people to new state institutions from the almshouses: young people were sent to orphanages, mentally ill people to mental asylums, people with physical or sensory disabilities to special schools, and non-disabled people to workhouses, leaving the elderly poor primarily in the remaining almshouses.[28]

Yet, despite the good intentions of reformers, the new state institutions replaced the old institutions as places of neglect, abuse, disease, isolation, and segregation.[29] These institutions were later supplemented by smaller institutions, such as nursing homes and homes for the aged, most of which were privately owned but financed partially by the states.[30] The first nursing homes were private residences during the Depression; women caring for their disabled husbands took in additional residents for a fee to help pay the bills.[31] In the

1940s, the number of elderly people in such smaller facilities increased by 38%.[32] The growth and medicalization of the nursing home industry were stimulated by public policies of subsidizing nursing facilities, first through the Hill-Burton program to pay for construction and later through direct payment for care under the Medicaid program.[33]

The de-institutionalization movement began in the early 1960s. It focused on closing the large state institutions for people with mental retardation or mental illness. Catalyzed by the media reports of abysmal conditions including filth, resident abuse and neglect at some state institutions, such as Willowbrook in New York, state legislatures acted rapidly in response to public disgust. In 1963, President Kennedy signed the Medical Retardation Facilities and Community Mental Health Centers Act of 1963, calling for a national policy of de-institutionalization, and the building of 2000 community mental health centers by the year 1980 and one per 100,000 population thereafter.[34] While de-institutionalization occurred according to plan, only about 400 of these outpatient facilities were ever built.[35]

The most significant results of the de-institutionalization movement have been the closing of many of the large state institutions, the discharging of thousands of people with mental disabilities into the community, and an associated growth in the number of homeless people with mental disabilities who are not receiving needed services in the community.[36] The number of patients in mental institutions in the country dropped from 559,000 in 1995 to 85,000 in 1994.[37] Critics argued that such de-institutionalization placed patients with mental disabilities at risk.[38]

People with the physical disabilities also were de-institutionalized, and many have been successful in making the transition to independent living. The following is the testimony of one individual about her experience before and after leaving the state institution:[39]

> I did not get to testify last Friday, but I wanted to express to you how I feel about State Schools and other institutions. I am disabled, I have cerebral palsy. Many of my friends lived in State Schools and now live in the community. I lived in a nursing home for 12 years, but now have been living in my own apartment with attendant services for almost 2 years. I would never go back. . . .
>
> When you're in a State School or other institution it's hell because your life is not your own. You are under constant

supervision. I don't care how old you are or how young. They treat you like you don't have a lick of sense. They speak for you. You don't get no respect. You got to go to bed when they say go to bed. You got to eat when they say eat—or you go hungry. If you get hungry after supper and you want a snack, they say 'sorry kitchen's closed.' Then you got to go hungry until the next morning. . . .

People laying in their own urine. You would go down the hall and you would see the bed patients half covered. You go up to them and feel on their leg or arm and they would be cold and wet and you would go and tell a nurse they need to be changed and they would say it's not time to change them yet. They changed on the two hour shift so they might not go back for hours to change that person. And to me that's a hell hole. . . .

Now that I'm living on my own I can do what I want and don't have to answer to anybody. I can come and go as I please and I have control over my life. (If I make a mistake so what? I like making mistakes. You learn from them.) I feel like a person not like a number or a puppy dog. In an institution somebody pats you on the head and says "oh you poor thing you're in here and we got control over you life." They may not say it in so many words but you can feel what they're thinking. I have a better feeling about myself because I'm making it on my own. I use attendant services and it's not always easy, but at the same time you have control of who you want and who you don't want. Like everything else you have to give and take, but that's everywhere; that's part of life. I would rather have that kind of worry than to be stashed away like a number.

To sum it all up, all institutions should be closed so we can get on with more productive and happier lives. . . .

In 1981, the establishment of the Medicaid section 1915(c) home and community-based services waiver program created a major impetus for states to transfer individuals with mental retardation and other developmental disabilities from institutions to community settings. Between 1993 and 1998, the number of these individuals living in intermediate care facilities for the mentally retarded decreased from 148,700 to 124,300 at the same time that the number of these individuals receiving home and community-based services increased from 86,600 to 239,000.[40]

Since the 1960s, most of the largest state-run institutions have been closed; the number of nursing homes has increased concurrently.[41] Those patients discharged from the state institutions who are deemed too mentally disabled to function in the community were moved to the smaller nursing homes. Others with physical or developmental disabilities, some of whom are deemed by the state not to have the capacity to live in the community and some of whom simply do not have the support necessary to live in the community, also reside in these institutions. Many indicate that they would prefer to live in the community if they had alternative options offering adequate supports.

In discussing the emergence of the nursing home as the central structure of our long-term care system and the lack of alternatives for elderly people to live in their communities, Holstein and Cole conclude that:

> By the 1970s, institutionally based structures would become the standard around which alternatives would be created. These alternatives were assessed principally in terms of their cost-saving potential. Only recently have many questioned if large, proprietary, and bureaucratically organized nursing homes best respond to the needs of the chronically ill aged; but for all the reasons noted. . . , that system is particularly resistant to change. Modern long-term care, to this day, uneasily and incompletely responds to the needs of chronically ill elders and their families.[42]

The same conclusion applies with equal validity to other disabled populations, including younger people with physical disabilities. The de-institutionalization movement until recently has served primarily to close down the largest and most egregious state institutions, with mixed results particularly for mentally ill individuals who have not received the support they need to live in the community. It has not resulted in a substantial reduction in the number of people in nursing homes who would prefer to live at home. This "second wave" of discharging nursing home residents to the community is starting to occur now largely as a result of some of the successes of the independent living movement.

The Normalization Movement

Closely related to the de-institutionalization movement is the movement for "normalization" of people with disabilities, which has been particularly important in the developmental disability community, particularly people with mental retardation.[43] The objective of these activists is to reverse the tendency to segregate and protect people with disabilities. However, this movement went beyond that of the de-institutionalization movement, in that it insisted that people with disabilities be subject to the circumstances that people without disabilities must face, including the risks of personal harm or failure. De-institutionalization advocates often were not willing to accept such risks, insisting instead on extensive community supports for the de-institutionalized individual.[44]

This notion that, to be treated as first-class citizens, people with disabilities must cast away their social protections and subject themselves to the risks of a "normal" life in the mainstream of society, is a central premise of the independent living movement. Professor DeJong summarized this idea as follows:

> The dignity of risk is what the independent living movement is all about. Without the possibility of failure, the disabled person is said to lack true independence and the mark of one's humanity—the right to choose for good or evil.[45]

THE INDEPENDENT LIVING MOVEMENT

In addition to the civil rights, de-institutionalization, normalization, and earlier disability rights movements, the independent living movement has also been affected by two other related movements. In the self-help movement, people with a variety of problems (e.g., drug abuse, gambling, smoking, alcoholism) attempted to assist themselves without professional assistance; in the de-medicalization movement, people with problems labeled "medical" have attempted to redefine themselves as "normal" people with problems that they can address themselves.[46] Independent living advocates borrowed from the strategies of these previous movements and built upon their successes. The independent living movement has also been affected by medical advances that allowed people with disabilities to survive and live independently out of institutions.[47] The result has been an unprecedented number of people with disabilities living in their communities, many with the services of personal assistants provided under the independent living model.

The general premise of the movement is that the individual's disability is not a primary impediment to the ability of the individual to live independently; rather, individuals are impeded primarily by barriers in the physical "built environment," such as stairs, and in the "psychosocial environment," such as negative attitudes and policies that discourage independence.[48] Consequently, Edward V. Roberts, a person with quadriplegia caused by polio, who is generally regarded as the "father of the independent living movement," made the following observation:

> I believe that the basic premise of the . . . movement is that everyone has potential to live more independently. Our experience shows that even the most severely and profoundly disabled individual can be independent—they may need all kinds of help—but that they can be in control of their lives.[49]

This apparent oxymoron—to be independently dependent—is at the heart of the philosophy of the independent living movement. Judy Heumann, generally considered the "mother of the independent living movement" and co-founder of the World Institute on Disability, expressed the driving spirit of the movement best in an early policy report: "To us, independence does not mean doing things physically alone. It means being able to make independent decisions. It is a mind process not contingent on a 'normal' body."[50]

Over time, the independent living movement has been successful in establishing a presumption in our society that individuals with disabilities should be allowed to make their own independent choices about their lives. After decades of political struggle, the ADA was enacted, demonstrating the progress and commitment of society in respecting the right of people with disabilities to exercise control over their lives in the mainstream of society. A fundamental principle of the independent living movement, embodied in the ADA, is that people with disabilities should receive their public services in the most integrated (i.e., least restrictive) setting appropriate.[51] For an increasing number of people with disabilities, that setting for long-term care services is their home.

The Beginning of the Independent Living Movement

The independent living movement had its early roots in the 1950s and 1960s. One of the first historic accounts of the movement explains that, in 1953, Los Angeles County discovered that it could take care of the needs of its 158 iron lung users with polio at a cost of only $10 per day using personal assistants, rather than the $37 per day it was paying to provide the same services at the Rancho Los Amigos Medical Center.[52] According to this account, Gini Laurie, one of the early independent living visionaries, claimed that, "This discovery was the start of the independent living movement."[53] Based on the insight that such services can be provided well by people who are not health professionals, the March of Dimes implemented a program of providing polio survivors $300 a month to live outside the hospital, the prototype of current day consumer-directed personal assistance programs.[54]

Later, in the 1960s, the concept of independent living was advanced when some individuals, primarily with physical disabilities, overcame the inaccessibility of college campuses to receive their degrees and thereby develop the financial wherewithal to live independently in their communities.[55] The University of Illinois established a small program for students with disabilities in 1950 and had 163 students by 1961.[56] In 1962, the University of California at Berkeley admitted Ed Roberts, thereby providing the educational training both in and outside the classroom that would help him to establish what would eventually become a worldwide movement of people with disabilities.[57] In 1968, Congress enacted the Architectural Barriers Act, drafted initially by Hugh Gallagher, which required among other things that new government buildings must be accessible to people with disabilities.[58]

Despite these early activities, the beginning of the independent living movement, as a national phenomenon, is generally considered to be in the early 1970s. In 1972, Roberts and his colleagues established the Berkeley Center for Independent Living (CIL), the first independent living center in the country.[59] Independent living centers are consumer-directed local organizations dedicated to meeting the independent living needs of people with disabilities. Their primary purpose is to allow the integration of people with a broad array of disabilities into the community so that they can live independently. One of the key services provided by the Berkeley CIL was the development of a personal assistant registry to help its consumers function using the independent living model of long-term care.

In 1973, Judy Heumann, who would later rise to be the top disability policy official in the federal government throughout the Clinton Administration, joined Roberts at Berkeley.[60] Although Berkeley is generally recognized as the birthplace of the movement, other important hubs developed in other areas of the country. Within a few years of the founding of the Berkeley CIL, similar centers were established in Boston, Houston, New York, Los Angeles, Columbus, Ann Arbor and eventually throughout the country.[61] Within 15 years, there were more than 300 independent living centers, at least one in every major city in the United States and many in small cities.

One of the first real tests of the early years of the movement was the effective advocacy for federal regulations for Section 504 of the Rehabilitation Act of 1973.[62] Section 504 was a relatively unnoticed provision of a funding bill for the federal vocational rehabilitation program. The provision, based on language from the Civil Rights Act of 1964, made it illegal for any federal agency, public university or other institution receiving substantial federal funding to discriminate against anyone "solely by reason of...handicap." The regulations were developed in draft form, but were not released by the Department of Health, Education and Welfare (DHEW) because of the high cost of compliance. Disability rights leaders in Washington, D.C., protested at DHEW Secretary Califano's home and office. Protesters in the San Francisco DHEW office held a 25-day sit-in, which ended only after the Section 504 regulations were signed by Califano.

The Maturing of the Independent Living Movement

Every social movement evolves through phases of development and maturity. By the early 1990s, the independent living movement had evolved from its early stage, focused primarily on the younger disabled population, to a more mature and flexible stage of reaching out to other populations and constituencies. Independent living advocates had become sophisticated in the art of political lobbying. This advocacy was best evidenced in the enactment of the ADA, in which a potentially fragile coalition of disability groups representing a broad array of different disabilities and other conditions held together in passing the most comprehensive civil rights law in a generation and the most encompassing disability law ever.[63]

The early stages of the independent living movement were characterized by a rigid orthodoxy to its fundamental principles of anti-paternalism and refusal to interact with the health care system or involve itself in health care policy issues. A small leadership developed, and had little tolerance for dissenting viewpoints. The tendency for such a fledgling movement to attempt to protect itself from compromising its principles is understandable, and such discipline was probably necessary to achieve its early goals. As the movement aged, it has become more secure in its survival. In recent years, the movement has further matured to the point in which it is now able to tolerate dissention within its ranks over controversial issues for which reasonable advocates may disagree.[64]

One issue for which there is a high level of consensus among advocates of the independent living movement is whether there should be enhanced access to consumer-directed personal assistance services under the independent living model. Dozens of articles have appeared in the specialized disability press by people with disabilities about their treatment in nursing homes and their demands to live independently in their communities. The following is one example of a common sentiment published in the *Resist* newsletter:

> I was in a nursing home for 12 years. I'd rather die than go back! It's like we were chanting [at an ADAPT Demonstration that] 'I'd rather go to jail than to die in a nursing home'. Hell I'd rather go to jail than to have anyone have to live in one.[65]

THE INDEPENDENT LIVING MOVEMENT AND ELDERLY PEOPLE

The independent living movement is primarily a social movement established and developed by the non-elderly population. It has focused primarily on the needs of working-age people with disabilities and younger disabled people preparing to establish their independence. In his seminal article on the early stage of the independent living movement, Gerben DeJong observed:

> The movement has concentrated its energies on a relatively few major disability groups: those with spinal cord injury, muscular dystrophy, cerebral palsy, multiple sclerosis, and post polio disablement. Moreover, the [inde-

pendent living] movement has concentrated its energies on a selected age group: the older adolescent and younger working-age adult... Notably absent from the movement's constituency are older persons with severe physical impairments resulting from stroke and other degenerative conditions. While the movement's philosophy may have direct relevance to older disabled persons, the movement has focused its concern elsewhere. The movement's present age bias is one that cannot last indefinitely. Medical science is not only enabling severely disabled persons to survive initial trauma but is also enabling severely disabled persons to live longer. Thus, as the movement's initial adherents grow older we can expect the movement to enlarge its present age focus.[66]

Although elderly people were not part of the independent living movement's initial core constituency, it was recognized fairly early in the movement that the lessons of independent living could have application to older people with disabilities.[67] Even before the establishment of the independent living movement, the goal of independence was recognized as an important value for the elderly population. Title I of the Older Americans Act, enacted in 1965, states that older people have a right to "free exercise of individual initiative in planning and managing their own lives."[68] Clearly, the fundamental American values of independence and autonomy stay with an individual throughout life, even if the individual's capacity to achieve such goals without assistance may diminish with age.

Several efforts have been advanced to develop a common agenda on independent living, to create a bridge across the generations. Two full issues of the aging journal, *Generations*, were dedicated to this issue, first in 1984 and later in 1992. These efforts have demonstrated significant similarities and differences between the younger and older populations with respect to independent living. A key similarity is that both clearly wish to maintain independent lifestyles. A substantial majority of elderly people indicate that they would prefer to receive care under some version of the independent living model.[69] Among the differences are that older people often have a poorer health status and cognitive capacity, as well as a greater psychological reliance upon health care professionals than younger consumers.[70]

THE INDEPENDENT LIVING MOVEMENT AND LONG-TERM CARE POLICY

Access to consumer-directed personal assistance services is perhaps the foundational policy issue of the independent living movement.[71] Achieving such access may also be conceptualized as a long-term care policy issue, in that personal assistance is the essential long-term care need of this population.[72] The demand for consumer-directed personal assistance services is consistent with the goals of inclusion, full participation, and independent living of the Americans with Disabilities Act of 1990 (ADA) and the Rehabilitation Act of 1973, as amended.[73]

Members of organizations such as ADAPT (Americans Disabled for Attendant Programs Today) and other independent living advocates have been very active in advocating for consumer-directed personal assistance services programs. These advocates have advanced the concepts of the independent living model through a variety of methods, including civil disobedience.[74] Due in part to their lobbying efforts, several states have established personal assistance services programs to provide greater options for persons with disabilities to meet their needs.[75]

Another indication of the movement's maturity was the establishment of the National Institute for Consumer-Directed Home-and-Community-Based Services in 1995. This federal institute, subsequently renamed the National Institute for Consumer-Directed Services, has served as a springboard for legitimization of the independent living model of long-term care. The Robert Wood Johnson Foundation, one of the largest and most influential health care foundations, developed a collaboration with the National Council on Aging for a research and demonstration initiative entitled Independent Choices: Enhancing Consumer Direction for People with Disabilities.

These initiatives would not have occurred without the effective advocacy efforts of leaders of the independent living movement. The power of the movement in the long-term care arena was also demonstrated in the 1993 debate over national health insurance. One key component of the Clinton Administration's National Health Care Security Act of 1993 was a series of long-term care provisions.[76] This was the first legislative effort to offer consumers a choice of consumer-directed personal assistance services under the independent living model.[77] The bill provided for a program of personal assistance services for low income people with disabilities, as well as a tax credit for other working people with disabilities. These provisions were never enacted into law because of the failure of the Clinton health reform plan.

Several years later, further legislation was developed by ADAPT, embodying the principle that government funding should follow the consumer and that the consumers should be allowed to choose the model and specific circumstances under which they receive long-term care services. The Medicaid Community Attendant Services Act of 1997 ("MiCASA") was introduced on June 24, 1997.[78] Subsequently, the Medicaid Community Attendant Services and Supports Act of 1999 ("MiCASSA") was introduced.[79] Recently, it was reintroduced in 2002, and will probably continue to be submitted until it will eventually be enacted into law.

The Olmstead Decision

On June 22, 1999, the U.S. Supreme Court decided in *Olmstead v. L.C.*[80] that two individuals with mental disabilities had a right under the Americans with Disabilities Act of 1990 to receive care in their communities, rather than in the institutions in which they were placed by the state of Georgia. The majority consisting of five of the nine Supreme Court Justices ruled that such individuals must be placed in the community "when the State's treatment professionals have determined that community placement is appropriate, the transfer from institutional care to a less restrictive setting is not opposed by the affected individual, and the placement can be reasonably accommodated, *taking into account the resources available to the State and the needs of others with mental disabilities.*" (Emphasis added.)

The *Olmstead* decision has obvious implications for access to long-term care services under the independent living model. Individuals who are institutionalized under state long-term care programs including Medicaid can use the decision for leverage to receive their long-term care in their communities.[81] However, the *Olmstead* decision will not implement itself; thus far, the implementation effort has proceeded fairly well, although it has been criticized by some advocates as too slow.[82] Long-term care recipients will need to assert their rights, and courts will have to enforce such rights. States that are intent upon providing care in institutions under the medical model will assert that they do not have sufficient resources to move individuals into the community. It will be important to track all cases in which rights are asserted under Olmstead.

SUMMARY

This chapter necessarily could only provide a cursory treatment of the history of the independent living movement. As indicated in the bibliography, full books and other publications have been dedicated to this topic and even to portions of the history, such as implementation of the Section 504 regulations and enactment of the ADA. The purpose of this abridged version of the history is simply to provide insight into what the independent living movement is and how it has evolved to affect the provision of long-term care for people with disabilities. Hopefully, it has demonstrated that people with disabilities who adhere to the independent living philosophy have been fighting for years to receive their long-term care services out of institutions and under their direction applying the independent living model.

4

Consumer Direction vs. Consumer Choice

Consumer direction and consumer choice, two key concepts in long-term care policy today, are important trends in the field of long-term care.[1] There is growing evidence that individuals who have feelings of real control and choice over important aspects of their lives derive therapeutic benefits, contributing to physical and emotional well-being.[2] Such autonomy is also associated with reduced risk of abuse and neglect, and increased satisfaction with one's care and life.[3] Although the concepts of consumer direction and choice are closely related, they must be distinguished from each other to understand the options that could be available to consumers. In examining different models of long-term care, it is important to keep in mind the general trends toward consumer direction and consumer choice. This chapter examines these issues and trends.

CONSUMER DIRECTION

The most commonly-used definition of consumer direction, developed by the National Institute on Consumer-Directed Long-term Care Services of the National Council on Aging (hereafter, the NCOA definition), states the following:

> Consumer direction is a philosophy and orientation to the delivery of home and community-based services whereby informed consumers make choices about the services they receive. They can assess their own needs, determine how and by whom these needs should be met, and monitor the quality of services they receive. Consumer direction

may exist in differing degrees and may span many types of
services. It ranges from the individual independently making all decisions and managing services directly to an individual using a representative to manage needed services.
The unifying force in the range of consumer-directed and
consumer choice models is that individuals have the primary authority to make choices that work best for them,
regardless of the nature or extent of their disability or the
source of payment for services.[4]

This good general definition encompasses the essence of the concept of consumer direction. The underlying idea is that people with
disabilities are the best judges of their needs and how to meet them
in a manner that reflects their personal values and preferences.[5]
These are the individuals who must bear the consequences of the
care and assistance they receive, and therefore they should have a
very substantial amount of control and choice over those services.
However, by merging the two concepts of direction and choice, the
NCOA definition compromises the value of identifying the distinct
contribution of each concept separately. For analytical clarity, each
concept should be considered and applied separately.

The following definition is both narrower and broader than the
NCOA definition: "consumer direction is the ability of consumers
within a specified system of care to exercise autonomy and control
over how, where, when and by whom they receive their care."[6] This
definition is narrower in that it focuses exclusively on the extent of
control exercised within the context of a specific system or model of
care (e.g., a specific home health agency), and not on choices among
different systems (e.g., different home health agencies) and models
(e.g., care under the medical model vs. the independent living
model). The definition is broader in that it is not limited to home-
and community-based care; consumer direction can even be exercised to some extent within an institution, although for structural
reasons, attempting to implement consumer direction in an institutional setting is often like swimming upstream. The nature of institutions is typically not conducive to real consumer direction; achieving consumer direction requires a very strong institutional commitment and conscientious effort by all involved, which are extremely
rare.

In her introduction as guest editor of a special issue of the journal, *Generations*, on issues concerning consumer direction in long-

term care, Robyn Stone, executive director of the Institute for the Future of Aging Services, states that:

> Consumer direction in long-term care starts with the premise that individuals with long-term care needs should be empowered to make decisions about the care they receive, including having primary control over the nature of the services and who, when, and how the services are delivered. Consumer control also assumes that long-term care is predominantly non-medical, focused on primarily low-tech services and supports that allow individuals with disabilities to function as independently as possible. Thus, the consumer should not be forced to rely on professionals to make key decisions about care and to be 'managed' by a formal system.[7]

Depending upon how it is implemented, any general model of long-term care can be oriented to a greater or lesser degree of consumer direction. The continuum of consumer direction ranges from consumer input in developing plans of care under the medical model to consumer control of services under the independent living model. *See* Figure 3 in Chapter 1 and Figure 8 in Chapter 5. The opposite of consumer direction is provider control, which is closely related to the concept of paternalism. As discussed earlier, the independent living movement was established largely as a reaction to the detrimental paternalism of physicians and the broader society in their treatment of people with disabilities.[8] Independent living advocates demand consumer direction and oppose the paternalism of provider control in all aspects of long-term care.

THE DEMAND FOR CONSUMER DIRECTION

Although the concept of consumer direction has a general meaning that is widely recognized, its application tends to be somewhat different in different populations and contexts. In particular, consumer direction obviously depends to some extent upon cognitive function and decisional capacity. However, inherent in the concept of consumer direction is the prerogative of the consumer to delegate decision-making authority to another person; this includes delegating authority to a surrogate who may act on the consumer's behalf in selecting service arrangements in the event that the consumer does not have the capacity to decide for himself or herself. *See* Appendix B.

Consumer direction emerged and evolved differently in the different populations of younger people with disabilities, older people with disabilities, and people with mental retardation and cognitive disabilities. Consequently, understanding the consumer's relevant population is helpful in understanding the consumer's desire and capacity for consumer direction. Generally, however, irrespective of age, impairment or disability, those individuals who are independent by nature are likely to be attracted to approaches to long-term care that offer a high level of consumer direction.

In one study, people with disabilities were tested for levels of psychological and psychosocial independence.[9] Individuals with high *psychologic independence* tended to live in relatively unrestrictive settings and have fewer communication problems than others.[10] Those with high social independence tended to have assertive, self-assured, and self-sufficient personalities, more education, and more earned income than others.[11] Both groups of highly-independent persons were likely to be outgoing, to perceive themselves as independent and hired attendants under the independent living model.[12]

Younger People with Disabilities

Consumer direction is a concept that emerged from the independent living movement. The young and working-age adherents with disabilities of this movement rejected the paternalism of the medical model of disability, in which people with disabilities are regarded as patients who were expected to follow the directions of their physicians.[13] Instead, they adopted what has been referred to as the "independent living model" of disability.[14] Under this model, people with disabilities are assumed to be consumers of the services they need and are capable of self-direction in all aspects of their lives.[15] In this context, the concept of consumer direction was fostered and has since expanded widely to other populations.

Among this younger population, efforts at achieving consumer direction in long-term care have focused almost exclusively on the independent living model, in which consumers hire personal assistants who are not health care professionals. These independent living advocates completely reject the medical model of long-term care.[16] Even the term "care" tends to be shunned among the younger disabled population because of its association with "medical care" and "health care." In its place, the term "personal assistance" is used to refer to virtually any assistance the consumer needs, even if it is in an area traditionally designated as health care. The advocates contend that independence cannot be fostered in any environment in which the medical model prevails, particularly an institutional environment.

Studies indicate that young and working-age people with disabilities strongly prefer consumer direction under the independent living model.[17] For example, a telephone survey of consumers under the Cash and Counseling Demonstration in New Jersey found that 57% of consumers under age 65 were interested in receiving a cash benefit so that they could direct their personal assistance services rather than receive agency-directed services.[18]

Older People with Disabilities

Elderly people have a very strong desire to receive their long-term care in their own homes, to the extent feasible.[19] The extent to which they want consumer direction in their long-term care is not entirely clear at this time; different studies yield different findings. For example, one survey found that only 18% of home health care recipients over age 60 indicated that they wanted "more involvement in determining the amount and type of services" than they receive.[20] Other studies suggest a more substantial interest in consumer direction among elderly people.[21] The New Jersey telephone survey found that 32% of consumers of ages 65 years and older were interested in consumer direction through a cash benefit, a smaller but still substantial percentage of consumers compared with younger population.[22] Much appears to depend upon the specific circumstances of the elderly individual (i.e., level of morbidity, disability and support) and what we mean by consumer direction. While many elderly consumers may not be interested in managing a personal assistance employment relationship, it appears that most would like to be able to determine when, how and by whom they receive their care.[23]

Consumer direction has been applied to the elderly population only relatively recently.[24] Even now, many providers of services under the medical model fail to acknowledge the right of elderly people to control their lives and their care. In dealing with the significant percentage of older people who have at least some cognitive problems, and related issues concerning decisional capacity, these health care professionals probably have a tendency to treat all or most elderly people in a paternalist manner. This paternalism is associated with the "elderly mystique," a cultural phenomenon of presumed dependency on the part of older elderly people with disabilities.[25] Because long-term care policy has focused primarily on the older population, paternalism is deeply ingrained in the service delivery system that treats all people with disabilities, not just those who are elderly.[26]

Younger people with disabilities also continue to be subject to paternalism, but they are more likely to react to such condescension in a confrontational manner. The older population has less of an ideological commitment to the concept of consumer direction, and has been more willing to apply it more flexibly to a wide array of long-term care contexts. Although advocates of elderly people have focused primarily on keeping older people with disabilities out of nursing homes, similar to the focus of the younger disabled population, there has also been a strong emphasis on making nursing homes, home health agencies and other traditional health care providers of long-term care incorporate opportunities for consumer direction into their approaches to service delivery.

In the younger disability population, working-age people with disabilities served as the primary disability rights advocates who provided the impetus for expanding consumer direction.[27] In contrast, expansion of the consumer direction concept in the older population has been spearheaded primarily by progressive professionals in the aging and long-term care fields.[28] Many of these professionals depend financially on the medical model of long-term care for their livelihood. One would not expect their advocacy to take the form of opposing the medical model or supporting the evisceration of the long-term care industry, as some of the younger disability rights advocates have supported.

People with Mental Retardation and Cognitive Disabilities

Among both the younger and older disabled populations are individuals with diminished decisional capacities.[29] In the younger population, people with certain developmental disabilities, such as mental retardation, as well as individuals who have brain injuries or diseases, experience cognitive limitations. In the older disabled population, many individuals have degenerative diseases associated with aging and dementia. In either case, the diminished decisional capacity has obvious implications for the potential for consumer direction.

However, contrary to some popular belief, consumer direction is important to many individuals with cognitive disabilities.[30] They developed their own separate version of the independent living movement in the 1990s, two decades after the establishment of the movement of younger self-directed people with disabilities. This movement, which was labeled the self-determination movement, has had a dramatic impact on the long-term care of people with cognitive disabilities.

By virtue of the nature of cognitive disabilities, consumer direction within the self-determination movement has taken on a somewhat different character than consumer direction in other contexts. In particular, people with cognitive disabilities must rely upon people they trust to help structure the choices that are available to them. Therefore, networks or "circles" of trusted individuals, sometimes referred to as "microboards," are key to the success of these individuals in achieving self-determination.[31] The consumer must be able to select members of their networks, and to eliminate members of their networks when the relationship of trust is damaged.

People with Psychiatric Disabilities

Perhaps the most neglected disability population with respect to issues of personal assistance is people with psychiatric disabilities. There has been a slow and evolving recognition that people with long-term mental illness also want to be able to control their lives, and that personal assistance services provide them with the potential to do so.[32] However, a recent study of state mental health administrators and consumers demonstrated a high level of confusion over what consumer direction entails in the context of meeting the needs of people with psychiatric disabilities; there is particular confusion about the meaning of consumer direction through personal assistance services as opposed to rehabilitation and case management services.[33] Consumers indicated a desire to have direct control over their personal assistance services, and mentioned transportation, emotional support, help with negotiating with social service agencies, and assistance with household needs as key areas of their lives in which they would like more control.[34]

The study concluded:

> Findings showed that psychiatric PAS [personal assistance services] is still in a nascent state in terms of policy and practice whereas there is ample consumer interest in

these services. The analysis of the WID [World Institute on Disability] data confirmed the findings of the policy review, that is, there is virtually no implementation of programs of psychiatric PAS per se. WID data demonstrates that to the extent that people with psychiatric disabilities are receiving PAS, it is primarily because they either qualify under criteria created for those with other disabilities or because psychiatric disability has been included in a roster of qualifying conditions along with other disabling conditions.[35]

CONSUMER CHOICE

As discussed above, consumer direction relates directly to control over services within a specific system of care. Such control, of course, equates to greater choice over how, when and by whom services are provided within that system. However, the concept of choice also operates at a broader level; consumers can choose to operate under a different system or model of care that allows more or less consumer direction.[36] Some people with a strong independent living philosophy may wonder why anyone would choose to have less control. However, different individuals have different preferences, and some may not wish to bear the burden of controlling their services.

Therefore, a model that offers the greatest consumer direction is not necessarily the best model for all consumers. Each consumer must decide the best model for himself or herself. This concept of choice, as distinct from direction, is essential. For some consumers, consumer choice may be more important than consumer direction. In other words, choice among models may be a higher priority than consumer direction within a model. However, consumer choice must mean real choice among alternative approaches that offer more or less consumer direction. Ideally, a full range of choices with varying degrees of consumer direction should be available to consumers.

One aspect of choice that is important but often ignored is that choice encourages personal "ownership" of the chosen option. In other words, when a consumer exercises choice among several possible options, he or she develops a personal stake in making that option work well. Conversely, when a single approach or model is imposed on the consumer, there is little incentive for the consumer to make it work. In fact, if the consumer resents the lack of choice, or resents the specific approach or model imposed, he or she could actually sabotage the approach in an effort to make other choices available. In our particular culture, choice is extremely important to many individuals.

THE TREND TOWARD CONSUMER DIRECTION

The growing demand for consumer-directed services is an important trend in long-term care.[37] There are numerous reasons for this trend. Some of the initial impetus came from the independent living movement, with increasing numbers of people with disabilities attempting to live independently in their communities. Currently, the trend is being fueled by the large number of people now growing into old age. As compared with the previous generation of older individuals, who were raised during the Great Depression when people gratefully accepted what they received, the new generation has had a lifetime of experience as demanding users of services.[38] Moreover, the current long-term care users from the previous generation are largely older women, many of whom do not have much experience controlling their lives, compared with the current generation that has much more experience in that regard.[39] The experience, attitudes and expectations of the current generation are already manifesting themselves in a growing demand for consumer-directed care.

In addition, there is a high and increasing level of awareness of the concept of consumer direction among administrators in state departments that address aging, Medicaid, vocational rehabilitation, mental retardation, and developmental disabilities.[40] From 1996 to 1999, the awareness of these administrators of this important concept increased from 92% to 96%.[41] The total number of consumer-directed programs increased from 103 to 185 programs throughout the country.[42] A substantial majority of administrators supported enhancing levels of consumer direction in their programs.[43]

The Commonwealth study considered several indicators of consumer direction in three state programs: Maryland, Texas and Michigan.[44] The indicators considered were whether the consumer: a) knew the personal assistant prior to hiring the individual; b) helps to schedule the services of the assistant; c) supervises the assistant; d) signs time sheets and/or paychecks; and e) handles changing assistants. Michigan's program was found to have the highest percentage of beneficiaries receiving services with the highest number of indicators of consumer direction. About 55% of consumers in Michigan were able to schedule their assistants, compared with 24% in

Maryland and 33% in Texas.[45] About 80% of Michigan consumers signed time sheets or paychecks, compared with 62% in Maryland and 14% in Texas.[46]

The Independent Choices Program, sponsored by the Robert Wood Johnson Foundation (RWJF) and the National Council on Aging, is a $3-million grant program that encourages the development of consumer-directed home- and community-based services through demonstrations testing new approaches to financing and delivery.[47] Currently, this program includes nine demonstration projects, including state initiatives in Missouri, Minnesota, Oregon and Ohio. In addition, one Independent Choices project, entitled Promoting State Policy Reform to Enhance Consumer Direction, conducted by the National Association of State Units on Aging, is assisting the national aging network to identify opportunities to increase consumer direction across the broad spectrum of home- and community-based services.[48] The assessment guide developed through this project is being used by numerous states.

Four research projects under the Independent Choices initiative have expanded knowledge about consumer direction. A project called Elder Preferences for Consumer Direction is being conducted at the Institute for Health Policy at the Heller School of Brandeis University. Another project entitled Factors that Influence Consumer Choice, conducted at the Florida Policy Exchange Center on Aging at the University of South Florida, examined issues of choice and control comparing older people living at home with those in assisted living centers. Still another Independent Choices project called Making Hard Choices: Respecting Both Voices, conducted at the Family Caregiver Alliance in San Francisco, examined control and choice for people with cognitive disabilities and their caregivers. Finally, the Evaluation of a Consumer-Driven Personal Care System, conducted at the Rusk Rehabilitation Center at the University of Missouri-Columbia, assessed a consumer-directed personal assistance program integrated into a Medicaid managed care delivery system for people with physical disabilities.

The Self-Determination Project was implemented to determine whether consumer direction is appropriate for people with cognitive disabilities.[49] RWJF awarded a three-year demonstration in New Hampshire to examine issues concerning costs, waiting lists and consumer satisfaction in a program that was based on the principle of self-determination: "The idea that people with disabilities will determine their own future, with appropriate assistance from families and friends." Based on this project, RWJF later funded a much larger $7-million grant program entitled *Self-Determination for Persons with Developmental Disabilities* based at the University of New Hampshire involving 29 states. Under this project, states have developed their own approaches to offering consumers with developmental disabilities self-determination, including the allocation of budgets for consumers to determine the services they want.

The trend in favor of consumer direction may be seen as a manifestation of several broader social forces, such as the independent living, deinstitutionalization, normalization, de-medicalization and self-help movements discussed in Chapter 3, and a general trend in the areas of health care law and ethics toward patient autonomy and self-determination.

THE TREND TOWARD CONSUMER CHOICE

In addition to the trend toward consumer direction, there is also a trend in favor of consumer choice. Again, this may be seen as part of a broader trend in the health care field toward greater choices for consumers in a competitive health care system, based on the theory of managed competition.[50] This theory is based on the economic concept that competition will encourage competitors to enhance the quality and reduce the cost of services. Although managed competition generally has been applied to competition among health care organizations in providing acute care services, analogous theories could apply to competition among providers and even models of long-term care. For example, providers of home health care under the medical model will be induced to enhance the quality of their services, as well as to enhance consumer direction, if consumers have the option to leave them and receive services under the independent living model.

The concept of consumer choice has been severely criticized by some with a communitarian ethic, who refer to it derisively as "consumerism."[51] They claim that the highly individualistic market-based approach can be very isolating for many people with disabilities. They advocate community actions, such as participation in groups for self-help, advocacy, and advice-giving. Although they acknowledge that the community is not a panacea, and that there can be "community failures" just as there can be "market failures," they contend that community action is more likely than the market to achieve favorable outcomes for people with disabilities.[52]

The problem with the communitarian critique is that it is not always clear how and what community activity will suffice to meet the long-term care needs of people with disabilities. This approach has been successful for some people with mental retardation, who rely upon "microboards," an informal group of trusted individuals in the community who have committed to assist the individual to live in the community. Relying primarily on community support seems less applicable to people with major physical disabilities who require extensive and often physically difficult or highly intimate personal assistance services, such as lifting and bowel and urinary care. Community assistance is not likely to be available for the provision of such services. Moreover, as a general matter, we must ask whether there is a sufficient "community" available at this time in our highly mobile and transient society to achieve the objectives of people with disabilities, and if not, whether it is feasible to establish such a community. The experience of people with mental retardation suggests this is feasible to some extent.

As with most policy-related issues, the answer probably lies not in the extremes, but rather in an accommodation of the available alternatives. Consumer choice is important. The market is an extremely powerful mechanism to achieve choice and satisfy consumer preferences. However, markets have imperfections, and are only as good as their participants (i.e., the suppliers and demanders of services, as well as intermediaries). For example, a market with an insufficient number of potential personal assistants obviously will not yield optimal outcomes.

Similarly, primary reliance upon the community will not offer optimal results if there is an inadequate number of community participants. Also, if the term community is used to mean volunteers, primary reliance on the community can result in a damaging form of dependence, even more problematic than primary reliance on family members because family members are more likely to remain available under adverse circumstances. The ideal situation for most consumers is probably primary reliance on the market backed up with strong community supports, such as the availability of emergency personal assistance services.[53]

The concept of consumer choice has already been applied to long-term care in a variety of policy contexts discussed throughout this book. It is being investigated in the Cash and Counseling

Demonstration, in which consumers are given choices between receiving their personal assistance services in kind or through cash payments that they control.[54] This demonstration, therefore, examines both the concepts of consumer choice and consumer direction. Moreover, choice is the central concept in recently proposed legislation designed to establish a national personal assistance program. In the Medicaid Community Attendant Services and Supports Act, consumers may choose among alternative approaches to receiving their services; the program's funding follows the consumer.[55]

SPECIAL ISSUES CONCERNING CONSUMER DIRECTION AND CHOICE

The exercise of both consumer direction and consumer choice presupposes at least some minimal capacity of consumers to make difficult decisions. Consumers must be able to understand the options available to them, determine which options are in their best interests, direct services under the preferred option, and monitor services and make corrections when necessary. These are all high-level cognitive functions. Consumers possess the capacity for these functions in varying degrees. Consumers with major cognitive deficits, such as senility, are not capable of self-direction in sufficient degree to control their care or choose their services independently. A substantial question under any model of long-term care is how to address the needs of these individuals.

Consumer Direction Through Surrogacy

The primary approach to addressing the needs of those without decisional capacity is to assign surrogate decision-makers, who are authorized to make decisions on behalf of the consumer in a manner consistent with the way the surrogate believes the consumer would have chosen. This issue is examined in depth in Appendix B.

Consumer Direction in Respite Care

For people who provide long-term care services to their family members or friends, and for the people who receive their services, respite care is a valuable service allowing them to have some time away from each other. Respite is particularly important for individuals caring for consumers who do not have decisional capacity, or who otherwise are not fully capable of self-direction. Increasingly, family caregivers are being considered legitimate beneficiaries of programs and approaches designed to provide long-term care services to their loved ones in order to provide them needed respite. As in all other aspects of long-term care, the concept of consumer direction has been applied to respite care. Several states have established respite care programs that offer families varying degrees of control over services.

One exemplary respite care program was established in California in 1979. Under the California Department of Mental Health, a statewide system of 11 regionally based Caregiver Resource Centers was created.[56] These nonprofit entities are staffed primarily by social workers, known as family consultants, and are designed to empower family caregivers. The consultants are trained to achieve the following objectives:

- Provide clear, easily understandable information in a variety of formats and languages;
- Offer a range of support services and delivery options;
- Respect the family caregivers' decisions even if they, the practitioners, would make different choices;
- Include family caregivers in agency planning in a meaningful way;
- Administer consumer satisfaction surveys and report findings to staff; and
- Use results from applied research to improve practice.[57]

The family consultants are responsible for providing information about all viable service options, which is essential to consumer direction. The ultimate goal of such consultation is for the consultant and family members to develop a plan of care, which includes a plan to link the family to all available services of the Centers and the community.

Each Center may authorize up to a maximum of $435 per month per consumer, but most Centers impose a lower cap; the average monthly cost in 1998-99 was $245.[58] Families are required to pay a small copayment. Altogether, on average, caregivers received seven hours of respite per week. Among the options available for respite care are in-home care, adult day services, overnight respite, weekend respite camps and caregiver retreats.[59] In-home respite services tend to be most popular, and may be received under two approaches: a) vouchers to purchase services from home care agencies (under the medical model) or b) "direct pay" vouchers to hire and manage their own respite workers, including family members and friends (under the independent living model).[60]

About twice as many families choose the direct pay approach to respite care under the program.[61] Families that choose this independent living model approach indicated they had a greater amount of control over day-to-day care decisions, such as who provides the respite services and under what circumstances.[62] They also received more hours of respite services, largely because such non-professional services were significantly less expensive than agency-based services.[63] Overall, these families also expressed greater satisfaction with their respite assistants.[64]

It appears that a substantial majority (67%) of family caregivers value the control associated with the direct pay model over the convenience of using an agency. Yet, this still leaves a significant number of caregivers (33%) who choose the agency approach. This supports the idea that consumers or their surrogates may exercise choice in a manner that allows less consumer direction than other available choices. Even if convenience and control were valued equally, it may be rational for families to select the agency model simply because the relatively small number of hours entailed in respite care may not justify the effort associated with locating, training and managing respite workers. Consumers who require many hours of assistance, or who value more control, may well come to a different conclusion.

There is growing consensus that the provision of respite care in a manner consistent with the values and preferences of the consumer, to the extent that they can be discerned, is likely to increase caregiver satisfaction and to reduce the emotional burden of caregiving.[65]

CONSUMER DIRECTION UNDER DIFFERENT MODELS OF LONG-TERM CARE

As indicated earlier, consumer direction can be achieved to some extent under any of the three major models of long-term care, and in almost any long-term care setting. The extent of consumer direction depends largely upon the commitment of the provider to honoring the autonomy of the consumer. While some independent living advocates recognize such possibilities, they stress that the independent living model inherently encourages consumer direction while the medical model inherently discourages consumer direction.

Others have stressed that, while formal mechanisms of consumer direction are most apparent in the independent living model, autonomy is achieved through informal processes in all models and settings of long-term care.[66] Specifically, they contend that independence is not an all-or-nothing situation, and that people with chronic conditions and disabilities negotiate different degrees of consumer direction and independent living in their lives. They conclude that:

> What emerges is the relativities in everyday negotiations involved as people assimilate or come to terms with the circumstances of disablement. A great deal of research by rehabilitation specialists and advocates of independent living makes use of an abstract notion of the individual and a categorical definition of independence. We suggest that through the subtle relativities individuals in fact sustain considerably more self-determination than is suggested by prevalent notions of independence. This state of affairs is more appropriately referred to as autonomy.[67]

Independent living advocates would acknowledge that such informal processes for achieving autonomy certainly occur even in institutions that are least amenable to consumer direction. However, such negotiations require time and energy on the part of the consumer. The onus is on the consumer to develop relationships that permit some degree of autonomy. Moreover, negotiations inherently involve an exchange of desired objectives; presumably consumers engaged in such informal processes must give up something of value in order to obtain autonomy. Even if all the consumer must exchange is acknowledgments of gratitude, the long-term consequence of having to thank people for allowing them what they should have in any event can affect one's self-esteem.

Under the independent living model, the amount of such informal negotiation is diminished substantially because the consumer is entitled to the services provided. Of course, there is an initial negotiation of the personal assistance agreement between the consumer and the personal assistant. There may be occasional renegotiations at different intervals of the employment relationship. However, these are negotiations between relative equals: a consumer who needs a good dependable assistant and an assistant who needs a job. There is no need to be constantly negotiating informally for autonomy. The consumer is not in the uncomfortable position of accepting charity, as in the case of care provided under the informal support model, or of being under the direction of professionals, as in the medical model.

SUMMARY

Consumer direction and consumer choice are two powerful concepts that represent trends in the long-term care field. Consumer direction can be achieved to some extent under any model of long-term care. However, it is most compatible with the independent living model. Ultimately, consumers should be given the choice to receive their care and assistance while exercising the level of direction they prefer. Consumers who cherish their autonomy, and who are willing and able to take responsibility for the management of their own care, may wish to receive care and assistance under the independent living model. Others who are less concerned about controlling their lives, or more concerned about the challenges of managing the independent living model, should have substantial options for consumer direction under the other two models.

—5—

Three Models of Long-Term Care

Chapter 1 briefly introduced the three models of long-term care: the informal support model, the medical model and the independent living model. This chapter considers these models in depth, including relevant evidence of their performance. The potential range of levels of consumer direction that can be achieved under each of the models is depicted in Figure 8.

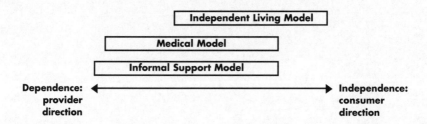

Figure 8: Ranges of potential consumer direction and independence under the three models of long-term care.

THE INFORMAL SUPPORT MODEL

Under the informal support model, the consumer receives long-term care services from family members and friends who are not paid for their services.[1] Care is provided under the direction of the caregivers. There is no formal plan of treatment, and no supervision by nurses or other health care professionals. Caregivers under this model receive no formal training. The role of the consumer in the informal support model depends upon the nature of the relationship, but it is often a role of dependency. The consumer is dependent upon the willingness and ability of the informal caregiver to provide services; he or she must accept services under the terms dictated by, or at least agreeable to, the caregiver.

The informal support model is therefore almost entirely private in nature; it is less subject to government regulations than the other models that involve payment, except to the extent that many states traditionally have imposed a responsibility for families to take care of their own; states also prohibit abuse or neglect under their criminal statutes.[2] Care under this informal support model is not covered under any government financing program, except for some available respite care to offer caregivers some relief from the obligations of caregiving. Also, because there is no payment for services, there is little accountability to any outside authority. This model raises difficult questions about what happens when the informal caregivers provide an inadequate quality of services. One consumer observed that it is not easy to "fire" one's family member or change the terms of the caregiving relationship after it has already been in place.

Another issue concerning this model is its ambiguous legal status.[3] The provision of care by family members could be construed as a violation of a state Medical Practice Act or Nurse Practice Act. Although such prosecutions are virtually never sought, the potential for legal problems exists in situations in which care involves sophisticated medical equipment such as respirators. Some states provide a clear legal exemption for care provided by family members and friends. Other states do not, and should clarify their laws to ensure that family members may perform these services. Any government effort to restrict informal support services by family members may violate federal and state constitutional prohibitions on the rights to liberty and privacy. This legal issue is discussed at length in Appendix A.

Critics of the informal support model often say that it results in an unhealthy dependence of people with disabilities on family members, and resentment by the family members who are not able to pursue their interests. Also, family caregivers tend to experience a higher level of emotional burden than outside caregivers.[4] The amount of consumer direction that is likely to occur under the informal support model depends upon the nature of the relationship between the consumer and the caregiver. Because the caregiver has the ability to withhold care, and the consumer does not control resources, the caregiver has all the leverage in controlling care. The consumer will therefore have control only if the caregiver yields control to the consumer. Although there are no data on this issue, largely because of the private nature of this relationship, it is reasonable to conclude that consumers who are not employed or have other resources are largely subject to the will of their caregivers.

Consumers and Providers under the Informal Support Model

The vast majority of consumers who require long-term care receive at least some services from family and friends under the informal support model, and many receive all their long-term care services under this model.[5] According to the 1990 Survey of Program Participants, about 83% of non-institutionalized individuals with disabilities on federal programs under age 65 relied exclusively on family members and friends for assistance; 73% of those over 65 relied exclusively on such informal care; only 9% of such individuals relied exclusively on care from health care professionals and other paid helpers.[6]

As many as 23% of all American households are engaged in informal caregiving. Over 27 million people served as informal caregivers in 1997, providing the economic value of $196 billion in uncompensated services.[7] About 75% of informal caregivers are women.[8] Some 41% of unpaid caregivers are the adult children of the consumer; 24% are spouses, 26% are other relatives, and 9% are non-relatives (e.g., friends and close acquaintances).[9] A typical profile of a caregiver is a woman in her 40s taking care of her parents; however, informal caregivers are represented in all adult age categories and many are over 65 years old.[10] Members of all social groups provide and receive care under the informal support model.

About two-thirds of caregivers are employed, and about half are employed full-time.[11] Informal caregivers often must forego economic and personal opportunities because of their caregiving responsibilities. Some develop health problems as a result of the physical and emotional burdens. However, according to one survey, less than 25% of caregivers considered caregiving to be a financial hardship.[12] Only about 6% of caregivers quit work entirely because of their caregiving responsibilities, but over half have to make at least one work accommodation to meet the demands of caregiving.[13] About 30% of caregivers indicate that they experience physical or mental problems related to caregiving.[14]

Most states prohibit payments to family members for services provided under their Medicaid programs. This prohibition has been criticized by some, contending that many consumers prefer receiving care from their family members, that this will increase the supply of home health workers, and that family members often provide a higher quality of service because of their personal interest in the consumer.[15]

The Future of the Informal Support Model

Despite being the dominant form of long-term care in this country, the informal support model has received less attention than either of the other models. Only recently have there been serious bipartisan legislative proposals to reduce the overall burden on family caregivers.[16] Due to the enormous demand for long-term care, the informal support model will always be needed, at least as a supplement to the other models. The majority of people who receive services under the medical and independent living models receive at least some unpaid assistance from friends and/or friends. In California, some 75% of individuals providing services to consumers were family members or friends.[17]

In other countries that provide services under both the independent living and medical models, a substantial number of individuals who are providing care and assistance are relatives and friends, many of whom are paid for their services. In the Netherlands, for example, 60% of such individuals were family members, friends and acquaintances.[18] In France, these individuals constitute about 30% of such workers.[19] In Germany, most participants in the system of cash payments regard this program primarily as a mechanism for supporting informal caregivers.[20] Only a relatively small number of family caregivers change their working or caregiving situations in response to the cash payments.[21] In Austria, about 10% reduced their working hours and 9% quit their jobs.[22]

One survey of the attitudes of Americans concerning public policies that assist informal caregivers found that, while only one-third of respondents supported paying family caregivers, almost 60% supported respite care to relieve family caregivers and over 70% supported tax credits to relieve the financial burden on these individuals.[23] Increasingly in this country, some government programs are authorizing payment of family members and friends who are providing care, in accordance with the demands of independent living advocates.[24] To the extent that this is occurring and is likely to expand over time, distinctions between the informal support model and the independent living model are likely to dissipate somewhat over time.

The likelihood that the informal support model will be absorbed into the independent living model entirely, however, is very remote because of fiscal concerns associated with the so-called "woodwork effect."[25] Policymakers are concerned that millions of people who are receiving care from family members and friends will "come out of the woodwork" to receive compensated care. This would obviously cost tens of billions of dollars. Others have contested suggestions that there would be a large woodwork effect. Whether, and the extent to which, the woodwork effect materializes will depend largely upon how the program under the independent living model is structured. For example, a broad definition of disability will allow many people currently receiving services under the informal support model to be eligible for compensated services.

To the extent that we continue to rely heavily on the informal support model, a key issue will be the availability of respite care to give caregivers an opportunity to get away from their caregiving responsibilities temporarily. Similarly, respite care gives consumers a welcome opportunity to get away from their regular caregivers for a while. Therefore, it is likely to be beneficial to the working relationship generally. Respite is an issue whenever the informal support model is used, but it is particularly important when this model is used exclusively and when the consumer has major cognitive problems like dementia (e.g., Alzheimer's disease). Taking care of a consumer with dementia can be extremely difficult emotionally and physically, and is often the equivalent of a full-time job.

The major advantage of the informal support model from the perspective of the consumer obviously is that it is affordable (i.e., free to the consumer). The major disadvantage is that it creates a strong relationship of dependency between the consumer and the caregiver, and may impose substantial harm to family relationships. Moreover, as indicated above, it may impose substantial physical and emotional costs on the caregiver. It also raises the essential question of who will take care of the consumer when the caregiver is no longer able to provide care. This is a growing problem as the population ages, and the average age of both consumers and caregivers is increasing.

THE MEDICAL MODEL

Under the medical model, long-term care services are provided in a variety of institutional and non-institutional settings, including the consumer's home, by and under the supervision of health care professionals.[26] Accordingly, providers control services to large extent. Nurses typically provide supervision to paraprofessionals known as nurses aides and home care aides, who are trained within the health care system and provide services directly to individuals. The individuals receiving care have the role of patients, who are supposed to follow doctors' orders. Providers are paid for their services by government programs, private insurers and patients; accordingly, the providers are assigned accountability under this model, and are heavily regulated at both the federal and state levels. Both nursing facilities and home health agencies must undergo certification processes and must abide by all applicable laws and regulations.[27]

Even though it is not the dominant model of long-term care in this country, the medical model has received by far the greatest attention and resources of our society.[28] The vast majority of long-term care services covered by the federal Medicaid program, as well as virtually all post-acute services provided by long-term care providers, are organized under the medical model.[29] The vast majority of policy proposals for long-term care have focused on services provided by health care providers under this model.[30]

Under the medical model, the individual's options for self-direction are often quite limited. The patient's role is fundamentally one of the dependence, despite a significant increase in rhetoric on patient autonomy and informed consent. Instilling substantial consumer control under the medical model is theoretically possible, and some providers have attempted to do so. In practice, however, it is very difficult to give large numbers of consumers greater control while attempting to fulfill all contractual and regulatory obligations under this model. Schedules for meals, bathing and other intimate activities are typically dictated largely or entirely by health care professionals employed by nursing homes and home health agencies.

One suggested advantage of the medical model is that agency workers receive significant formal training.[31] Another is that this model is theoretically capable of offering backup workers in the event that the primary agency worker assigned to a consumer becomes unavailable. Home health agencies, with numerous aides in their employ, have a major advantage in terms of providing services on demand. However, this does not guarantee that such services will be available. Consumers in the California program who receive agency services indicated that they believed a backup worker would not be available from their agency in the event of such an emergency.[32] Based on the early experience of the Cash and Counseling Demonstration, there are indications that consumers in other states are having similar problems in attaining backup assistance from home health agencies under the medical model.[33]

The extent to which consumer direction can be instilled in the medical model depends largely upon whether providers are willing to recognize consumer rights. One of the key autonomy rights under the medical model is the right to informed consent. As discussed in Chapter 4, informed consent is a right of negative autonomy; the consumer only has the option to accept or reject the interventions proposed by medical professionals.[34] It is theoretically possible to achieve rights of positive autonomy under the medical model; consumers would determine for themselves how, when, where and by whom they receive their services, but this would require substantial flexibility by health care professionals.[35]

In practice, such positive autonomy in the form of true consumer direction is rarely if ever achieved under the medical model. Even negative autonomy in the form of informed consent often is implemented without real commitment as "a bothersome administrative afterthought following design of the treatment plan by the physician."[36]

Consumers and Providers under the Medical Model

Services provided under the medical model may be divided into two general categories: a) institutional care and b) non-institutional care (including home and community-based services, such as home care and other ambulatory care on an outpatient basis). Long-term care services are provided in a variety of institutional settings such as nursing homes, intermediate care facilities for the mentally retarded (ICF-MR), and psychiatric hospitals.

In the area of home and community-based services, a distinction is often drawn between "agency-directed" home health care services under the medical model and "consumer directed" personal assistance services under the independent living model.[37] Currently, elements of these two approaches are often blended in state programs.

Traditionally, however, agency-directed services have featured the following: care delivered through a provider agency by caregivers who are supervised by medical professionals; case management to coordinate services; and public regulation of providers to assure quality.

Until recently, almost all home-based long-term care services provided through government programs have been organized under the medical model.[38] Service decisions are often made by the agency's case manager or professional staff. Critics of the medical model contend that it has significant shortcomings, particularly with regard to diminished control of disabled individuals over their lives. A variety of home care services are provided under the medical model. These services include:

- Personal care and assistance, such as assistance in the ADLs and IADLs;
- Chore services (e.g., housekeeping, cooking, laundry, driving and escort assistance);
- Routine nursing and health maintenance activities (e.g., assistance with medications, general monitoring, and palliative assistance);
- Supervision and oversight;
- Rehabilitation services to increase functional abilities, and
- Management assistance.[39]

The primary provider of home care under the medical model is the home health agency, although many practitioners provide home services independent of agencies. The services of home health agencies have been depicted according to the following categories: rehabilitation services, convalescence services, hospice care, ongoing care for recurrent and routine needs, and respite care to provide relief for families.[40]

Payors under the Medical Model

Medicare is not officially a long-term care program; it does not generally cover personal assistance services or other "maintenance care" in an institutional setting or elsewhere. However, it will pay for such long-term care services when they are part of a Medicare beneficiary's post-hospitalization nursing facility or home health services. In other words, such services are covered if they are needed by a patient who is discharged from a hospital with medical needs substantial enough to warrant care in a nursing facility or at home through a home health agency. In recent years, both the extent and duration of such services have increased, thereby making Medicare a de facto long-term care program to some extent.[41]

Medicare covers nursing, physical therapy, occupational therapy, speech therapy, medical social work, and home health aide services provided by certified home health agencies under specified circumstances.[42] In particular, skilled services must be deemed medically necessary. Medicare also covers home hospice services, including pain relief and symptom management, provided by certified hospices for individuals who are terminally ill (expected to die within six months) and agree to forego life-prolonging therapies.[43] The Medicare home care program has been subject to substantial fraud, abuse, negligence and other problems by unscrupulous home health agencies and practitioners.[44]

In contrast with the Medicare program, the federal Medicaid program officially covers long-term care, including home care. States have great flexibility in deciding which specific services to cover, and vary substantially with respect to which types of agencies qualify for payment under their Medicaid plans. Although they have the option to cover consumer-directed personal assistance services under the independent living model, most states continue to provide the vast majority of long-term care services under the medical model. (Chapter 8 further discusses the strong bias in favor of the medical model.)

The Future of the Medical Model

The medical model of long-term care will always be with us. A multi-billion dollar long-term care and home health industry has evolved with a broad array of powerful institutional and professional providers and a strong lobbying capability. The medical model will always attempt to perpetuate itself. Some consumers simply prefer to receive their care under the medical model. Others, who may otherwise prefer consumer direction, are too sick to have the energy or decisional capacity necessary to control their own care. Some may not have anyone available to serve as a surrogate to assist in decision-making on their behalf. As the demand for long-term care services grows, the demand for care under the medical model will grow significantly, challenging the capacity of our health care system to answer that demand in a manner that ensures quality.

THE INDEPENDENT LIVING MODEL

Under the independent living model, consumers hire their own personal assistants and direct their care. *See* Table 2. Personal assistants are trained and supervised by consumers, not by health care professionals. Although some individuals who are employed as personal assistants may have had previous health care experience, such experience is relatively rare and not a necessary qualification for the job. Many consumers actually prefer that their assistants have not had health care training, in part because they believe assistants with a health care orientation are less likely to provide services in accordance with the consumer's directions.[45] Under the independent living model, there is no formal plan of care. To the extent that services provided under this model are covered under government programs, such services are heavily regulated to ensure financial accountability. However, services ideally should not be subject to the same command and control regulation as other health care services. Consumers are ultimately accountable for the quality of the services they receive.

The key feature of the independent living model is that consumers control the circumstances under which their care is provided. Consumer-directed personal assistance services are intended to allow informed consumers to assess their own needs, determine how and by whom these needs should be met, and monitor the quality of services received.[46] Under some state programs, consumers also have the flexibility to choose other ways to meet their needs for personal assistance (e.g., home modifications and assistive devices).[47] Although differing degrees of consumer direction may be built into different personal assistance services programs, the unifying principle underlying all programs under the independent living model is that the individuals receiving the services have primary authority to make choices that work best for them.[48]

Typically, the consumer places an advertisement in a local newspaper and proceeds to interview those who respond to the ad. Obviously, there are security risks associated with allowing complete strangers to enter one's home.[49] However, there are no available statistics on the occurrence of harm caused by personal assistants (or prospective personal assistants). Some variations on the independent living model, such as the hiring of personal assistants through private agencies, independent living centers, or local government agencies, could reduce the security risk. Although there is nothing

Table 2: **Employer-Related Tasks Associated with the Independent Living Model**

1. Personal assistant recruitment and hiring
develop a job description and written agreement (i.e., contract)**
advertise job description or otherwise identify potential candidates***
develop an interview protocol*
interview potential candidates**
screen and evaluate candidate qualifications (e.g., reference/criminal background checks)**
develop candidate selection criteria*
select assistant and notify other candidates***
determine/negotiate wages and benefits for new assistant***
supervise submittal of employment forms (e.g., verification of alien status)***
arrange for emergency/backup assistants, if possible**
2. Payroll management and disbursement
obtain an employer identification number***
authorize assistant timesheets and/or vouchers**
withold and deposit state and federal taxes, if requested***
withold and deposit Social Security and Medicare taxes (i.e., FICA)***
withold and deposit federal and state unemployment taxes (i.e., FICA, SUTA)***
purchase and manage witholding for mandatory benefits, if applicable***
purchase and manage witholding for non-mandatory benefits, if applicable***
comply with all federal and state labor laws (e.g., minimum wage)
generate and issue paychecks***
issue IRS W-2 forms annually***
inform assistant about Earned Income Credit provision*
issue pay increases and/or bonuses when appropriate and possible*

Table 2 (continued)

3. Personal assistant supervision
ensure that assistant receives any state-required training if applicable***
develop and discuss with assistant a list of tasks and issues (e.g., no smoking)*
develop and discuss with assistant specific work schedules*
orient and train personal assistant*
evaluate assistant's performance and provide regular, periodic feedback to assistant*

4. Termination of general assistant relationship
assess and discuss problems*
determine whether problems require resolution, notice or immediate termination**
if resolution is indicated, attempt to negotiate solution**
if notice is indicated, provide according to contract or otherwise reasonable notice***
if immediate termination is indicated (e.g., neglect, abuse, theft, etc.) include rationale***

***mandatory task under federal or state law or otherwise necessary task

**highly suggested task, may be mandatory under some state laws and programs

*suggested task, advisable to avoid problems

Much of the information in this table was provided in Flanagan, S. A. & Green, P. S. (1997). Consumer-directed personal assisted services: Key operational issues for state CD-PAS programs using fiscal intermediatry service organizations. Cambridge, Massachusetts, MED-SATA, Inc, at 10-11.

inherent in these organizations that will protect consumers, they may reduce risk to the extent that these organizations are better able than individual consumers to conduct security checks on and otherwise assess prospective applicants for personal assistant positions.

The success of the independent living model depends largely upon the ability of the individual with a disability to manage the personal assistance relationship. This, in turn, depends on the knowledge and skills of the consumer concerning the nature of the relationship, including an understanding of the independent living model on which it is based. Managing a personal assistance working relationship can be extremely challenging, involving the following tasks:

- Recruiting, hiring and training personal assistants;
- Delineating responsibilities and developing work schedules;
- Supervising assistants;
- Managing payroll and associated taxes/reporting requirements;
- Providing disciplinary measures and discharging assistants, if necessary.[50]

Personal assistants are generally treated by the Internal Revenue Service as employees, not as independent contractors.[51] Accordingly, consumers have certain legal responsibilities, as discussed at length in Appendix A. One of the most challenging aspects of the independent living model for consumers, and the one for which they would most want assistance, pertains to payment of personal assistants and management of employment taxes.[52] Specialized organizations called Intermediary Service Organizations (ISOs) have been established specifically to meet this demand. Chapter 6 addresses the various models of ISOs.

Federal Medicaid regulations prohibit consumers from hiring and paying "legally responsible" relatives (e.g., spouses to care for spouses, parents to care for minor children). Most states examined in the Medstat study limited the hiring of relatives in some way.[53] However, several states have decided to interpret the federal regulations in a manner that allows the hiring of some family members.[54]

Consumers and Providers under the Independent Living Model

Under the independent living model, the individual with the disability requiring long-term assistance is considered a self-directed active recipient of services capable of recruiting, selecting, training, and directing his or her own personal assistant. This raises obvious questions concerning which consumers have such capacities for self-direction, and what can be done for consumers who do not have these capacities. The concept of surrogacy, whereby individuals capable of self-direction make decisions on behalf of the consumer based on their understanding of what the consumer would have wanted under the circumstances, has been applied to allow people with cognitive deficits to receive care and assistance under the independent living model.

Proponents argue that approaches based on the independent living model increase consumer satisfaction and autonomy,[55] improve health,[56] and enhance independence.[57] The independent living model has become the model of choice by most working-age people with disabilities, ages 18-65.[58] It is particularly attractive to individuals seeking to maintain gainful employment, who require the model's flexibility.[59] The ability to maintain employment may require the employee to work during unusual hours or travel. Providers under the medical model typically are not able to provide the flexibility needed by these consumers, at least at an affordable cost. However, this model is also becoming increasingly popular with people older than 65 years because of financial necessity.[60]

Although personal assistants do not receive the formal training of agency workers, it is reported that they often receive training informally from family physicians, home health nurses and other health professionals, as well as from consumers and their families.[61] This training is typically much more specific to the particular consumer who is being served than the general training received by agency personnel. Such specific training may to some extent explain the greater satisfaction of consumers.[62]

The relationship between the consumer and the provider of services tends to be closer emotionally under the independent living model than under the medical model. In California, approximately 75% of personal assistants knew the consumers they work for prior to being hired, whereas only 7% of agency workers knew the consumer first.[63] The average agency worker was responsible for providing services to about 4 consumers, compared with only 1.4 consumers for personal assistants providing services under the independent living model.[64] This smaller ratio of consumer-to-provider allows for more time together, and the opportunity for a closer personal relationship. In the Dutch independent living program, 90% of personal assistants indicated they have positive personal relationships with their consumers and positive feelings about their work environments.[65]

On the other hand, some have raised criticisms of the independent living model, contending the following: quality of care could suffer as a result of non-professionals providing care; there will be a great increase in the number of people applying for benefits; frail consumers will have difficulty in resolving the myriad of legal liability and employee benefit issues associated with managing one's own care; and some consumers or their family members may spend benefits inappropriately if provided in cash. To the extent that these concerns have been considered valid, the states are beginning to address them successfully in current state programs through such means as program design, counseling and fiscal intermediary services. *See* Chapter 9.

Another concern under the independent living model is the need to make arrangements for backup assistants in the event of emergency. As discussed earlier, a primary personal assistant could, at any time, become ill, incapacitated or have a family emergency. Without adequate backup, consumers could have no way to get in and out of bed, which can have catastrophic medical implications in terms of bedsores and other problems. In California, approximately one of every six consumers under the program indicates that they have nobody available for backup assistance.[66] At least one emergency backup program has been established in this country to address the problem.[67]

Some independent living advocates support the concept of direct cash payments to consumers with disabilities for their personal assistance services.[68] Others prefer services provided directly "in-kind" through the program with no cash going to the consumer.[69] Still others prefer that consumers receive a cash equivalent, such as a voucher or a tax credit, with which to purchase services. The specific form of the program and method of payment has substantial implications for program accountability, as discussed in Chapter 6.

Researchers and advocates have proposed or supported the establishment of a national personal assistance services program or policy in this country.[70]

Payors under the Independent Living Model

In state long-term care programs, the independent living model offers some significant advantages to states. By giving consumers more responsibility for their own care, states are relieved of some day-to-day responsibilities of managing services or overseeing providers.[71] Through consumer-directed personal assistance services, states may reduce their overhead costs, and may even be able to reduce the size of public sector programs through privatization of government functions.[72] A number of states, including Michigan, Wisconsin, and Colorado, are currently using state funds to make the general concept of consumer-direction one component of their long-term care systems.[73] Similar approaches are being used by several European countries, including the Netherlands, Germany, France, Norway and Austria.[74] *See* Chapter 12.

The Future of the Independent Living Model

Interest in the independent living model is rising in this country because national and state government officials are looking for innovative and cost-effective approaches to meet the long-term care needs of a growing disabled population. As relative newcomers to the long-term care scene, independent living advocates have to make up much ground in placing the independent living model on an even footing with the medical model. Despite major advances in the understanding of the independent living model among policymakers in recent years, this model is still not well known by the American public.

The likelihood that the independent living model will be adapted by the states in their Medicaid and other programs will depend upon a variety of factors, including the political clout of the nursing home and home health industries in each state.[75] Some authorities in the field believe that these industries are threatened by this model.[76] It is reasonable to expect that they will oppose it rigorously. These experts also indicate that other significant impediments to adopting the independent living model pertain to policymakers' concerns about the safety of consumers, and the liability and accountability of all parties for the services provided and the resources allocated.[77]

Some of these appear to be exaggerated concerns raised by health care providers who are threatened economically by the independent living model. Some criticisms of the model are unfair, in that they do not recognize that the other models have similar shortcomings. For example, while it is true that abuse can occur under the independent living model, it also has been documented under the informal support and medical models. Still other criticisms of the independent living model have some legitimacy, in that every model of long-term care has strengths and weaknesses. Therefore, it is essential that the three models be analyzed and compared on an evenhanded basis.

SUMMARY

This chapter provided an overview of the three models of long-term care. Each model has apparent advantages and disadvantages that must be assessed from the perspective of the consumer. The model that is best for any particular consumer depends largely upon the specific objectives and circumstances of that unique individual. No single model is for everyone, and often the optimal situation for many consumers is a combination of two or more models. For example, many consumers who demand autonomy would benefit substantially from receiving their assistance under a combination of the independent living model and the informal support model, thereby offering them both freedom and security.

6

Variations of the Independent Living Model

The independent living model has taken many specific forms, depending in part on whether it is being implemented by the federal or state government or by an individual consumer who is not covered by any government program. In considering the various possibilities under this model, there are several key dimensions: whether the consumer is allowed to control the funds; whether the consumer is allowed to hire family members; whether the consumer has assistance in conducting administrative responsibilities; and whether the consumer is ultimately responsible for quality and financial accountability. This chapter discusses the various forms of the independent living model that have been adopted.

CONSUMER-FUNDED PERSONAL ASSISTANCE SERVICES

There appears to be a misconception in our country that all people with significant disabilities receive government financial assistance for their medical care and personal assistance services. There are strict financial eligibility criteria for all state Medicaid programs. To be eligible for Medicaid, applicants with disabilities must have extremely limited financial assets and income, based on requirements set by their states. To be eligible for Medicare, which is not fundamentally a long-term care program, applicants with disabilities must have completed at least 40 quarters of qualified employment contributing to the Social Security System. To be eligible for personal assistance services under the Veterans' program, applicants must have service-related disabilities.

Therefore, there are many people with disabilities who do not qualify for these programs and must finance their personal assistance services out of their own funds. One potential way in which to plan for the costs of personal assistance services is through the acquisition of long-term care insurance. However, the private long-term care insurance market is very poorly developed, constituting only about 5% of all payments for long-term care.[1] Also, very few of the existing long-term care insurance products explicitly cover personal assistance services under the independent living model, although some provide cash benefits that can be used to purchase services under that model.[2] Therefore, private long-term care insurance, as currently structured, provides only part of the relief needed from the financial burdens of paying for consumer-directed personal assistance services. Moreover, it provides such relief only for those individuals who had the foresight and resources to purchase and maintain such coverage before they require such services.

Many individuals who fund their own personal assistance services use the independent living model to satisfy their needs for assistance. Since such self-funded services are not part of a government program, they have not been subject to the study that government-financed personal assistance services have received. A primary distinction between the independent living model as used by people who fund their own services and the model as used by those under government programs is that self-funded individuals have much greater flexibility in adapting the model to their specific needs. There are no regulations limiting the services available to these consumers, or mandating these consumers to conduct themselves in a specific manner. Of course, these consumers are required to file and pay relevant taxes and to comply with applicable employment and other laws, as discussed in Appendix A. The nature of the relationship is defined by the oral or written contract between the consumer and the personal assistant.

Due to the flexibility of the independent living model as applied to self-funded consumers, it takes on many variations based upon the needs and preferences of consumers. Some consumers use a single assistant; some use two or more. Some use live-in assistants; most use live-out assistants. Some require that the assistant provide household services (e.g., shopping, cleaning the house), services in the workplace and/or transportation services (i.e., driving the consumer's vehicle). Every consumer is unique; therefore, each personal assistant relationship is somewhat unique. Although many of the variations used by self-funding consumers are also found in state programs, consumers in these government programs typically have fewer options from which to choose. Therefore, research should consider the broad spectrum of possibilities used by self-funded consumers.

THE VETERANS' PROGRAM

Interestingly, with the exception of the larger states like California and Michigan, the agency of government that can offer the most insight on the independent living model is the Department of Veterans Affairs. Although the veterans' health system has been subject to much criticism over the years, it has been very responsive to the health care needs of disabled veterans, particularly paralyzed veterans with war-related injuries and extensive long-term care needs. For over three decades, this federal agency has provided a personal assistance cash benefit to eligible disabled veterans under the Aides and Attendants Allowance program.

Under this innovative and pioneering program using the independent living model well before that model had a name, veterans have enormous flexibility in using their cash benefits to meet their daily needs, including the need for personal assistance services. While government officials typically have concerns about the accountability of consumers for using these resources in an appropriate manner, the veterans' department has concluded that these particular consumers have earned this benefit by their sacrifices to the country.

Unfortunately, the Aides and Attendants Allowance program has never undergone a formal evaluation. Consequently, we do not have the advantage of the many lessons that could be learned from decades of implementation of the independent living model under this program. Nevertheless, we do know based on this program that it is possible to implement this model on a large scale throughout the country over an extensive period of time.

STATE-FINANCED PERSONAL ASSISTANCE SERVICES

Many states cover personal assistance services under the independent living model in their Medicaid plans either under the personal care optional benefit or under the Medicaid waiver program. One key issue under the Medicaid program is whether family members can be paid for providing personal assistance services. Technically, "relatives" cannot be paid under federal Medicaid regulations, but states have been able to get around this requirement to some extent by being allowed to define "relatives" narrowly, such as including only spouses in their state definitions.[3] Under the waiver program, states are given additional flexibility in developing personal assistance services programs. For example, states may choose to target specific groups under the waiver program. *See* Chapter 8.

In addition, states may provide personal assistance services under their Social Services Block Grant programs under title 20 of the Social Security Act and programs under the Older Americans Act.[4] Using such social services funding offers some additional flexibility because these funds are not encumbered by the medical model. On the other hand, the total amount of these social service funds is far more limited than the money available for long-term care services under Medicaid.

Overall, states have many options for covering consumer-directed personal assistance services, and virtually every state does so to some extent. However, they vary substantially as to how they do this. The following are a few of the more prominent state-sponsored programs. It is important to recognize that government programs change their policies over time; therefore, any program descriptions may not reflect the current policies of a particular program. The purpose of the descriptions is not to document the status quo, but rather to illustrate the various approaches taken at different points in time.

California

California's Medicaid long-term care program offers three different sub-models under which counties may run their personal assistance services programs:
- The independent living model (referred to in the state as the "independent provider model"), in which consumers hire their personal assistants on their own;
- The agency model, in which consumers hire their assistants through a county-qualified agency;
- A supportive independent living model, in which the county offers supports such as training, and backup); or
- A combination of these options.[5]

One study found that consumers in California who received their care under the independent living model exercised substantially more control and choice than consumers who received their care under the medical model.[6] They also experienced a high level of satisfaction with the technical and interpersonal aspects of their care, and they assessed the quality of their lives as better than medical model consumers assessed the quality of their own lives.[7]

About 200,000 individuals in California received Medicaid personal assistance services in 1997; 55% of these individuals were over age 65.[8] California's program, which has been considered a model program due to the combination of consumer choice and the consumer direction it offers, has been evaluated over an extensive period of time; it has demonstrated that consumer-directed services can be provided successfully to people with a wide variety of disabilities, including people with very substantial disabilities, in a large-scale state program.[9]

Massachusetts

The Massachusetts program was also established and implemented with substantial input from independent living advocates.[10] As one of the earliest programs organized under the independent living model and established in 1976, it has served as a model for other states. It is one of the more generous programs, in terms of paying assistants above the minimum wage. Also, it was one of the first and only state programs to provide training to consumers in managing a complex personal assistance services relationship.[11] In addition, independent living centers in the state have been incorporated into the program and receive payments for administrative services provided to assist consumers.

Michigan

Michigan also developed a program focused on enhancing consumer direction, although its program was equally focused on strong cost containment with a relatively low monthly cap on payments for most consumers.[12] It has used a two-party check system, whereby the consumer must sign the check to authorize payment. This key feature of the Michigan program is designed to give the consumer leverage in controlling the services provided. A study of the Michigan program found that about 40% of the state's consumers under the program indicated that they were able to exercise substantial control over their lives compared with about 4% of consumers in Maryland and Texas, which had programs under the medical model.[13]

Virginia

Virginia's consumer-directed personal assistance program conducts a determination of the assistance needed by consumers through home visits.[14] A standard allotment of time is allocated for most tasks required, with additional time determined and allocated for special tasks. The consumer's home, school and work environments are taken into consideration to determine whether additional assistance is necessary because of environmental barriers. Funding for certain home modifications and assistive devices is available. Based on the total number of assistance hours allotted, consumers may schedule hours as they desire. They recruit, hire, train, and manage one or more assistants, who may provide assistance with any tasks identified in the state's needs assessment. No certification or licensure of assistants is required. Consumers pay a co-payment based in part on income and expenses, with disability-related expenses taken into consideration. The state's centers for independent living provide support services, including training in personal assistance management, periodic recruitment of potential assistants, and maintenance of assistant registries.

An assessment of outcomes under the Virginia program, comparing a group of people with disabilities who received consumer-directed personal assistance services with a group on the waiting list for such services, revealed that those receiving consumer-directed services:

- Had higher levels of preventive health care;
- Had lower levels of emergency room use, hospital days, skilled nursing facility days, and doctors office visits due to a medical condition;
- Exerted greater control over their lives than the comparison group of consumers not receiving personal assistance services;
- Were substantially more likely to be living in a home setting, rather than an institutional setting;
- Were more likely to be employed; and
- Were more productive.[15]

These positive outcomes occurred for those receiving personal assistance services even though they had more substantial disabilities than the comparison group. Finally, the group receiving personal assistance services was more likely to be satisfied with their long-term care services.[16]

Other States

Virtually every state has developed an approach to providing consumer-directed personal assistance services. Different states vary substantially as to their approaches, including the extent to which they conform strictly to the independent living model, who may provide services, which services are covered, how services are paid for, whether fiscal intermediary services are available to assist consumers, and an array of other issues. Some states are much more generous than others in their personal assistance coverage and payment policies. Alaska and New Hampshire allow consumers to draw upon a budget in deciding how to meet their needs. Many states, such as Oregon, cover personal assistance services under a home and community-based waiver.

THE CASH AND COUNSELING DEMONSTRATION

In implementing the independent living model, many independent living advocates support the use of direct cash payments to the consumer, or the equivalent of such cash payments, such as vouchers, tax credits or medical savings accounts.[17] The Cash and Counseling demonstration is evaluating a variation of the independent living model that uses cash payments as part of an overall package that many believe offers the ultimate form of a consumer-directed program under the independent living model.[18] Consumers receive cash payments that they may use to purchase a variety of support services; they may purchase personal care services from a personal assistant, a home care agency or a friend or a relative (to the extent that the consumer's state allows family members to be compensated).[19] In addition, they may use the money to make home modifications or buy assistive devices that could, to some extent, reduce their future need for personal care. Consumers make the decisions concerning which combination of services or other acquisitions maximize their satisfaction and their ability to live as they wish in their communities.[20]

Along with the cash, consumers may receive information, advice, and training on how to access and manage their own personal assistance services.[21] Counseling may include a variety of supportive activities including the following: assistance in hiring, training and supervising workers; maintenance of a registry of workers available to provide backup support; assistance in handling tax and accounting responsibilities; and other forms of assistance.[22] Sources of counseling services may include independent living centers, other public or private disability organizations, and individuals with interest and expertise in independent living.

A key reason for the Cash and Counseling program is to provide adequate demonstration and evaluation of a large-scale personal assistance services program. It has been recognized that establishment of a national personal assistance services program, particularly one that provides cash to consumers, will not be achieved until such evaluation takes place. The Cash and Counseling program is currently undergoing such a major assessment sponsored by the U.S. Department of Health and Human Services, the Robert Wood Johnson Foundation and the states of Arkansas, New Jersey and Florida.[23] This approach emerged as a culmination of about 20 years of research sponsored by the federal government and private foundations on consumer direction, the independent living model, and home-and-community-based services.[24] Dr. Pamela Doty, the project officer for the demonstration, concluded:

> Cash and Counseling represents a highly visible test of the effects of maximizing consumer choice and control over the supportive services that elderly and younger people with disabilities need to meet their needs for assistance in the community. However, Cash and Counseling also represents a hopeful effort on the part of its federal sponsors to move beyond the impasse at which the policy debate on home-and community-based services has seemingly been stuck for nearly two decades. Cash and Counseling is an experiment that puts the responsiveness of public programs to the needs and preferences of low-income people with disabilities front and center, instead of defining the main or only value of home-and community-based services in terms of providing cost-effective 'alternatives' to institutional care.[25]

There is growing evidence that significant numbers of people with disabilities in this country would like to receive services under the Cash and Counseling sub-model of personal assistance services.[26] Cash and Counseling or similar approaches are being used by several European countries, including the Netherlands, France, Germany, and Austria.[27] National and state government officials have become interested in the independent living model and the cash payment approach because they are looking for innovative and cost-effective approaches to meet the needs of a society that is rapidly growing older and more disabled.

On the other hand, there are some who are extremely critical of a cash approach.[28] They claim that much of the support for this approach is based on the experience of a few European countries with relatively small numbers of consumers, and that this experience is not sufficiently representative or extensive to draw conclusions for this country. Even among those who accept the goals of consumer control and choice in long-term care, some are wary of the capacity of the market to achieve true control and choice.[29] They emphasize market failures, such as limitations in the quality and amount of information consumers have in making highly complex and potentially risky decisions.[30] They also question whether the market will supply a sufficient number of qualified workers to meet the demand for services.[31] They claim that extensive regulation will be necessary to make markets work and protect consumers.[32]

Still others recognize the challenges of implementing a cash approach, but conclude that it is worth pursuing.[33] Robyn Stone concludes:

> Several demonstration programs in the United States and experience from other countries suggest that many persons prefer cash to a defined set of services, even when the payments are greatly reduced relative to the service package. The implementation issues...are challenging but not insurmountable and in most respects are no more complex than those raised by the care/indemnity model. Policy makers and private insurers need to recognize the value of the [independent living model using cash payments] to many consumers and should further examine the costs and benefits of this approach to the public coffers, the private market, and persons who want more flexibility and responsibility.[34]

Arkansas IndependentChoices Program

The early experience of the Arkansas Cash and Counseling Program, entitled IndependentChoices, is encouraging.[35] The program offers individuals who are eligible for Medicaid personal assistance services the opportunity to receive a monthly cash allowance instead of traditional services. For purposes of evaluation, eligible individuals who indicated that they are interested in receiving the cash allowance were assigned randomly to the treatment group that received the cash allowance or to the control group that did not receive a cash allowance and continued to receive traditional Medicaid personal assistance services from agencies.

Recipients of the cash benefit were primarily elderly people (73%), in poor health (54%), and with high levels of disability (over 70%), contradicting the belief that only young people with physical disabilities and others with relatively mild disabilities will be attracted to this model.[36] However, older consumers did disenroll at substantially higher rates than younger consumers (40% disenrollment for participants over age 65 versus 14% for participants under age 65).[37] Prior personal assistance services users were less likely to disenroll than new users (14% vs. 40%).[38]

Some 92% of all participants had at least one paid caregiver. Of those with paid caregivers, 60% had one paid caregiver, 27% had two and 13% had three or more.[39] About 59% of participants who had paid caregivers hired relatives.[40] Interestingly, the vast majority attempted to hire family members, friends or neighbors, and very few hired people they had not known previously: about 75% tried to hire a family member; 37% tried to hire a friend, neighbor or church member; and only about 8% published or posted an advertisement.[41] About 26% of consumers with paid caregivers had live-in assistance; the remainder had visiting assistance. Most consumers used both paid and unpaid caregivers.

The number of hours of paid care varied substantially among participants: 34% received between 10 hours and 20 hours of care over a two-week period; 40% received between 21 hours and 40 hours of care; and 15% received more than 40 hours over the two weeks.[42] Uses for such services varied as well: 95% paid for assistance with light housework; 90% for assistance with bathing; 80% for assistance in preparing meals; 62% for assistance in getting in and out of bed; and over 55% for assistance taking medications or with other routine health care needs.[43]

In addition to providing resources for direct care and assistance, the program offered consumers the financial flexibility to pay for other needs that affect their independence. About 26% of consumers modified their homes to be more accessible to them, and 9% reported that they used their program funds to do so. About 33% obtained or repaired equipment for other personal activities, communication or safety, and 10% used their program allowance to do so.[44]

Approximately 96% of consumers were satisfied with their overall care.[45] Virtually all (99%) were pleased with the way in which their assistants fulfilled their duties and with their relationships with their assistants.[46] About 82% of participants receiving the cash allowance indicated that it has improved their quality of life; 79% said that it improved a great deal, and none reported that quality of life had diminished.[47] Explanations for improved quality of life focused on issues concerning flexibility, choice and control of services.[48] Still, many consumers who reported significant unmet needs: 41% needed more assistance with meal preparations and housework; 33% had unmet transportation needs; 33% had unmet personal care needs; and 27% needed more assistance with medications and routine health care.[49]

The other states participating in the Cash and Counseling Demonstration are still being assessed, but outcomes appear to be consistent with the Arkansas results.[50]

EMERGENCY BACKUP UNDER THE INDEPENDENT LIVING MODEL

As discussed earlier, a major concern under the independent living model is the need to make arrangements for backup assistants in the event of emergency. If a consumer's primary assistant becomes ill, incapacitated or otherwise unavailable without adequate notice, a consumer may be left in a precarious situation. If we can generalize from the situation in California, about 15 percent of consumers do not have emergency or backup assistants available to them.[51]

At least one emergency backup program has been established in this country to address this problem.[52] In Oakland, California, the Rapid Response Worker Replacement system has been providing around-the-clock home care replacement services since 1999.[53] It employs eight home care workers, most of whom do not have health care training or credentials.[54] Calls from consumers are answered by a contracted community-based agency during weekday business hours, and by an answering service during other hours. All calls requesting assistance result in the dispatching of a worker to the consumer's home within an hour of the call; most calls are completed within three hours.[55] Consumers are limited to using the service four times a month. Approximately 53% of calls relate to replacing a regularly scheduled home care worker, while the remaining 47% relate to urgent situations that could result in emergencies if not addressed immediately.[56]

For the independent living model to expand substantially throughout the country, a more extensive response to the problem of lack of emergency backup will be needed. Although the Oakland program is laudable, it is a single program in a single locality. Some additional backup programs probably have been established by independent living centers throughout the country, but they have not yet been documented in the literature for others to learn about their successes and failures. Clearly, many people with disabilities receiving their personal care and assistance under any of the three models of long-term care have no emergency backup whatsoever or very limited backup.

INTERMEDIATE SERVICE ORGANIZATIONS

Many consumers who prefer to receive their services under the independent living model have difficulty conducting the many tasks necessary for this model to work well. As discussed earlier, these tasks include the following:

• Recruiting, hiring and training personal assistants;
• Defining duties and work schedules;
• Supervising personal assistants concerning the performance of specific tasks;
• Managing payroll functions, including paying assistants and filing tax forms; and
• Disciplining and discharging personal assistants.[57]

Organizations known as intermediary service organizations (ISOs) have been established to assist consumers with these responsibilities. An ISO is "An entity that acts as an interagent between a consumer-directed personal assistance services program and eligible consumers for purposes of disbursing public funds and assisting consumers in performing tasks associated with the employment of personal assistance services attendants."[58] However, ISOs may also be used by consumers who are not eligible for public programs, if they are willing to incur the costs associated with ISO services. The Medstat study found consumers wanted the following supportive services:

- Service assessment and/or case management and service monitoring;
- Peer counseling and support;
- Access to employer management skills training;
- Access to technical skills training for assistants;
- Access to training regarding employer-related fiscal skills;
- Access to criminal and certification (e.g., nurse aide registry) checks;
- Access to personal assistant registry; and
- Access to emergency/backup personal assistance services.[59]

In different states, one or more of these support services are incorporated into the state's program. Thus, each program is to some extent a unique sub-model of the general independent living model.

INFORMAL ARRANGEMENTS UNDER THE INDEPENDENT LIVING MODEL

In addition to formal programs of consumer-directed personal assistance services, less formalized approaches to providing such services and addressing the burdens of management have been developed. For example, as indicated earlier, an innovative arrangement in British Colombia called a microboard involves the collaboration of several households to meet the needs of a person with a developmental disability.[60] Consumers who fund their own personal assistance services develop their own informal arrangements both explicitly through the employment agreements they develop and implicitly through the manner in which their interpersonal relationships develop with their personal assistants. Therefore, in a sense, each consumer develops his or her unique sub-model of the independent living model.

SUMMARY

There are countless variations of the independent living model, probably almost as many as the number of consumers who receive care and assistance under this model. However, there are several key issues that differentiate several key sub-models. One of these issues is whether consumers may receive direct cash payments to obtain their own consumer-directed personal assistance services. The Cash and Counseling demonstration is based on the concept of giving consumers maximum control through cash payments. The final results of this major evaluation will provide substantial insight into variations of the independent living model.

7

Criteria for Assessing Long-Term Care

The various models of long-term care should be evaluated as objectively as possible using appropriate criteria derived from the legitimate goals of consumers and other relevant stakeholders. There is a tendency for policymakers and the public who are aware of the different long-term care models to prejudge and dismiss a model based upon its most apparent weaknesses. However, the models should not be judged against a standard of perfection, which is not attainable. Instead, each model should be compared with the other available models, which represent the real options available to consumers. In analyzing the models, we must recognize that no single model is perfect, and no single model is appropriate for everyone. We must take into consideration the very different circumstances of consumers who are eligible for public versus private sector long-term care coverage, and consumers who are not eligible for any coverage and must pay out-of-pocket. This chapter examines the goals and objectives of long-term care, developing and applying specific criteria by which to assess the models against one another.

THE GOALS OF LONG-TERM CARE

In attempting to conduct such an evaluation of various long-term care models, it is necessary to identify the goals of long-term care and derive specific criteria from those goals. Different participants in the long-term care process, such as consumers, family caregivers, paid service providers and payors, have different goals concerning long-term care.[1] The current analysis focuses primarily on the goals of the consumer, which are shared to greater or lesser extent by other participants. Although the goals of other participants are important, the consumer is the reason the services are being provided, and the consumer's goals must be considered paramount. Of course, if the legitimate interests and needs of other participants are not satisfied, the consumer's interests will be compromised in the long run.

Among the goals concerning consumers that have been considered in the literature are the following:
- Improve or maintain health;
- Improve or slow deterioration of functional abilities;
- Meet needs for care and assistance;
- Enhance psychological well-being;
- Maximize independence and autonomy;
- Allow the consumer to live in the least restrictive setting feasible; and
- Promote a meaningful life.[2]

Although these general goals are useful conceptually, they are less helpful analytically in making comparisons among the models from an independent living perspective. First, these are not all entirely independent living goals. Even the goal of improving functional abilities may not be consistent with the independent living goals of a specific consumer. An individual with low-level quadriplegia, with the ability to use arms, but not legs or fingers, may be able to operate a manual (i.e., non-motorized) wheelchair with great effort. This individual's ability to use the manual wheelchair could be enhanced over time with exercise and therapy. However, this does not mean that such exercise and therapy are indicated from an independent living perspective. This activity may require so much time, effort and energy that the individual's ability to live independently is actually diminished. An independent living perspective may suggest that such an individual should obtain a motorized wheelchair to conserve essential resources.

Of course, some optimal level of functional ability is useful to be able to achieve independence. The individual in the example should ideally attempt to maintain sufficient function to be able to use the manual wheelchair when it is needed, such as when the motorized wheelchair is in disrepair or when the motorized wheelchair would be less convenient (e.g., a visit to a house with stairs or airline travel). The point is that an independent living perspective often involves a tradeoff between different independent living objectives (i.e., conserving time and energy versus attaining maximum functional status).

Similarly, the seemingly self-evident goal of improving health may conflict to some extent with an independent living perspective. Often, people with disabilities are placed in situations in which they must make choices involving a calculated risk in order to achieve independent living objectives. A working-age person with a disability may risk developing a decubitus ulcer (i.e., bedsore) in order to complete job responsibilities that require the individual to sit in his wheelchair too long. The ADA requires employers to make reasonable accommodations to satisfy the needs of people with disabilities, which may include the need to alter working hours to reduce certain physical risks. However, as a practical reality, virtually all workers including those with disabilities encounter job responsibilities that require longer hours than usual; most workers with disabilities will work under such circumstances despite the associated physical risks.

Enhancing health also may entail significant time and effort requirements that conflict with independent living goals. For example, many people with disabilities would benefit from physical therapy interventions on a regular basis, but most cannot afford to undergo such therapy because it requires too much of their valuable time and/or it requires financial resources that would be better used for alternative purposes (e.g., acquiring personal assistance services or assistive technologies). On the other hand, improving health may also entail improvements in diet, which are entirely consistent with independent living objectives. Ultimately, the goal of maintaining health, or improving health to the extent consistent with other independent living objectives, is a better way to characterize the goal from an independent living perspective.

For the purpose of analyzing and comparing different models of long-term care, analytical criteria must be constructed.

CRITERIA FOR LONG-TERM CARE

The following are specific criteria for the evaluation of different models of long-term care. Admittedly, these criteria are relatively crude, and are intended to permit comparisons at the most general level. Moreover, these criteria and their levels of priority must be tested empirically on large representative samples of people with disabilities and other long-term care stakeholders. Such individuals should ideally determine how they would prioritize these criteria. We ultimately need to know which criteria consumers weigh more or less heavily. However, at this stage of theory development, it is valuable to develop unweighted general criteria that appear conceptually sound and apply them against different models of long-term care. To date, such a comprehensive theory has not been developed explicitly from an independent living perspective.

The proposed criteria, presented in alphabetical order and without any intended suggestion concerning prioritization or weighting, are as follows:

- *Accountability:* The extent to which the allocation of resources for care is satisfactory to the funding source, including absence of fraud and financial abuse.
- *Affordability:* The extent to which the costs of care, including out-of-pocket costs to the consumer, are reasonable and do not impose a financial burden on the average consumer.
- *Autonomy:* The extent to which the consumer may control how, where, when and by whom he or she receives care.
- *Manageability:* The extent to which legal, regulatory and paperwork requirements are not unduly burdensome and are acceptable to the consumer.
- *Security:* The extent to which the consumer is free from unreasonable physical and emotional risks, as well as risks of theft and financial abuse.
- *Quality:* The extent to which the consumer receives competent assistance, and the process and outcomes of care are satisfactory to the consumer.

ANALYSIS OF THE MODELS

In applying the various criteria to the three models, drawing conclusions often is not straightforward. Each of the models encompasses a broad array of sub-models and variations on the themes. Therefore, the criteria are applied in a manner considering the range of options available under each model. Making the analysis even more challenging, the empirical research that has been conducted on issues of long-term care and personal assistance services uses inconsistent and often vague definitions concerning the criteria of interest. Therefore, often the best that can be done is to discern general trends and overall consistency of results and findings among the various studies.

Finally, no attempt was made in the current analysis to prioritize and weigh the importance of the specified criteria. Clearly, each criterion should not be given equal weight in considering and comparing the various models. For example, most independent living advocates would weigh autonomy more heavily than accountability or security. Conversely, most payors would probably weigh accountability and security more heavily. Further operationalizing, prioritizing, and weighing of criteria will be important objectives of the research agenda concerning long-term care issues.

At a recent national conference, one commentator alluded to this discrepancy in priorities between consumers and payors by drawing an analogy to his personal situation with his son. He said, "When my son asks to borrow the car, his primary objective is autonomy. My primary objective is safety." Although this analogy was offered to graphically illustrate different priorities, the commentator did not appear to recognize the paternalistic nature of his statement. Most of the consumers we are considering are not children; they should be allowed to make adult decisions about tradeoffs between different criteria.

There is no objective way in which to determine the appropriate weight of a particular criterion. The weight that was assigned to a criterion depends upon the particular values and interests of the evaluator. Future research ideally should examine the priorities and weights applied by different stakeholders to these criteria or whatever other criteria are adapted to evaluate models and programs of long-term care. For purposes of the current analysis, the reader is encouraged to apply his or her own relative weights to the various criteria.

ACCOUNTABILITY

Accountability is the extent to which the allocation of resources for care is satisfactory to the funding source, including absence of fraud and financial abuse. Unlike the other criteria, which are focused primarily on the consumer, accountability focuses primarily on the needs of the payor. Still, accountability is an extremely important criterion with respect to assistance provided to recipients of public programs. Perhaps the single most substantial impediment to expansion of public personal assistance programs is the concern among policymakers that societal resources will be used in an irresponsible manner.

Accountability is clearly a legitimate and essential factor for policymakers to consider. Policymakers have an obligation to the public to serve as the trustees of government revenues paid through the taxes of hard-working citizens. Each tax dollar should be scrutinized carefully to ensure that funds are used wisely and efficiently, and constitute the best use of scarce resources. This effort requires serious analyses concerning how, where, how much, and by whom long-term care is best provided.

Unfortunately, in the long-term care context, such real analysis of the use of resources often takes a back seat to pretenses of accountability. Policymakers like to have professionals to blame in the event that something goes horribly wrong, such as a consumer being harmed or resources being used for totally inappropriate purposes (e.g., alcohol or drug abuse). To the extent that incentives can be created and applied to ensure accountable behavior, both in terms of positive reinforcement for compliance with appropriate standards and sanctions for irresponsible conduct, real accountability can be achieved through the use of accountable providers.

Yet, more often, provider accountability is considered as an afterthought once problems have occurred. Such pretenses may be worse than having no accountability mechanism whatsoever. They can create a false sense of security that someone is being held accountable, thereby reducing the scrutiny of everyone else who could be ensuring real accountability. Interestingly, the consumer is often in the best position to ensure accountability, in that the consumer is often the only individual other than the direct provider of services who knows precisely what care or assistance was provided and how it was provided. Ironically, under some models of long-term care, the consumer is given little or no responsibility or even incentive to ensure accountability.

Informal Support Model

As the only model of long-term care that does not entail compensation, the informal support model does not have any formal mechanisms for ensuring financial accountability. To the extent that family members are providing care and assistance, any accountability issues would exist at the family level. The only real accountability issue that might arise is over family members not meeting their obligation to take care of the consumer, such as when grossly inadequate resources are provided to the family member requiring long-term care and assistance.[3] Such neglect or abuse could result in prosecution against family members, which may be construed as an accountability mechanism.[4] However, such prosecutions are rare.

Medical Model

Advocates of the medical model often contend that the other models of long-term care do not have adequate mechanisms for ensuring accountability. The medical model has many such mechanisms, including very extensive paperwork requirements and severe penalties for misappropriation of program funds.[5] A variety of federal and state statutes have been enacted and are designed specifically to ensure that providers are qualified and accountable and to deter and punish individuals engaged in fraudulent and other illegal activities.[6] Penalties include felony incarcerations, severe financial penalties and possible permanent exclusion from federal and state programs (e.g., Medicare and Medicaid).[7]

Despite these safeguards against misuse of public and private sector insurance funds, fraud and other financial abuse amount to billions of dollars a year;[8] long-term care and home-based care in particular have been subject to rampant fraud and abuse.[9] Such abuse is posing a major challenge to Medicaid programs in virtually every state.[10] Medicare home health care, which has grown dramatically in recent years, is similarly plagued with tens of millions of dollars of fraud, including the billing for services never provided and over-billing for services rendered.[11]

In recent years, efforts have been made to recruit consumers as agents of fiscal accountability through whistleblower statutes that allow consumers to retain a share of resources recovered as a result of their informing authorities about fraud and other financial improprieties by their providers.[12] While these efforts have had some success, they are not likely to be as successful as when the consumer is placed directly in a position of accountability. As long as the provider is considered the primary agent of fiscal accountability, we will always have the proverbial situation of the "fox watching the chicken coop."

Although most providers maintain high ethical standards, there will always be a minority willing and able to take illegal advantage of a system that largely offers the equivalent of blank checks to providers without having the capacity to verify the services provided.

This approach was more problematic during the earlier years of the Medicare and Medicaid programs when providers were reimbursed retrospectively based on costs incurred; however, today, providers continue to commit fraud now under prospective payment systems.[13] The amount of payment permitted has been limited substantially to a specified dollar amount per case irrespective of costs actually incurred, but the specifics of coding patients that determines how much payment is permitted remains based largely on an honor system in which providers request payment for services.

In view of the lack of adequate financial accountability in every federal and state program operating under the medical model, contentions by medical model advocates and practitioners concerning the lack of adequate accountability in other models cannot be taken very seriously.

Independent Living Model

To the extent that the independent living model has been used in public programs, such as state Medicaid programs, mechanisms of accountability have been adopted.[14] However, these programs are much smaller in scope and number of beneficiaries than programs operated under the medical model. Also, these programs have a much shorter history than the medical model programs, particularly because they have only grown in number substantially in the past decade or so. Consequently, we know much less about the amount of fraud and abuse that occurs under the independent living model.

As discussed above, claims by medical model advocates that the independent living model lacks accountability should be regarded with great skepticism. On the other hand, any claim by independent living advocates that we do not need to be concerned about accountability under the independent living model should also be challenged. Any system in which money is provided by some remote government agency (or by a remote private agency for that matter) is potentially subject to fraud and abuse. There is little reason to believe that consumers with disabilities are any more or less honest than others in the population. As we have seen in the context of food stamps and refundable tax credits, some consumers will engage in fraudulent activities.

There is strong reason to believe, however, that putting funds in the hands of consumers rather than providers will result in greater accountability. It is important to remember that these consumers rely on these personal assistance programs for their very existence. Therefore, engaging in fraud is like biting the hand that feeds them. If they are caught, they have compromised their very lifeline. Although the same could be said to a lesser extent of providers of long-term care services under the medical model, in that they may be heavily dependent on their jobs for economic survival, they are not dependent on such programs for life itself and could presumably get some other job in the economy.

Different versions of the independent living model address issues of accountability differently and to greater or lesser extent. The most controversial version is the cash model. Many policymakers have reservations about providing cash to consumers; they are concerned that a cash benefit can be spent in any number of ways that are not accountable to taxpayers.[15] While this is a general concern with cash payments, policymakers appear to draw distinctions between the "deserving" working disabled population and the "non-deserving" non-working disabled population; they are particularly reluctant to provide cash to the recipients of welfare programs such as Medicaid. Policymakers are more likely to be comfortable with a cash benefit to working individuals with disabilities in the form of a tax credit. This approach raises important issues concerning horizontal equity among different people with disabilities.

Overall, financial accountability is likely to be as great under the independent living model as under the medical model, and possibly more so.

AFFORDABILITY

Affordability considers the extent to which the costs of care, including out-of-pocket costs to the consumer, are reasonable and do not impose a financial burden on the average consumer. Affordability is a key criterion in that most would agree that access to even the best long-term care is not a positive outcome if consumers must impoverish themselves to gain such access. One of the strongest criticisms of our current "system" of long-term care is that consumers must spend down almost all of their resources before they can be eligible for Medicaid, the primary government program that covers long-term care. Once eligible, consumers may have very limited options available to them depending upon their state of residence. Clearly, the cost of care is a key issue for all entities involved in the financing of long-term care. What is not recognized by the public is that consumers and their families are among the most significant payors of long-term care. Yet, most Americans do not recognize this stark reality until they are faced with such out-of-pocket costs when considering nursing home or other long-term care for themselves or their family members. *See* Chapter 8.

Informal Support Model

The strongest advantage of the informal support model is that it does not entail direct financial costs to consumers and their families. For those consumers who are fortunate enough to have relatives or friends willing and able to assist them, this model offers the possibility of a relatively normal life in which their resources are preserved. Those resources that otherwise would have to be spent on paid assistance can therefore be used for other needs of consumers and their families, such as housing, nutrition, health care, and recreation.

However, it cannot be said accurately that the informal support model has no economic impact on consumers and their families, only that there are no direct financial costs. This model does impose what economists call "opportunity costs" on the providers of care; that is, families under this model incur the cost of foregone benefits associated with lost opportunities. In other words, the amount of time and effort the informal caregiver spends in providing care and assistance to the consumer could be spent in other compensated, productive activity. One estimate of the value of these services is $196 billion per year.[17]

In addition to opportunity costs, the informal support model also may entail significant indirect and/or intangible costs, including physical injuries, emotional stress, and damage to family relationships and friendships. There can be substantial physical or emotional costs associated with taking care of a loved one, particularly if no respite care or other opportunities for occasional relief is available. With some exceptions, such respite care is often unavailable, or if available, is often inadequate to provide the full relief needed.[18]

Medical Model

The medical model is by far the most expensive of the three models, in that it relies upon highly-trained health care professionals who are subject to extensive and costly licensure, certification and accreditation requirements and other regulations. Nursing home care can be particularly expensive. The average cost of a year of nursing home care was about $50,000 in 1997; the average private pay rate per day rate at nursing homes was $125 per day.[19] Such costs are expected to continue to rise rapidly as demand continues to expand. Home health care under the medical model also is spiraling out of control.[20]

One reason for the high costs associated with the medical model is that agency providers receive somewhat higher wages than personal assistants. One early survey in 1988 found that, while neither type of provider tended to receive fringe benefits under most state programs, agency-based medical model providers received an average of $6.02 per hour as compared with $4.59 per hour for personal assistants under the independent living model.[21]

A more significant reason for the higher costs of the medical model is that it involves numerous "middlemen" who do not directly provide care, but whose incomes and costs must be reflected in the overall costs and charges of providers under the medical model. These middlemen include a broad array of administrative people employed by nursing homes, home health agencies and other medical model providers. Case studies indicate that, irrespective of wages and benefits paid to long-term care workers, the medical model entails a significant amount of administrative overhead and profit.[22] Even in the direct provision of services, the medical model is extremely labor-intensive in that it requires supervision of para-professional health workers by nurses as well as extensive documentation of all care provided.[23]

Whether the costs of this model are borne by consumers and their families depends upon what types of insurance or government program eligibility they have. Middle class consumers with no long-term care insurance, or with inadequate coverage, are in the worst position. They have too much money to be eligible for Medicaid, but not enough money to pay the substantial costs of long-term care.

Consequently, many middle class families have developed legal mechanisms to transfer the assets of consumers in such a manner as to allow them to qualify for Medicaid. Some of these mechanisms are legal and others are not. Overall, consumers and their families pay a substantial share of the long-term care bill; the vast majority of this out-of-pocket expense is for care provided under the medical model. *See* Chapter 8.

Independent Living Model

Care and assistance provided under the independent living model generally is substantially less expensive than that provided under the medical model. The independent living model relies on non-professional personal assistants who are trained by the consumer (or by a surrogate on behalf of the consumer). The amount of money paid by the consumer for personal assistance services depends upon the job requirements, including the nature of the work, the number of hours entailed, the labor market in the area, and the financial situation of the consumer. Consumers who are professionals, or who have resources available from other sources (e.g., a lawsuit), can afford to pay more than the minimum wage, and often do so to attempt to attract more qualified and dependable workers.

Several studies provide some insight into the relative affordability of services under the independent living model as compared with the medical model. As already discussed, the WID study found that wages for personal assistants are somewhat lower than for agency workers.[24] Conversely, the study found that more hours of personal assistance services were available under the independent living model: 22 hours for personal assistants compared with 15 hours for agency workers.[25] Another study found that consumer-directed personal assistance services are significantly less costly on a per capita basis than nursing home care or care by a home health agency.[26] The researchers concluded:

> Although those who used an independent [living] model of care-giving received significantly more hours of paid assistance, the average annual cost of care was significantly lower for each individual. In addition to reducing the financial burden on the individual and society, self-managed care seemed to diminish the emotional burden borne by these individuals.[27]

Generally, whatever the consumer spends for personal assistance services will be significantly less than would be spent for comparable services provided under the medical model for several reasons. First, as suggested above, professionals and para-professionals expect to be paid more than non-professionals for their services. The costs associated with education, training, certification, licensing, and compliance with other regulations must be compensated. The major question concerning these expenses is whether the consumer derives additional value from the services of those who have incurred these expenses. Consumers under the independent living model often contend that they prefer not to have workers with such training and certification, even if these credentials did not come at an additional cost.[28]

Second, the independent living model eliminates the expensive "middle man" who absorbs substantial resources under the medical model. As noted above, nursing homes and home health agencies have large administrative costs that are passed on to the consumer. The independent living model entails a significant amount of "sweat equity," whereby consumers and surrogates conduct the management functions such as locating and hiring workers that nursing home and agency administrators typically conduct. The independent living model therefore rates relatively low on the "manageability" criterion. Of course, to the extent that consumers under the independent living model use intermediary organizations to reduce their management burden, expenses will be accordingly higher and may approach the costs of the medical model.[29]

The actual financial burden on the consumer depends upon the consumer's specific circumstances. Those consumers who are employed and not eligible for health care coverage under government programs must pay all personal assistance and other long-term care expenses out-of-pocket. Depending upon the consumer's needs, and whether any supplemental assistance is available from friends and family members under the informal support model, this situation can be very expensive, running into the tens of thousands of dollars. However, it is still likely to be significantly less expensive than similar services under the medical model.

AUTONOMY (CONSUMER DIRECTION)

Autonomy, also referred to as self-determination, considers the extent to which the consumer may control how, when, where, and by whom he or she receives care. Ethicists have conceptualized autonomy as having positive and negative dimensions.[30] Negative autonomy encompasses the right to accept or reject recommended options, such as the option to accept or reject a recommended medical intervention in the case of informed consent. Positive autonomy "encompasses proactive participation in the actual design and implementation of options selected by the individual, such as the design and implementation of a personal service plan in the case of consumer-directed services."[31] Another distinction has been drawn between "decisional autonomy," concerning the cognitive capacity to express preferences, and "executional autonomy," concerning the ability to carry out one's choices.[32]

The autonomy criterion adopted here relates to positive decisional and executional autonomy, i.e., consumer direction. Chapter 4 is dedicated exclusively to the topic of consumer direction and the related concept of consumer choice; for this reason, these concepts are not addressed at length here. Suffice it to say that control is extremely important to most consumers of all ages and demographic categories. As indicated earlier, control is associated with good health, reduced risk of abuse and neglect, enhanced satisfaction with care and life, and overall well-being.[33]

The amount of control that consumers are able to exercise depends largely on individual factors, such as the personality of the consumer and the relationship between the consumer and the provider. However, the model under which a consumer receives care and assistance will have strong influence on how much control may be exercised. Different models have specific characteristics that lend themselves to greater or lesser extent to consumer control.

Informal Support Model

Under the informal support model, the amount of control that consumers can exercise depends on the nature of their relationship with the family members or friends who are providing care and assistance. Some of these relationships are well-balanced, with each party providing input on the schedule of care and other key issues. More often, though, one party has greater power and control than the other. This type of relationship often results in resentment on the part of the individual with less power and control, strained family relationships, or compromised friendships.

As might be expected, the individual with the greater power is typically the caregiver; the caregiver has the ability to withhold or ration care in any way. In such situations, consumers may have very little control over their care and their lives. If they do not have adequate resources to purchase external assistance services, and they are not eligible for Medicaid or any other program that covers or directly provides long-term care, they may have no choice but to accept the care and assistance they receive in the manner they receive it from friends and relatives.

Medical Model

Under the medical model, the amount of control consumers can exert also varies considerably based upon the philosophy of the providers and the assertiveness of the consumers. Although there is now much rhetoric about patient rights and control, the extent to which consumers actually control their care depends upon their knowledge of their rights and their ability to advocate for themselves. Virtually no data are available on the amount of control exercised by consumers under the medical model.

Some features of the medical model, however, suggest optimal autonomy will not be achieved. Independent living advocates opposed to the medical model often claim that the environment in nursing homes is so inherently coercive that consumers are dissuaded from self-advocacy; such assertive actions could result in retribution by an over-worked staff. Moreover, health care providers will abide by their professional standards, and are not likely to comply with consumer requests that they interpret as being in conflict with their standards. Therefore, although consumer control has definitely expanded under the medical model in recent years, particularly in the context of negative autonomy through informed consent, consumers are not likely to achieve substantial positive autonomy under this model. *See* Chapter 3 on de-institutionalization.

Independent Living Model

Theoretically, the independent living model offers consumers the greatest amount of control over their long-term care. By allowing consumers to select, train, and manage the personal assistant, this model provides substantial positive autonomy at all levels of consumer assistance and care. In the event that consumers are dissatisfied with the care received, they may terminate the employment relationship. Among the various sub-models of the independent living model, the cash model, in which the consumer receives a cash benefit that can be spent on any of a wide variety of personal assistance and assistive technology services, is the most flexible and offers the greatest amount of positive autonomy.[34]

Empirical evidence from states and countries that have adopted versions of the independent living model indicate that consumers have substantially greater control under this model. In the 1988 WID study, five indicators of control, labeled client direction, were identified:

- Having known the aide prior to employment;
- Helping in scheduling aides;
- Supervising the aide;
- Signing time sheets and/or paychecks; and
- Being involved in changing aides.[35]

States with programs that conformed closely to the independent living model had higher scores concerning consumer direction. For example, almost 40% of consumers in Michigan, which has a model based on consumer-directed personal assistance services, indicated four or five of the above indicators, compared with only about 4% of consumers in Maryland and Texas with agency-based systems.[36] Over half of Michigan consumers indicated that they helped in scheduling the assistant, compared with 24% in Maryland and 33% in Texas.[37]

In California, individuals receiving consumer-directed care reported considerably more control and choice than consumers who receive care from agencies.[38] In Germany, 85% of respondents under their program using the independent living model indicated a major advantage: they may decide how to use their cash benefits. Only 27% of respondents who received agency services under the medical model reported such an advantage.[39] Similar results are reported in the Netherlands.[40]

The presentation of these findings is not intended to suggest that autonomy is guaranteed under the independent living model. Particularly in situations in which the consumer does not have any alternative personal assistants available, and where the consumer's personal assistant is negligent or abusive, autonomy may be sacrificed altogether. However, such circumstances appear to be relatively rare. Overall, the independent living model offers by far the greatest amount of positive autonomy to consumers. Of all the criteria, the independent living model is supported most strongly by the criterion of autonomy.

MANAGEABILITY

Manageability refers to the extent to which legal, regulatory and paperwork requirements are not unduly burdensome and are acceptable to the consumer. This criterion may be important to consumers depending in part upon their abilities to manage a complex personal care relationship. Like many domestic employment relationships, the personal assistance relationship can be highly complex; it often involves a combination of job responsibilities, personal friendships, and sometimes unusual hours. In addition, unlike business employers, who can hire accountants and attorneys to assist them in complying with regulatory, tax and other legal requirements, much of which requires substantial paperwork, consumers typically do not have such professional assistance. The obligations of consumers can be very considerable. For this reason, manageability can be a key criterion for some consumers, particularly those who are less concerned with autonomy than with living their lives without bureaucratic frustrations. *See* Appendix A.

Informal Support Model

Under the informal support model, manageability is not a major concern. This model does not use either an independent contractor or an employee, and consequently does not have any legal paperwork requirements. This is an enormous advantage to the consumer because such legal requirements, including tax reporting and payment, can be extremely burdensome. Like any model of long-term care, the informal support model entails the inherent challenge of managing a working relationship. This challenge is exacerbated by the additional emotional issues for consumers associated with relying upon uncompensated care and receiving such assistance from relatives and friends. The difficulty of managing this relationship depends largely on the nature of the relationship with the person providing assistance and care without compensation.

Some innovative approaches to addressing the burdens of management have been developed under the informal support model.

The Microboards in British Colombia involve the collaboration of several households to meet the needs of a person with a developmental disability.[41] Such assistance in addressing manageability issues can be invaluable, particularly for people with cognitive problems resulting in diminished decisional capacity. *See* Appendix B.

Medical Model

Manageability is a somewhat greater concern under the medical model. The extent of the challenge depends upon whether consumers are covered by private long-term care insurance, Medicaid or some other payor, or are paying for care out-of-pocket. Those consumers who have private insurance or are paying from their own resources have the greatest paperwork burden. Completing insurance forms for payment of long-term care expenses and tracking such expenses for insurance and tax purposes can be extremely burdensome.

There is little burden associated with managing the care relationship under the medical model. The health care provider basically does all the work. To the extent that consumers want to exercise control over their care, the consumer burden will be increased accordingly. However, this burden does not compare to the substantial burden on consumers under the independent living model. In a French demonstration of long-term care options, 66% of survey respondents indicated that avoiding the burden of management tasks is an advantage when using agency services under the medical model.[42]

Independent Living Model

Under the independent living model, consumers have a very considerable burden in managing the employment relationship and complying with all legal requirements. This burden should not be underestimated. It is only a small exaggeration to say that consumers are treated like small businesses by the federal government and many states. Consumers are responsible for filing all relevant federal, state and local tax and regulatory requirements; failure to comply may result in significant penalties. These requirements are discussed at length in Appendix A.

Consumers indicate that the management of payrolls and employment taxes is particularly challenging to them, and that this is the single area in which they would most want assistance.[43] Some states provide the services of fiscal intermediaries to assist consumers with such requirements; these organizations address such functions as invoicing and disbursing funds and managing employment taxes.[44] Some intermediaries provide additional tasks including paying non-labor-related expenses, addressing workers' compensation issues, addressing health benefits, and dealing with other paperwork.[45]

Studies in other countries confirm that bureaucratic barriers can pose substantial impediments to consumer autonomy under the independent living model. In the Netherlands, consumers complained that the fiscal agent responsible for paying workers created problems by not paying on time.[46] Of course, this is not a fair criticism of the independent living model, in that late payments can occur under the medical model as well. However, under the medical model, nursing homes and home health agencies are likely to have substantially more resources than individual consumers to pay for their workers while waiting for payments from a program.

In France, there is considerable criticism of the bureaucracy of their consumer-directed system.[47] Again, this should serve as an admonition that bureaucracy should be kept to the minimum feasible level for this model to work effectively. The four European countries that have been reported as having programs under the independent living model–Austria, Germany, France and the Netherlands–all provide assistance to consumers in management areas such as recruiting, training, supervising, and paying assistance.[48] However, all have been criticized as providing insufficient assistance.[49] In France and the Netherlands, the primary assistance is in the form of fiscal agents that address payment of workers and relevant taxes on behalf of consumers.[50]

In addition to the substantial paperwork and regulatory requirements, the independent living model entails an extremely complex employment relationship. Mastering the management of this relationship in a manner that ensures the satisfaction of both the consumer and the assistant often takes several years of experience. Consumers typically learn through trial and error which strategies work and how to structure responsibilities and benefits. Even with the best planning, consumers may face some trying moments in which personal assistants do not show up for work or resign without notice. If not managed skillfully, the very human nature of this relationship can result in misunderstandings, bad feelings and abrupt terminations. Unless the consumer has adequate backup, severe consequences can occur.

SECURITY

Security is the extent to which the consumer is free from unreasonable risk of physical and emotional abuse, as well as risks of theft and financial abuse. Although security is clearly a key criterion concerning long-term care, security is by no means the only criterion or even necessarily the most important criterion. Different consumers have different levels of tolerance for risks of abuse. There are often tradeoffs between security and other key criteria such as autonomy and affordability. Ultimately, consumers should be allowed to choose their own level of security, taking into consideration all of their values, goals and criteria. We should not impose a standard of high security on consumers who are more concerned about other issues.

Having said this, security obviously is an important issue, and some assurances of security are necessary, particularly for government programs using public funds and for consumers who are vulnerable to harm or exploitation (e.g., those with cognitive problems). Elder abuse is a serious problem in our society.[51] Between one million and two million instances of elder abuse occur each year, affecting about 5% of the elderly population.[52] Abuse occurs in both home and institutional settings; perpetrators and victims are members of all races, ethnic groups, genders and socioeconomic backgrounds.[53] Only one in every eight cases of elder abuse is reported to authorities.[54] Senior citizens are reluctant to report abuse for a variety of reasons, including feelings of powerlessness and embarrassment, and fear of future mistreatment or abandonment. Even when elder abuse is reported, the offender is seldom prosecuted because of problems of proving guilt.

Elder abuse is growing at an alarming rate. This situation has become particularly evident in states with large numbers of senior citizens, such as California and Florida. According to the California State Association of Counties (CSAC), reports of abuse and neglect of adults rose more than 116% between 1984 and 1993.[55] The California Department of Social Services reported approximately 44,700 cases of elder or dependent adult abuse in 1996; it estimated 180,000 instances of abuse went unreported that same year, for a total of roughly 225,000 incidents.[56] One of the reasons that much elder abuse is not reported is that many of the abuse seniors are concerned that their family members would put them in a nursing home.[57]

Younger people with disabilities are substantially less vulnerable to abuse than elderly disabled people. Younger people tend to have fewer and less significant cognitive and communication problems and are therefore more able to protect themselves. Still, abuse among the younger disabled population is also a problem, particularly among the more vulnerable elements of the population, such as people with mental retardation or mental illness.[58] Abuse of women with disabilities of all ages is also a substantial problem.[59]

Therefore, security is clearly an important issue concerning the provision of long-term care. The challenge is to incorporate security assurances without compromising the other beneficial aspects of a long-term care model, and to do so in a manner consistent with the desires of the consumer. Each consumer's personal situation, including level of vulnerability, should be considered on an individual basis in considering and addressing issues of security.

Informal Support Model

The level of security under the informal support model for consumers depends entirely on the relationship between the consumer and the caretaker, and whether the caretaker is an abusive person. We may assume that most care provided under this model is provided in a safe and supportive manner. However, we also know that there is a large amount of child and elder abuse in residential settings.[60] There is every reason to expect that at least the same rates of abuse exist in relationships involving the provision of long-term care services.

The primary social mechanisms for detecting and addressing abuse are reporting requirements whereby certain types of professionals, including virtually all health care professionals, are mandated to report suspected abuse. Such mechanisms are probably least effective in providing protection under the informal support model. Under this model, care is provided in the home where abuse is less likely to be subject to detection by outsiders. Moreover, to the extent that the consumer is completely or largely dependent upon family caregivers, the consumer may be in a particularly vulnerable situation in which he or she may not be willing to report abuse.

Medical Model

The medical model contains several safeguards to ensure the security of the consumer. These safeguards include extensive credentialing of providers, including licenses for health care professionals, certifications for para-professionals, and accreditation of long-term care facilities.[61] Health care organizations are required to conduct security checks on their prospective employees. Extensive health care regulations at the federal and state levels, as well as the threat of civil lawsuits, are designed in part to reduce the threats of physical and emotional injury to the consumer. All these safeguards significantly increase the cost of long-term care under the medical model.[62] The question is whether such increased costs are justified by reduced risks to the consumer.

Allegations by supporters of the medical model that the other models are subject to extensive abuse would be more credible if not for the extensive documented abuse under the medical model.[63] One national study estimates that one-third of all nursing homes have been cited for abuse or neglect.[64] The industry claims that it has significant safeguards preventing abuse, such as professional supervision of para-professional home health workers. However, in California, it has been reported that approximately 37% of agency workers report that they have very little or no supervision.[65]

One measure of abuse in nursing homes is contained in reports of complaint investigations filed by residents under the Long-Term Care Ombudsman Program of the Older Americans Act (OAA).[66] The 1995 report of this program indicated that 162,338 complainants filed a total of 218,455 complaints with the 52 national Ombudsmans' Offices.[67] Some 86.7% of the complaints related to nursing homes.[68] Of the 28 state Ombudsmans' Offices that provided a detailed breakdown of complaints, 47,343 of 54,305 total complaints (87%) pertained to nursing facilities; 30% of these complaints were directly from the residents.[69] Of the 82,442 complaints pertaining to nursing homes, 24,587 pertained to residents' rights, 6,128 of which were for abuse, gross neglect, and exploitation.[70]

Independent Living Model

Security concerns under the independent living model are similar to those under the informal support model. Because care is provided at home under both models, there is little opportunity for outsiders to detect abuse. However, the additional control by consumers under the independent living model gives policymakers some reason to be somewhat less concerned about abuse in that context. Yet, the risk clearly exists, and examples of abuse have been documented under the independent living model.[71] However, we do not know the extent to which abuse occurs under the independent living model, and further research is needed on these issues.[72] Based on such research, additional security mechanisms could be built into any program based on the independent living model.

QUALITY (CONSUMER SATISFACTION)

Quality considers the extent to which the consumer receives competent assistance and the process and outcomes of care are satisfactory to the consumer. Obviously, this definition is not the only possible way to define quality; there are actually dozens of approaches to defining and measuring quality in long-term care.[73] This definition is adopted here specifically because we are analyzing quality from an independent living perspective. The definition contains both an objective and a subjective component. Objectively, we want to ensure that care and assistance provided meet at least minimum standards of competence. To independent living advocates, however, the greatest concern is whether the care meets the subjective needs of the consumer as defined by the consumer. Quality also may be defined from either a positive or negative standpoint. Positive quality is associated with positive outcomes of care, such as the ability to live independently, and satisfaction with the process. Negative quality entails the lack of adverse experiences or outcomes, such as absence of errors in the provision of care. *See* Chapter 10.

Informal Support Model

Negative quality issues of concern raised about the informal support model involve allegations of negligent, reckless or other incompetent care. Like similar allegations concerning security, health care providers and other advocates for the medical model claim that any model that does not rely upon professional health care providers will place consumers at an unreasonable risk. Again, there is very little evidence of the extent to which mistakes resulting from negligence, recklessness or other incompetence occurs under the informal support model, or whether such problems occur more or less frequently than they occur under the medical model. The informal nature of the informal support model makes monitoring of quality extremely difficult.

Medical Model

Many of the same regulatory safeguards for ensuring security under the medical model also apply is ensuring quality. Licensing, certification, accreditation, and other regulations pertaining to government financing of long-term care are designed to ensure at least some minimum level of quality.[74] Long-term care facilities, like other health care provider organizations, are required to review the National Practitioner Data Bank to ensure that facilities do not hire practitioners who have been guilty of malpractice or ethical violations. Again, an important question is whether the increased costs associated with these regulatory requirements are justified by enhanced quality of care and accordingly reduced risks to the consumer.

The medical model does not perform optionally in addressing the criterion of quality.[75] Just as consumers under the medical model have been subject to extensive documented abuse, they have also been subject to extensive negligence and incompetence.[76] The record of the health care industry generally, and long-term care providers specifically, is far from stellar despite all the safeguards built into the system.[77] One review of nursing home care in Oklahoma found that 1,000 people had died since 1990 from preventable malnutrition, bedsores and other causes.[78] In Missouri, 19 people died over a two-year period as a result of "abysmal treatment or indifference."[79]

Another recent study of deficiencies identified in state survey reviews of nursing facilities found that about 23% of all such facilities were cited in the year 2000 for at least one deficiency resulting in harm or significant risk to a patient.[80] Although this percentage is somewhat lower than in previous years, it is still alarming.[81] Of the top 10 reasons for deficiencies, almost all related to quality of care problems: food sanitation, accidents, pressure sores, housekeeping issues, professional standards, and assistance in the activities of daily living.[82] Some 17% of facilities were cited for failure to prevent pressure sores.[83]

Table 3: Comparison of the Three Models
of Long-Term Care

Criteria/Model	Informal Support Model	Medical Model	Independent Living Model
Accountability	0	+	+
Affordability	++	--	+
Autonomy	-	-	++
Manageability	++	-	--
Security	+	+	-
Quality	0	+	++

Legend

-- very negative   - negative   0 neutral   + positive   ++ very positive

Accountability—The extent to which the allocation of resources for care is satisfactory to the funding source, including absence of fraud and financial abuse.
Affordability—The extent to which the costs of care, including out-of-pocket costs to the consumer, are reasonable and do not impose a financial burden on the average consumer.
Autonomy—The extent to which the consumer may control how, where, when and by whom he or she receives care.
Managability—The extent to which legal, regulatory and paperwork requirements are not unduly burdensome and are acceptable to the consumer.
Security—The extent to which the consumer is free from unreasonable physical and emotional risks, as well as risks of theft and financial abuse.
Quality (consumer satisfaction)—The extent to which the consumer receives competent assistance, and the process and outcomes of care are satisfactory to the consumer.

Like nursing facilities, home health agencies also have been criticized for providing an inadequate quality of care.[84] The objective of documenting these quality problems is not to indict all medical model providers of long-term care. In fact, ensuring quality of care in a long-term care environment is extremely challenging under any model and any set of providers. For example, preventing pressure sores in consumers who have extremely limited mobility and sensitivity is extremely difficult. While any model of long-term care must be held accountable for breaches of quality resulting in pressure sores, no model or set of providers will be able to avoid all such sores in every year of operation. The point of documenting these quality problems is to demonstrate that the medical model is subject to the same quality problems as the other models. Whether the medical model is more or less subject to such problems is an empirical issue that should be assessed further. Some comparisons between quality under the medical model and the independent living model have been conducted, as discussed below.

Independent Living Model

As with security, quality concerns under the independent living model are similar to those under the informal support model. Again, the additional control by consumers under the independent living model gives policymakers some reason to be somewhat less concerned about quality in that context. If consumers are truly concerned about quality, they have the ability to terminate their personal assistants under this model.

An assessment of California's In-Home Support Services program, which offers both agency-based services under the medical model and consumer-directed services under the independent living model, reveals that consumers receiving care under the independent living model feel more empowered in their service relationship; they are also more satisfied with both the technical and interpersonal aspects of their care.[85] They rate their overall quality of life as better than consumers under the medical model rate their lives.[86] The higher satisfaction with technical aspects of care under the independent living model is interesting, considering that workers under the medical model received substantially more formal training than personal assistants.[87] Other studies support these findings, concluding that there are lower levels of hospitalization and higher levels of life satisfaction for consumers under the independent living model.[88]

Analysis of the early stage of the Arkansas Cash and Counseling demonstration suggests that consumers experience a high level of satisfaction under this version of the independent living model.[89] All respondents expressed satisfaction with their relationships with paid caregivers who assisted them; virtually all (99%) were pleased with the way in which their assistants fulfilled their duties.[90] Approximately 96% of consumers were satisfied with their overall care.[91] Some 82% of participants who received the cash allowance indicated that it improved their quality of life; 79% said that it improved a great deal; and none reported that quality of life had diminished.[92] Over 90% of participants, including those who disenrolled and those whose family members responded on their behalves because they died during the demonstration, would recommend the Independent Choices program for people who wish to exercise control over their personal care.[93]

The Commonwealth Study similarly found that knowing a personal assistant prior to working with the individual is closely related to consumer satisfaction.[94] Consumers who knew their assistant previously were about three times more likely to be highly satisfied.[95] This finding is an important because, between the two models of long-term care that involve paid assistance, consumers are most likely to have known the personal assistant previously under the independent living model. This is because consumers have much greater control over hiring under the independent living model. Under the medical model, in which an agency would typically hire the aide, it would be a rare coincidence that the consumer knew the personal assistant previously. Of course, the independent living model does not guarantee that the consumer and assistant knew each other previously. Particularly in states that do not allow relatives to be hired as personal assistants, consumers and assistants are less likely to have known each other, resulting in a lower probability of consumer satisfaction.[96]

Other factors found to be statistically significant to a high level of overall satisfaction with an assistant are whether the consumer helps to schedule the assistant and whether the consumer supervises the assistant.[97] Consumers who reported that they supervise their assistants were twice as likely to be highly satisfied.[98] Moreover, there appears to be a synergistic effect whereby the more indicators of control and choice that are incorporated in a state program, the more satisfied is the consumer. Consumers who reported that their state program has four or five indicators were significantly more likely than others to be very satisfied.[99] In a study of the Virginia program operated under the independent living model, a comparison of people with disabilities receiving consumer-directed personal assistance services with those on a waiting list to receive such services found that those receiving the services were more likely to be satisfied with their long-term care services.[100]

SUMMARY OF EVALUATIONS

Table 3 presents an overall summary of the assessment of the three general models of long-term care based on the established criteria. The table shows that there are tradeoffs among the various models. No single model is for everyone; consumers should choose the model under which they receive their long-term care based upon those criteria that are most important to them. Consumers who value autonomy, and who are not unduly concerned with security and manageability issues, may wish to choose the independent living model. Those who do not wish to contend with the challenging issues concerning managing a personal assistance services relationship, and who desire the security of having professional health care providers available, may choose the medical model. Under either of these models, quality will depend largely on the specific provider of services and that provider's relationship with the consumer.

Consumers who have family members or friends willing to assist them for free will benefit from having at least some of their care provided under the informal support model. Most would not want to rely primarily on this model unless they have no financial resources available to pay for assistance under either of the other models. If resources were available and no restrictions were placed on hiring family members (as currently occurs in several states and European countries), many consumers would choose to continue receiving care from their family members but would pay them, thereby giving the consumer greater leverage in controlling their care. Financing issues, which directly affect the criteria of affordability and accountability, play a major role in structuring the choices actually available to consumers.[101]

—8—

Financing

$\mathbf{T}$he single most important prerequisite to the expansion of consumer-directed personal assistance services under the independent living model is the establishment of a long-term care financing system that supports this option. Long-term care expenditures constitute approximately 12% of total personal health expenditures, a threefold increase since 1960.[1] The vast majority of long-term care services are provided under the medical model of long-term care.[2] This chapter considers the sources of financing for long-term care.

A BIASED SYSTEM

In 1998, over $117 billion was spent on long-term care, including nursing home and other institutional care and home health care services not affiliated with hospitals.[3] Long-term care is funded in approximately the following proportions: Medicaid, 39%; Medicare, 17.8%; private health insurance, 7.4%; out-of-pocket 29.5%; and other sources, 6.3%.[4] In 1994, 81% of the Medicaid program's $45.6 billion in long-term care spending was spent on institutional care; 61% was spent on nursing homes and 20% on intermediate care facilities for people with mental retardation.[5]

Thus, there is a strong traditional bias in favor of institutional care under our long-term care system. A key reason is that policymakers are politically risk-adverse; they are often so concerned about very bad "career-ending" outcomes (e.g., abuse or neglect of consumers) that they avoid new approaches, even approaches with strong potential benefits. To the extent feasible, policymakers like to delegate responsibility and financial accountability to providers whom they can blame if anything goes wrong. The result is that much of federal health care policy is directed at shifting financial risk to health maintenance organizations (HMOs) and other managed care organizations (MCOs). Policymakers hesitate to delegate responsibility to consumers, concerned that some may misuse funds or be harmed. When something goes wrong, there is nobody except the consumer and the policymaker to be held accountable. The prospect of prosecuting a program recipient with a major disability for misappropriation of funds is not as politically attractive as prosecuting a health care organization responsible for the individual's care. Even less attractive to policymakers is a television expose showing consumers who are harmed, and reporters asking about the lack of safeguards to protect the consumers.

The institutional bias of the long-term care system has been strongly criticized by disability rights and independent living advocates.[6] With the evolution of the independent living movement and the growth of consumer direction, this bias has decreased gradually over time.[7] Still, it persists to a considerable extent. The financing of long-term care services continues to be biased against the independent living model, particularly the cash version of the independent living model.

PRIVATE FINANCING

Most analysts begin their treatment of the financing of long-term care services with a discussion of the various public financing programs, such as Medicaid and Medicare. This approach, while justified based on actual dollars spent, provides a misleading impression both economically and historically. Historically, the public funding of long-term care is a relatively recent development, with very little federal funding prior to 1965. Prior to that year, state funding was concentrated almost exclusively on institutional care of citizens with the most substantial disabilities. Public financing developed largely in response to a failure of private sector markets to meet the long-term care needs of these citizens who had limited resources and family support.

Economically, as a result of this historical evolution, private financing continues to dominate the financing of long-term care, but only in a very unconventional sense. The private sector dominates primarily through the provision of uncompensated care under the informal support model, enormous out-of-pocket spending by consumers and their families, and a relatively small amount of private long-term care insurance. In aggregate, these financing mechanisms dwarf the total amount of public financing for long-term care. In other words, most of the economic burden of long-term care in this country is borne on the backs of consumers and their families.

Personal Resources

A large percentage of paid long-term care services are financed out-of-pocket by consumers. Some $35 billion was spent out-of-pocket in 1998, representing almost 30% of spending on nursing facilities and home health care.[8] For elderly people, who pay about 14% of all medical expenditures out-of-pocket, about 42% of long-term care expenditures are financed out-of-pocket.[9] They incur such expenses because very few public or private insurance programs cover long-term care, and those that do provide coverage have substantial restrictions. Typically, it is not until consumers require long-term care that they also determine that they have no coverage or inadequate coverage for it. Often, the consumers then pay for such care until their resources are exhausted, at which time they may become eligible for Medicaid long-term care.

Little financial relief is available to consumers and their families who pay for long-term care out-of-pocket. Congress has recently clarified that long-term care expenses qualify for the federal health care tax deduction. However, that tax deduction is subject to a limitation of 7½% of adjusted gross income. Therefore, only those individuals who itemize their federal tax returns, and only those whose combined health care and long-term care expenses are above the limit, even qualify for the relief. This provision substantially reduces the relief available to the vast majority of long-term care consumers. Moreover, this approach is inequitable in that it particularly benefits those consumers in the highest tax brackets, who may therefore deduct their expenses at a higher rate.

One way in which to relieve the financial burden on consumers and their families would be to replace the tax deduction with a tax credit for long-term care expenses. A tax credit would benefit anyone who incurs long-term care expenses and has a federal tax liability against which the credit would apply. Moreover, such a credit would provide an identical dollar benefit to people in different tax brackets. However, it would not provide relief for low-income people who have no tax liability, and therefore nothing against which the credit would apply. For such individuals, only a refundable tax credit, in which the credit would apply to provide a cash benefit irrespective of a tax liability, would provide financial relief for long-term care expenses.

To date, tax credits have been proposed for long-term care expenditures, such as the long-term care tax credit proposed in the Clinton administration's national health care reform proposal.[10] No proposals have been debated seriously for a refundable tax credit for long-term care. Among the reasons for political resistance to such a tax credit are the large cost to the federal treasury, and concerns about fraud and abuse.[11]

Informal Support

Even more significant economically than out-of-pocket payments is the uncompensated care and assistance provided by family members. The estimated $196 billion in uncompensated services provided each year for the long-term care and assistance of consumers exceeds the estimated $117 billion spent on all long-term care paid directly to compensated providers in 1998.[12] Of course, the total amount of uncompensated long-term care and determining its monetary value are issues that are subject to debate. What is clear is that millions of consumers who are not eligible for any public programs and with very limited financial resources require long-term care services and receive such services in some manner.

Due to the uncompensated and unregulated nature of such services, we will never have as complete an understanding of the extent of these services as we have of services provided under the medical model, or to a lesser extent, under the independent living model. It has been estimated that approximately 80% of people who require long-term care, or over 7 million people, receive assistance from relatives under the informal support model.[13] These consumers receive their care from a variety of caregivers in approximately the following proportions: 41% of unpaid caregivers are the adult children of the consumer; 24% are spouses; 26% are other relatives; and 9% are non-relatives (e.g., friends and close acquaintances).[14]

Determining the value of such services depends upon specific assumptions concerning the appropriate hourly wage to apply, the number of hours, and the value of benefits and other foregone economic opportunities for the caregiver. The estimate of $196 billion in uncompensated services provided each year for the long-term is based on relatively conservative assumptions.

Private Long-Term Care Insurance

Before 1985, there was virtually no market for private long-term care insurance.[15] Experts in the field questioned whether long-term care could even be considered an "insurable event." The idea was that the purpose of insurance is to protect against risks (i.e., the probability of a negative outcome), and the issue was whether long-term care constitutes a risk with a fairly dependable set of probabilities that care will be needed at different age intervals, or a certainty for the vast majority of individuals. Typically, private insurance markets do not develop to protect against fairly certain negative events. In recent years, experience has demonstrated that the need for long-term care is a risk that private insurance markets can address.[16]

The market for private long-term care insurance currently is very small, but growing rapidly, particularly in response to encouragement by the federal government. The Health Insurance Association of America has claimed a growth in long-term care policies of about 21% per year between 1987 and 1997.[17] By 1998, more than 5.8 million long-term care policies had been sold.[18] However, this represents only about 7% of total long-term care expenditures.[19] There are real limits to the potential size of this market; only people with significant wealth or relatively high incomes can afford the high premiums of private insurance.[20] Moreover, even those who can afford such insurance at one point in time may not be financially able to maintain their policies over time until they need the benefits. Insurers expect that half the policies they sell will lapse in 5 years, and 65% will lapse in 10 years.[21]

An important question that has not received much attention is to what extent private insurance is covering services under the independent living model. A study of long-term care insurance claimants reveals that about 77% have at least some informal support.[22] About 67% of their formal care is provided by home health aides, and 7% is provided by nurses.[23] In aggregate, over 74% of formal care paid by private insurance is being provided under the medical model by home health aides and nurses. The remainder is being provided under the independent living model by other non-medical providers. At least two major insurance companies, UNUM and Aetna, pay a cash benefit for consumers who have sufficient disabilities to be eligible.[24]

PUBLIC FINANCING

Several federal programs provide funding for long-term care services. These programs include Medicaid, Medicare, the Veterans' health care program and various smaller programs authorized under the Social Security Act and the Older Americans Act. Although government pays a substantial share of the long-term care bill, most is spent on care provided under the medical model; a disproportionate share is spent on institutional care. Consumers bear a large share of the financial burden. Consumers who wish to live at home receiving services under the independent living model often do not have that option.

Medicaid

The Medicaid program is by far the largest source of federal funding for long-term care. Medicaid is a joint federal-state financing program, in which the federal government provides matching funds to states that comply with its general program requirements. States administer the program within the parameters of the federal requirements. Altogether, in 1997, Medicaid paid approximately $59 billion for institutional and home- and community-based services; 73% of such expenditures were for care in nursing homes and intermediate care facilities for the mentally retarded.[25] Again, this demonstrates the strong bias of the Medicaid program in favor of institutional care. In every state except Oregon and Vermont, over 50% of Medicaid long-term care expenditures are allocated to institutional care.[26]

Under federal Medicaid rules, coverage of nursing home services is mandatory for all states, but the states may determine how and how much to pay for such care. State per capita spending on institutional care varies enormously, from $50 in two states to between $300 and $450 in two other states and Washington D.C.[27] Similarly, states must provide physician-ordered home health services. In addition, since the early days of the Medicaid program, states have had the option to provide personal care services prescribed by a physician; 32 states had authorized this "personal care services option" in their Medicaid plans by 1994.[28] Total Medicaid expenditures for the personal care services option was just under $3 billion that year, making Medicaid the single largest source of financing for home- and community-based long-term care.[29]

States have complained that a problem with Medicaid funding of long-term care services generally is that rigid federal requirements have stifled state creativity and innovation. As an optional benefit, the personal care option has allowed states some flexibility, and has greatly increased access to consumer-directed personal assistance services. Surveys by the World Institute on Disability in 1984 and 1988 found that these optional programs were organized either exclusively or predominantly under either the independent living model with personal assistants or the medical model with agency-employed aides.[30] By 1988, 13 of these programs were organized under the medical model, and 9 were organized primarily under the independent living model.[31] Yet, even those programs under the independent living model often had features that limited consumer control, such as not allowing consumers to train or participate in paying assistants.[32]

Medicaid Home- and Community-Based Waivers

The most important development concerning consumer direction in Medicaid long-term care was the establishment in 1981 of the optional Home- and Community-based Care Waiver Program, Section 1915(c) of the Social Security Act. Under this program, states could establish a system of home- and community-based care that deviates from the rigid federal rules of the traditional Medicaid program. However, to gain this flexibility, states must first demonstrate to the federal government that savings will be achieved from avoided institutionalization. States must request a specified number of waiver slots and comply with regulations on informing recipients of their rights and options, as well as other applicable regulations.

By 1993, Medicaid expenditures for home -and community-based care under the section 1915 (c) waivers exceeded spending under the optional personal care benefit.[33]

Yet, it should be emphasized that over three-quarters (76.7%) of this funding is allocated to people with mental retardation and other developmental disabilities.[34] Another 21.3% goes to people who are elderly or disabled and are not included in the developmentally disabled category.[35]

In 1998, the average annual spending on people with mental retardation or other developmental disabilities receiving services under the home- and community-based services waiver program was $30,782; average annual spending was $78,369 for those receiving services in an intermediate care facility for the mentally retarded.[36] While these disparate figures cannot be compared directly, because presumably most of those receiving services in the community have higher levels of functioning and fewer health problems than the institutionalized individuals, the much lower figure for home- and community-based care suggests the potential for substantial savings for those capable of living in the community.

States may choose which benefits they cover under the waiver program. Among the most popular benefits are case management, respite care, habilitation services and personal assistance services. Therefore, different states have structured their programs to conform more or less to the independent living model or the medical model. In addition to programs under the federal waiver program, 39 states have indicated that they have at least one home- and community-based services program that is funded exclusively by the state, and therefore not subject to federal requirements.[37] States spent over $1.2 billion on these state programs.[38]

Although Medicaid continues to have a strong institutional bias, this bias has been reduced somewhat as a result of the increased emphasis on home- and community-based services.[39] Between 1992 and 1997, Medicaid spending for services under the waiver program almost quadrupled from $2.2 billion to almost $8 billion, reflecting a reallocation of resources away from the largest institutions and toward care in the home and community.[40] In this period, the number of Medicaid recipients served by the waiver program increased from 236,000 to 562,000, with the greatest increases among the mentally retarded/developmentally disabled population (from 58,150 to 216,570) and the aged and disabled population (from 167,779 to 326,615).[41]

Shortcomings of Medicaid as a Long-Term Care Program

Because Medicaid serves as the principal federal program designed to finance long-term care services, it is important to identify any key weaknesses of this program. Medicaid's eligibility coverage and pay-ment policies for long-term care have been severely criticized.[42] A major shortcoming of Medicaid as a source of funding for long-term care is that it has very restrictive eligibility rules. Only children and adults who are blind, disabled and/or age 65 and older who meet their state's income and asset tests are eligible.[43] To be eligible for home- and com-munity-based services under the Medicaid waiver program, an individ-ual must satisfy all the basic criteria and also otherwise require institu-tionalization.[44] The system has also been criticized for presenting con-fusing choices to consumers and coordinating care poorly with related service systems.[45]

Due to the eligibility criteria, even if an individual who requires long-term care lives in a state that provides excellent coverage of long-term care services under the model of care that the individual prefers, such care will be available only if the individual satisfies all the state's eligibility criteria. Some states are more generous than others in terms of who qualifies for Medicaid coverage, but in all states people in the middle class typically would not qualify. Many consumers of long-term care are not able to qualify for Medicaid until they have exhaust-ed so much of their resources as to be considered indigent. About 25% of consumers admitted to nursing homes as private pay patients impoverish themselves as a result of their long-term care costs.[46] The program has been severely criticized for requiring such individuals to become destitute to become Medicaid-eligible.[47]

With respect to coverage policy for long-term care services, Medicaid has strengths and weaknesses. By requiring all states to cover certain basic long-term care services, Medicaid ensures that eli-gible recipients in every state will have at least some access to long-term care. However, by imposing no significant standards as to how much of these services must be available, it allows the promise of long-term care to become a mere pretense in those states that want to limit their spending on this expensive budget item. Moreover, to the extent that states are concerned that residents of other states will migrate to them in response to generous long-term care benefits, it has been asserted that the flexibility of federal Medicaid coverage policy creates a "race to the bottom" among states competing to discourage new disabled residents.

This concern is exacerbated further by federal flexibility concern-ing Medicaid payment policy. In an effort to contain program costs, states have devised payment systems that provide very low rates of payment for Medicaid long-term care. The result, of course, has been to limit the number of long-term care providers who are willing to accept Medicaid recipients. Such low payments have been the basis of criticisms of the Medicaid program generally. Low payments are particularly problematic in the long-term care context in that such payments continue for each consumer over a long and often indefinite time period. While acute care providers may be willing to accept a certain number of Medicaid patients as part of a strategy of obtaining a diversified payor base, long-term care providers may be more hesitant to accept low payments for an extended period of time.

Finally, the major criticism of Medicaid long-term care as disproportionately institutional and medically oriented in nature is slowly being addressed through the section 1915 home- and community-based services program. There has been an enormous growth in home-based long-term care in recent years, including care and assistance provided under the independent living model. Due in part to the optional and flexible nature of these home- and community-based service programs, there is great variation among the states as to whether their citizens may receive consumer-directed services. Some have criticized the system as inequitable because different people with disabilities receive different benefits based on where they live, their age, and their specific disability.[48] According to the Urban Institute, average annual spending per waiver recipient ranged from $2,800 for the aged to $29,200 for people with traumatic brain injury.[49]

Medicare

The Medicare program does not officially include a long-term care program, but does cover certain services provided by the traditional providers of long-term care. It finances institutional and home-based services focused on skilled nursing and therapy rather than the non-medical custodial and personal assistance services that people with disabilities need to live independently. Specifically, Medicare Part A, the mandatory portion financed primarily through payroll taxes, covers certain skilled nursing facility services: services provided at a nursing home that meets specific Medicare skilled nursing requirements and home health services provided by certified home health agencies. Such coverage is not designed for the type of long-term maintenance care required by many people with disabilities. It is specifically intended for post-hospitalization recovery typically after an operation or injury, and is limited to 100 days following hospitalization for skilled nursing care.[50]

Despite the stated goals of Medicare that do not include the provision of long-term care, analysts have concluded that Medicare pays a significant share of long-term care costs. Altogether, about 10% of Medicare expenditures were spent on skilled nursing facility and home health care in 1998.[51] Medicare finances about 55% of acute care expenditures for elderly people, and about 18% of their long-term care expenditures.[52] It covers about 14.4% of the $107.8 billion of all long-term care services in 1993.[53] Moreover, the incentives inherent in Medicare's coverage and payment policies have strong implications for the financial circumstances of beneficiaries who require long-term care.

Medicare's fastest growing benefit is for home care.[54] The Council on Scientific Affairs of the American Medical Association has concluded "The goal of home care is to make the patient and family self-sufficient."[55] The Medicare home care benefit is designed primarily for acute care purposes, not long-term maintenance care. Altogether, Medicare home care expenditures have grown from $2.8 billion per year in 1988 to $15 billion per year in 1995.[56] One substantial concern about Medicare home health services is that such expenditures have been subject to a very high rate of Medicare fraud.[57]

Like Medicaid, Medicare has strict eligibility criteria. Generally, one must be age 65 or older or have a documented disability and also have contributed payroll taxes to the Social Security retirement system for a requisite number of quarters of employment. Therefore, there are many consumers who require long-term care services who do not qualify for Medicare. On the other hand, some consumers are jointly eligible for both Medicare and Medicaid, and have the most comprehensive coverage available to them.

Overall, the traditional Medicare program consisting of Medicare Parts A and B has contributed to meeting the long-term care needs of people who are eligible, but cannot be considered adequate as a long-term care program. This finding is not surprising in that Medicare was not, and is not designed to meet the long-term care and assistance needs of the population. To the extent that any component of Medicare has the capacity to satisfy such needs, it is likely to be authorized under Part C, the program of alternatives to the traditional Medicare program. Therefore, while Medicare is not technically a long-term care program, it is clearly an important component of the financing of long-term care in this country.

Veterans' Health Care

The Department of Veterans Affairs is not a large payor of long-term care services compared with Medicaid or Medicare. However, it is an important payor because its Housebound and Aides and Attendant Allowance Program has been providing cash payments to disabled veterans for over 50 years.[58] Specifically, veterans with service-connected disabilities may receive between $1,500 and $2,200 per month for their personal assistance services, or even more under certain special circumstances in which there is a "need for a higher level of care."[59] Paid assistance provided by family members is explicitly permitted. This program is probably the oldest and longest enduring program of consumer-directed long-term care services under the independent living model in the world, having been established in 1951 soon after World War II and about 20 years prior to the beginning of the independent living movement.

It is instructive to ask how such a progressive program could have been established so long before its time. Apparently the traditional reluctance of policymakers to offer an unencumbered cash benefit for consumers to use as they deem appropriate was overcome by the desire to provide a high level of satisfaction to consumers who became disabled in the service of their country. Although this program offers a valuable operational model for providing services under the independent living model, it does not provide insight into the political difficulties of making such a model available to the general public.

Other Federal Funding Sources

In addition, limited funding for long-term care is available under the Older Americans Act (OAA),[60] Social service block grants under the Social Security Act,[61] and initiatives financed using state revenues exclusively.[62]

GENERAL ISSUES

There are some issues that cut across financing sources and programs.

Health Care vs. Social Service Funding

One fundamental issue is whether the financing of long-term care services is best achieved through health care financing systems, such as Medicare and Medicaid, or through social service financing systems, such as the Social Service block grants and programs under the OAA. Basically, there tend to be tradeoffs among these approaches. On the one hand, Social Service financing programs do not generally have the trappings of the medical model; therefore, there is often more flexibility to provide services under the independent living model without major restrictions. On the other hand, Social Service funding is typically much more restricted than health care financing, which is more likely to provide an entitlement with few limitations to covered services.

The ideal resolution of this issue from an independent living perspective is to eliminate the trappings of the medical model in the more generous health care financing systems. Slowly, over time, this liberalization of programs such as Medicaid and Medicare has occurred to some extent through the establishment of waiver options and other administrative flexibility. Still, there remain substantial vestiges of the medical model in many of these programs, and in practice consumers are often limited in their ability to direct their personal assistance services. Further reform of the health care financing systems will be necessary to achieve the goals of consumers who wish to operate under the independent living model.

Eligibility Issues

Long-term care is relevant to everybody, because anybody could possibly develop a major disability at some point in life and require personal assistance services or other long-term care services. However, most Americans will find that they do not have adequate long-term care coverage at that time, or that they do not have any coverage at all because of the restrictive eligibility criteria of the federal programs that cover long-term care. The current policy of the United States on long-term care coverage appears to be to encourage people to impoverish themselves to become eligible for Medicaid. Although some incentives have been provided to purchase long-term care coverage, only people with substantial financial assets to protect are likely to purchase such expensive insurance. Clearly, reform of the eligibility rules for the various programs is needed. Eligibility should ideally be based on a sliding scale of income and assets, allowing people with significant assets to be eligible for assistance with significant co-payments.

Coverage Issues

Closely related to issues concerning health care vs. social services funding are issues concerning which services are covered and who may provide them. As discussed throughout this book, the independent living model contemplates the provision of a broad array of services by non-professional personal assistants under the supervision of the consumer. Therefore, under an ideal long-term care program from an independent living perspective, any service that the consumers would otherwise be able to provide for themselves, if not for their disabilities, should be covered and should be allowed to be provided by anyone hired by the consumer, including family members and friends. Different states have different coverage rules, some of which are more or less consistent with the independent living model. A key issue concerning the financing of long-term care will entail reform of the coverage rules to allow consumers to use consumer-directed personal assistance services under the independent living model.

Cash vs. In-Kind Benefits

Currently, most long-term care services are provided in kind; rather than providing a cash benefit to consumers, the programs provide the services directly through payments to certain providers.[63] However, the fact that in-kind personal services dominate at the current time does not mean that these services must be or should be provided in kind.[64] If all other factors were equal, people with disabilities presumably would prefer a cash benefit to an in-kind benefit of equal value; cash benefits offer far greater flexibility to pursue their independent living goals. For a variety of reasons, however, many consumers and policymakers prefer that benefits are provided in-kind rather than in cash.[65]

Policymakers, who are accountable to the taxpayers financing these programs, are often concerned that a cash benefit does not provide the assurance that the money will be spent in a manner that would satisfy taxpayer concerns, which is critical to ongoing political support for the program. Although a cash benefit might be used rationally by a beneficiary for better nutrition or housing, taxpayers may resent this use of program funds if they believe that they have paid for personal assistance services, not a higher standard of living generally. Far more damaging from the perspective of policymakers is the worst case scenario: consumers using the cash for entirely unjustifiable purposes, such as the purchase of alcohol or illegal drugs. Although such circumstances appear relatively rare, they can jeopardize support for a program.

Consumers also may be concerned about the use of an equivalent cash benefit for at least two reasons. First, a cash benefit may not guarantee the ability to purchase the service previously obtained through the in-kind benefit. This situation is most likely in a tight labor market in which the cost of personal assistance services is rising rapidly. Second, even if the cash benefit is set adequately at the outset, there will be a political tendency over time for it to fall below the level necessary to obtain adequate services. This problem is particularly likely in periods of economic downturn and tight government budgets, but it may even occur in relatively good times when the political clout of long-term care consumers is overwhelmed by other political interests.

The concept of using a cash benefit, in conjunction with counseling services available to the consumer, is currently being tested in the Cash and Counseling Demonstration and Evaluation Project. An alternative to the strict cash approach that may better satisfy the concerns of some policymakers is a model based on "cash equivalents." A system based on vouchers, Medical Savings Accounts (MSAs)[66] or tax credits that would provide a cash equivalent limited to the purchase of specified services will satisfy the accountability needs of many policymakers. The feasibility of this cash equivalent approach will depend largely on whether it can be structured to satisfy the significant concerns of consumers and policymakers. Assurances would be needed that the voucher, MSA or tax credit would be sufficient to obtain the needed service over the long term and that it would not be unduly subject to fraud and abuse.

Specialized vs. Generic Approaches—Social HMOs

One key issue concerning the financing and delivery of long-term care is whether people with disabilities should be addressed in the general health care system or whether special systems of financing and delivery should be established. Generally speaking, it appears preferable to address the needs of these individuals within the general health care financing system, rather than carving them out of the general system and thereby reducing the incentives for policymakers to make these systems more amenable to the needs of people with disabilities over time.[67] However, while the needs of these individuals should be addressed within the general financing system, specialized systems of delivery may be particularly useful for this population.[68]

The term "Social Health Maintenance Organizations" (Social HMOs or SHMOs) has been applied to general systems designed specifically to meet the long-term and acute care needs of people with different disabilities.[69] One of the first and most prominent Social HMOs is On Loc in San Francisco's Chinatown. The founders of this community-based program established a comprehensive set of benefits, including community-based long-term care services for the frail elderly population. They used an innovative combination of Medicaid, Medicare, private insurance and other financing programs to provide care for this population.

Based on this program, The Robert Wood Johnson Foundation provided seed money to expand the Social HMO model to provide care to a variety of populations of people with disabilities throughout the country under its PACE initiative. As a result, Social HMOs addressing the needs of younger, working-age, elderly and special populations (e.g., people with AIDS) have been established throughout the country. Also, other specialized models of integrated delivery systems for meeting the needs of people with disabilities, including long-term care needs, have been established and have been providing services effectively for years.[70]

SUMMARY

An examination of our long-term care financing system reveals a strong bias in favor of the medical model and against the independent living model. Independent living advocates have called for a correction in this imbalance. The bias is being corrected slowly through the Medicaid waiver program and other recent innovations. If the funding for consumer-directed personal assistance services is made available, the services will necessarily follow and will reflect the coverage and payment policies of the financing mechanism. For example, if the financing mechanism prohibits or discourages the provision of care by non-professionals, the result will be a medical model long-term care system. If, on the other hand, the financing mechanism places no restrictions on who may provide services, a substantial number of consumers will hire friends and relatives, which is likely to result in a high level of consumer satisfaction.

───9───

Work Force Issues

One issue that is obviously key to the success of the independent living model, as well as any other model of long-term care, is whether an adequate work force will be available to meet the needs of consumers. This complex issue requires analysis of the demand and supply of workers who are capable of providing long-term care services, including compensation, benefits and working conditions. This chapter examines the job market for personal assistants and other long-term care workers, and the prospects for meeting the growing demand for long-term care using the independent living model.

DEMAND FOR LONG-TERM CARE WORKERS

The effective demand for workers who can provide care and assistance to people with disabilities is based on the need for such services and the financial capacity to pay for them. Chapter 2 provides some estimates of the need for personal assistance services. Altogether, over 9 million people of all ages require personal assistance services to carry out daily activities, and this number is likely to increase dramatically over the next few decades.[1] This need may potentially be satisfied under any of the three models of long-term care, or under a combination of them.

Whether a consumer may receive services under one of the models entailing paid services—the medical model or the independent living model—depends largely upon the individual's personal resources or eligibility for a public program. These financial requirements significantly reduce the number of individuals who currently demand services under a paid model. Presumably, those individuals who are sufficiently disabled to require personal assistance services and do not have access to private or public resources are either receiving services under the informal support model from friends or family members, or they are simply not receiving the services they need. As discussed in Chapter 5, the vast majority of consumers receive their long-term care services entirely or partially under the informal support model.[2]

In considering any policy to expand access to paid personal assistance services, we must attempt to estimate the "induced demand" in addition to current demand. Under any new personal assistance services program, policymakers must be concerned about the substitution of paid personal assistance services for informal, unpaid services previously obtained under the informal support model. This notion of induced demand is closely related to the "woodwork effect," whereby individuals receiving informal support services come "out of the woodwork" to receive formal care under a new program.

SUPPLY OF LONG-TERM CARE WORKERS

Long-term care workers come in a variety of different ages, ethnicities and backgrounds. However, these workers are disproportionately female members of racial minorities with limited education and resources.[3] For many, it is the only job available; many get burnt out and leave the field as soon as another job opportunity becomes available. There is already a substantial shortage of long-term care workers, and this shortage will be exacerbated in the coming years as demand continues to grow.[4] The inability to locate competent individuals to provide such services has been reported as causing a deterioration in the quality of care and substantial harm to many consumers.[5] Some have observed somewhat cynically that:

Recruiting, training, and retraining nursing home aides and home care aides to provide responsible, high-quality care is an ongoing problem for which no easy solutions are in sight; it is a problem shared by all industrialized countries. The functions performed by this work force are, on the whole, distasteful, boring, and physically and emotionally exhausting. Wages are low—worse than those of hospital aides[6]—and fringe benefits are generally unavailable for home health aides. These front line workers have little opportunity for advancement.[7]

This statement may offer an overly harsh assessment of the supply situation. Whether one believes that the jobs of personal assistants and other long-term care providers are "distasteful" or "boring," compared to other occupations and jobs available to these individuals, is a matter of taste and personal values.[8] Some individuals do not have the aversion to dealing with bodily functions that many Americans seem to have. Some actually enjoy the personal nature of a caring one-to-one relationship, particularly under the independent living model in a non-institutional home setting.

Moreover, some individuals are not looking for a career position with opportunities for advancement. Some people, such as students who are working to get through school and retired people who are interested in supplementing their retirement incomes, simply want a regular paycheck without substantial decision-making responsibility. Whether the pay for providing long-term care services should be considered "low" depends upon what other opportunities for higher pay are available to the worker, and whether those jobs are more attractive to the worker than the personal assistance job.

The general point of the commentators is well-taken, however; a certain percentage of individuals will not be attracted to this type of employment. There is also a high level of burnout for workers who provide personal assistance and other long-term care services, with a turnover rate that has been estimated as high as 50% per year.[9] This estimate is probably related to the intense nature of the job, which is often physically and emotionally exhausting, particularly if there is little or no back-up assistance or respite care available.[10] This finding is likely to have a major impact both in the market for para-professional workers under the medical model and personal assistants under the independent living model. Efforts have been made to reduce burnout through training.[11] Several structural factors explain the shortage, including the following:

Low Wages of Personal Assistance Services

Most personal assistance services jobs pay at or around the relevant minimum wage, typically the federal minimum wage except in states and localities that have enacted a higher minimum wage. State Medicaid programs, in particular, rarely pay significantly above the relevant minimum wage of the state, because of the restrictions of state budgets and the relatively low priority of personal assistance services programs for many governors and state legislators. Those consumers who pay out-of-pocket and are financially able to pay above minimum wage have a substantial advantage in the market in attracting the most dependable, capable personal assistants.

There is a general belief that personal assistants are paid less than agency workers, although it is difficult to prove this empirically because of inconsistencies in available data. The WID studies suggest that, in 1988, agency providers received $6.02 per hour compared with independent providers who received an average of $4.59 per hour under state programs.[12] The somewhat lower wages for independent providers allows some states to cover more hours of personal assistance services.[13] In the Netherlands, research on the wages of personal assistants under their independent living program and agency workers under their medical model program did not reveal significant wage differences.

However, the pay for personal assistants varies significantly from program to program and from consumer to consumer, and much depends upon the specific circumstances. Some consumers pay their assistants more than the average agency worker. Also, it is important to recognize that such comparisons are sometimes misleading, in that the jobs, working conditions, and benefits may be very different.

Lack of Benefits of Personal Assistance Services

Very few personal assistant jobs offer the broad range of benefits one might receive working for large corporations, such as health care coverage, pension plans, paid vacation, paid sick leave, unemployment insurance and workers' compensation insurance. Many of these benefits are extremely expensive, and they may not even be affordable to employers who wish to purchase policies for one or two employees. In comparison, about 40% of health agency employees reported that they received paid health benefits, sick leave and vacations; some 60% received paid holidays and compensation for travel costs.[14]

Even in countries known for their generous employment benefits, personal assistants do not necessarily qualify for benefits. In the Netherlands, consumers who employ assistants for less than 12 hours per week are not required to pay certain social security taxes that qualify these employees for benefits.[15] These employees also may not receive the benefits of collective bargaining agreements that ensure agency employees access to certain benefits such as disability insurance.[16]

In Austria, a "gray market" exists, in which consumers confronted with high taxes for employees have hired low-cost workers underground, thereby avoiding the taxes.[17] This is the other side of mandating benefits. For some consumers, the cost of employing a personal assistant legally becomes so high that there is a strong incentive to break the laws. The same issue has arisen in the United States with respect to payment of social security taxes.

Working Conditions

The working conditions of personal assistants under the independent living model versus agency providers under the medical model depends largely on the specific agency or consumer serving as employer and the related environmental circumstances. For example, it has been contended that many immigrant workers in long-term care are subject to bad working conditions.[18] Some agency employers are tyrants just as some consumer employers are tyrants. However, as a generalization, consumer and provider relationships appear to be better under the independent living model than under the medical model. In the Dutch independent living program, 90% of personal assistants indicated they have positive personal relationships with their consumers, as well as positive feelings about their work environments.[19] Dutch workers who have worked under both models indicate that they have more control of their work under the independent living model.

About 75% of personal assistants in California knew the consumers they work for prior to being hired; this finding may be compared with only 7% of agency workers who knew the consumer first.[20] The average agency worker provided services to about four consumers, compared with only 1.4 consumers for personal assistants providing services under the independent living model.[21] The smaller ratio of the independent living model gives providers more time to do their jobs, and gives consumers and providers more time to develop good personal relationships with consumers. The other side of this friendly personal relationship is that about 61% of personal assistants provided at least some unpaid assistance.[22] This situation probably occurs because of inadequate payment for services, and it results in a lower effective average hourly wage for personal assistants. Another downside of this model is that some assistants report feeling isolated, compared with agency workers who were more likely to have peer support, supervision and emergency backup.[23]

MATCHING SUPPLY AND DEMAND

Over time, the disequilibrium between supply and demand is likely to increase. The ratio of caregivers to elderly people will decline every year for the next 30 years as the baby boom population advances into old age.[24] This trend has ramifications throughout the long-term care system for care provided under all three models. As fewer and fewer family caregivers are available under the informal support model, the relative demand will increase for paid caregivers under both the medical model and the independent living model. According to economic theory, such disequilibrium is typically resolved over time through the price mechanism. In this case, wages should increase and working conditions should improve over time to attract more workers to this field. Whether this will, in fact, occur will depend in large part on how government policy makers respond to the shortage of workers.

Supporters of the independent living model argue that expansion of this model could decrease pressures on supply, attracting individuals to serve as personal assistants who would not otherwise be attracted.[25] They claim that many programs organized under the independent living model allow consumers to choose from a wide variety of personal assistants, including neighbors, friends or even family members.[26] As discussed at length in Chapter 12, consumers under European programs rely heavily on care from family members. To the extent that individuals who normally would not apply for positions as long-term care workers are attracted to such work as personal assistants under the independent living model, this increases the overall supply of long-term care workers.

Claims of "Exploitation"

Some critics of the independent living model have alleged that workers are subject to exploitation under this model.[27] Some have reacted negatively to descriptions by independent living advocates of personal assistants as "extensions of the bodies" of consumers with disabilities. This analogy, which depersonalizes human beings providing valuable services who have real feelings and needs, is not productive and may reflect negative attitudes by some people with disabilities concerning their dependence on others. However, it does not validate the contention that personal assistants are exploited by the independent living model. This contention requires serious critical analysis.[28]

Allegations of exploitation must be based upon some reasonable definition of exploitation. Yet, these critics do not offer specific definitions. Instead, they offer a variety of concerns about working conditions, ranging from low pay and lack of benefits to long hours and physically demanding job requirements. Although these concerns are sometimes legitimate, we must question whether they rise to the level of exploitation, which suggests actual abuse of the worker. Although such abuse certainly occurs in some cases, which is also true of other forms of domestic work and non-domestic work for that matter, it is usually considered criminal behavior on the part of the employer and may be prosecuted.

Most circumstances likely to be labeled "exploitation" by critics are really more a reflection of the critic's ideal society in which workers are paid what they consider to be a living wage, as well as comprehensive benefits, and working conditions are ideal. However, using this standard to judge the working circumstances of personal assistants and other long-term care workers is not fair. These are basically unskilled positions held primarily by individuals with very limited skills and education. There are, of course, exceptions to this generalization such as students and retired individuals attempting to supplement their incomes. The general point, however, is that the alternative jobs available to most of these individuals provide similar levels of pay, benefits and working conditions. Therefore, the criticisms are not really criticisms of the independent living model, but rather criticisms of the treatment of low income workers in the United States generally.

Some critics have recommended a code of working conditions for home care workers. A general code calling for safe working conditions, mutual respect, and adherence to all aspects of the agreement between the consumer and the assistant, including prompt payment for services, may be good idea as long as it is provided to offer helpful guidance rather than to impose intrusive regulations on a very private and personal relationship. Even if such a general code is not developed, consumers would be wise to establish such a code for their personal assistance relationship. This code, which would be adopted voluntarily, could be incorporated into a written agreement to clarify obligations and to avoid the potential for misunderstanding in this complex relationship.

However, some have gone beyond suggesting such a general statement, and have recommended a code of working conditions incorporating their own political agendas. One commentator suggested a code including "adequate wages to enable workers to support their families"; access to health benefits for themselves and their children; access to full-time work, if desired; training in areas that preserve safety and health of both workers and consumers; access to proper and maintained equipment; access to mediators to manage communication or conflict; advancement possibilities as mentors or trainers; and access to needed supports such as transportation and child care.[29]

Most of us would agree that these are conditions we would want if we were serving in the capacity as personal assistants, and that prudent consumers would offer assuming they have the financial capacity to afford them. To the extent that consumers offer generous pay and benefits, they will be more able to attract and retain dependable, high quality workers than consumers who do not or cannot offer comparable benefits. Therefore, it is in the interest of consumers to offer an attractive set of benefits and working conditions, if they are financially feasible and affordable. Moreover, presumably workers will not accept employment unless some minimum level of pay and other benefits are provided.

The vast majority of family members providing care under the informal support model are women. There appears to be a division among feminists as to whether payment should be available under independent living model programs for informal caregivers. According to Leutz:

> . . . the large majority of family caregivers are women,
> who may already have other family obligations and who
> often make career sacrifices to provide care. Some feminists
> oppose encouraging family care (as would be the case if cash
> were allowed to pay family members), but others value
> women's caring nature, accept that their caring opportunities/obligations will present themselves at various points in
> peoples' lives and focus on how fairly to support caring with
> adequate programs.[30]

Therefore, it appears that some feminists would oppose payment of family members on the basis that it will encourage family care, which they claim is inherently exploitative. Others support an "emancipation policy" that ensures fair wages, benefits, limits on informal care, and favorable working conditions.[31] The weight of opinion appears to favor programs that permit payment of relatives and treat them well.[32]

As is always the case, the outcomes of any program depend largely on how the program is designed and implemented. In one social experiment with payment of family caregivers in Canada, the outcomes were negative: long hours, high rates of burnout, and very low wages.[33] On the other hand, a study in the Netherlands found that informal caregivers valued the gesture of being compensated as much as the compensation.[34] A survey of caregivers in New York City found that social and emotional supports, such as homemaker services, medical care, and respite care, are more important to them than payments for their services. This response may have been in part because the cost of the desired supports exceeded the value of their expected compensation.[35]

LABOR ISSUES UNDER THE INDEPENDENT LIVING MODEL

A variety of issues concerning the broader labor market affect the supply, pay, benefits and other factors affecting the provision of personal assistance services.

Training and Certification

Some states require that personal assistants must have mandatory training or certification.[36] Most independent living advocates object to mandatory standardized training claiming that every individual consumer is unique in his or her needs, preferences and techniques; they contend that consumers are the most qualified individuals to provide training to meet their needs.

Mandatory certification, in particular, is likely to reduce the supply of available personal assistants at any point in time and over time. When a consumer is advertising for a personal assistant, only those who have already undergone certification and training in states where this is mandatory will be available. Over time, fewer assistants would be available than if certification and training were not mandatory because many individuals who otherwise might be attracted to the position will be unwilling to expend time and money in order to qualify for a job that does not pay a large salary. Conversely, those who do make such an investment legitimately expect a higher salary as a result, thereby imposing higher costs on consumers who do not necessarily value the certification or training. Many consumers prefer to train their own assistants.

Advocates of mandatory certification and training argue that it insures that all assistants have at least a basic set of skills, and that particularly older consumers who have not undergone medical rehabilitation are not aware of safe and appropriate methods of providing service.

Fiscal Intermediaries—Intermediary Service Organizations

Fiscal intermediaries are agencies that perform administrative functions on behalf of employers in assisting them to meet their legal obligations with respect to employment. In the context of personal assistance services, they are called intermediary service organizations (ISOs). These intermediaries have a variety of fiscal responsibilities, including distributing paychecks, reporting to tax and regulatory authorities, and ensuring other regulatory compliance.

States that implement programs based on the independent living model must achieve a balance among several competing factors:

- The desire of consumers for autonomy and choice;
- The duty to ensure compliance with federal and state tax and labor laws and regulations;
- The duty to ensure proper administration of program funding;
- State desire not to be the employer of record;
- State duty to ensure health and safety of beneficiaries.[37]

States have contracted with intermediary service organizations for a variety of fiscal, administrative and support services to enable consumers with diverse desires, needs, and abilities to manage their personal assistance services. Consumers who are not beneficiaries of state programs may also contract with such organizations, but the cost of doing so on an individual basis may be prohibitively expensive.

Among the services ISOs can provide are payroll, taxes, fringe benefits, attendant registries, criminal background checks, training personal assistants, management, emergency backup, consumer assessments, and case management.[38] Six models of ISO s have been identified:

- The fiscal conduit model, in which the ISO disburses funds on behalf of consumers, who serve as the employers of record;
- IRS employer-agent model, in which a government entity acts as a fiscal agent on behalf of consumers who serve as employers of record for the purpose of preparing and filing employer-related taxes (and sometimes also address payroll issues);
- The vendor fiscal ISO model, which is basically the same as the IRS employer-agent model except that the contractor is a private sector entity;
- The supportive ISO model, in which the ISO provides support services to consumers such as conducting training, background checks, emergency backup plans;
- The agency with choice model, in which an agency is the employer of record of personal assistants, and consumers are considered managing employers responsible for managing the day-to-day activities of the personal assistant; and
- The spectrum ISO model, in which an ISO provides a broad array of administrative and management services to consumers, who may or may not serve as employer of record.[39]

The Medstat Group conducted a study, funded by the Office of the Assistant Secretary for Planning and Evaluation, DHHS, to examine issues concerning ISOs, including best practices. The study found that state administrators should focus on the desire and ability of consumers to perform a wide variety of employer-related tasks. These desires and abilities vary substantially across disability groups. Even individuals may vary in their desires and abilities over time. Working age people with physical disabilities prefer to be the employer of record, while people with developmental or cognitive disabilities are less concerned about that. The majority of consumers generally prefer to distribute their personal assistants' paychecks, claiming that it is empowering.[40] There appears to be a strong symbolic aspect associated with the check coming directly from the consumer, whether or not the consumer is actually the employer of record. This symbolism reinforces the role and authority of the consumer as managing employer.[41] Despite this, many Medicaid programs require that ISOs distribute the checks, thereby tacitly undermining the authority of the consumer.

The study found that only the most motivated consumers with the greatest capacity for autonomy and self-direction should use the fiscal conduit model. Many consumers, even those who are fully capable of functioning without administrative support, indicated that they would like the services of ISOs. At the very least, most consumers would want the services of ISOs under the IRS Fiscal Agent model or vendor fiscal ISO model in paying taxes on their behalf. However, many consumers identified the desire for other services as well. The most requested supportive service was back-up assistance in the event that the primary personal assistant is ill or otherwise unavailable.[42]

Finally, the study concluded that even ISO services provided under the Agency with Choice model, in which personal assistants are officially employees of the agency and not the consumer, substantial autonomy, control, choice and satisfaction could be achieved if the agency has a philosophy reflecting the goals of the independent living movement.[43] Those ISOs that conform most closely to the independent living philosophy had the highest rates of consumer satisfaction.[44] Accordingly, it has been recommended that one of the bases on which ISOs is evaluated is commitment to principles of consumer direction.[45]

Personal Assistance Registries

Registries are organizations that help to develop an employment market for personal assistants. Their basic function is to serve as a matching service between consumers and prospective assistants, although some registry organizations provide additional support services, such as orientation, training, communication, problem solving and conflict resolution. Orientation services, for example, can introduce prospective assistants to the general philosophy of independent living and the various aspects of consumer-directed personal assistance services under the independent living model. Many independent living centers serve as personal assistance registries.

Such registries can be very helpful to consumers. Certain economies of scale are associated with them. For example, the cost of placing an ad in the newspapers can be extremely expensive for many consumers, particularly those with low-income jobs or those receiving public assistance. However, the same ad can potentially produce enough assistants to meet the needs of dozens of consumers. A negative aspect of registries is that they sometimes become subject to preferential treatment for friends of those running the registry. However, such problems can be addressed by sound policies that prevent such preferences, possibly through systems of random selection. Overall, registries provide valuable services which consumers can choose to use or not to use.

Unionization

The question of whether domestic workers should be unionized is highly debatable at this stage of our history. Significant legal safeguards are in place to protect such workers, in part due to the past lobbying successes of organized labor. On the one hand, union representation could be helpful in situations involving actual illegal exploitation against assistants and in negotiating with states for better pay and benefits. On the other hand, such membership can be expensive for low income workers and may not be justified in terms of likely benefits. It is questionable whether unions could negotiate a better deal for workers than they could achieve for themselves as a result of economic conditions in the supply market.

In Alameda County, California, the independent living model is the only option available for their consumers. Personal assistants in this county are represented by the Service Employees International Union, Local 616.[46] The consequences of this representation have not been studied adequately at this time.

IMPLICATIONS OF WORKER SHORTAGE

Long-term care is extremely labor intensive. The essence of long-term care, as discussed in Chapter 1, is the provision of personal assistance services and other services to people with disabilities. Therefore, the demand for long-term care may be met by virtually anyone who is willing and able to provide such services. It does not require people with health care training and credentials. It does not require someone with extensive formal education. It does require someone with at least the minimum physical and mental capacity to provide competent care and assistance and the responsibility to always show up on time and provide the services that were agreed upon.

Therefore, the so-called shortage of long-term care workers is not really a shortage in the conventional sense; that there are an insufficient number of qualified individuals able to provide the services needed.

That type of shortage typically requires several years to remedy, as government or corporate policy create incentives for individuals to derive the necessary education or training to fulfill the unmet demand. A certain amount of time is required to get these individuals through the pipeline to the consumer. In the case of personal assistants and other long-term care workers, the pool of workers exists at any point in time, and the challenge is to attract these qualified individuals to serve in this capacity. The reason that the long-term care industry is always facing a "shortage" is that its working conditions and compensation packages deter individuals from serving in long-term care positions.

Some practitioners under the medical model appear to be concerned that expansion of the independent living model will make their supply situation even worse. This situation may occur to the extent that some workers under the medical model may decide that they are tired of the stress and depressing environments of many institutions, and choose instead to provide consumer-directed personal assistance services at the home or homes of one or more consumers. What is more likely to occur on a broader scale is that individuals who would not otherwise be attracted to providing such services will be attracted by the independent living model. The competition between the two models for qualified workers could induce an improvement in working conditions and compensation for workers under the medical model. Ultimately, as demand expands dramatically, there will be a necessity to tap the pool of workers who are available in any way that is financially feasible.

SUMMARY

This chapter has examined the market for personal assistants and other long-term care workers, concluding that our nation will face a major challenge in meeting the growing need and demand for long-term care and assistance. Use of the independent living model will help in the effort to meet this demand. It is likely to attract individuals who otherwise would not have considered being long-term care workers, including retired people who need additional income, family members and friends of consumers, and others who enjoy helping other people but who do not want to obtain health care credentials or to work in a health care setting. Resolving these workforce issues, and attracting an adequate long-term care workforce, will be essential to ensuring the ongoing quality of long-term care.

——10——

Quality Assurance

$\mathbf{A}$ key objective of any long-term care program is to define and measure quality and to develop and implement effective mechanisms to ensure quality. Among the tasks are developing and implementing a system for the reliable measurement of quality and examining issues concerning recruitment, retention, and quality of a work force that includes people with a broad range of skills, from highly-skilled professionals to unskilled workers. The challenge of achieving these objectives under the independent living model of long-term care is to ensure quality without imposing the extensive top-down regulatory mechanisms typically used under the medical model, which are incompatible with the independent living model. This chapter considers appropriate mechanisms of quality assurance under this model.

THE CHALLENGE OF QUALITY ASSURANCE

Assuring quality has always been one of the most difficult goals of health care policy. Quality assurance is particularly challenging now in the midst of the managed care revolution and its powerful incentives and mechanisms for cost containment.[1] To a much greater extent than containing costs and enhancing access, quality is a highly nebulous concept that is extremely difficult to measure, and even harder to attribute to specific interventions.[2] While containing costs is often largely a matter of rationing resources and enhancing access is largely a matter of expanding or reallocating resources, quality may be improved or deteriorated irrespective of the level of resources allocated. Quality depends specifically upon how and by whom the resources are used.

Increasing resources for inappropriate care results in poor outcomes and poor quality; even enhancing access to appropriate care subjects consumers to risks.[3] "Iatrogenic medicine" is a term used to describe health problems resulting from the medical or health care process. One example of this is "nosecomial infections," which are infections obtained from germs in health care facilities. Simply providing long-term care in an institutional setting imposes health risks on consumers related to the germs, diseases or even violent tendencies of other consumers and staff members.[4] This situation raises serious issues concerning clinical quality in any institutional long-term care setting.

Of course, providing long-term care in any setting poses certain health risks to consumers relating to communicable diseases and germ control. However, the risks are much greater in institutional settings, where consumers are exposed to the germs of multitudes of people, many of whom have compromised immune and/or respiratory systems.[5] The risks of infection in a home setting under the informal support or independent living model are substantially smaller. The consumer is likely to develop a greater tolerance for the germs of the relatively few caregivers involved. Home care under the medical model, although theoretically less risky than institutional care under that model, still imposes higher risks than care under other models because the consumer is exposed to the germs that the provider receives from other patients. This concern could also apply to care under the independent living model to the extent that some personal assistants provide care to more than one consumer. Generally, however, personal assistants provide care to far fewer consumers than do home health aides under the medical model.

Understanding quality is a challenge in the acute care context; it is even more so in the long-term care context and particularly home-based long-term care. Unlike acute care, in which there is often a very specific intervention and a very specific goal, such as an operation intended to increase blood flow, long-term care involves a multitude of more general interventions and more general goals. Like institution-based long-term care, home-based care "encompasses a wide variety of procedures and services delivered to a diverse range of consumers by diverse health and social service agencies, independent vendors, and families."[6] Unlike institution-based care, in which the patient is almost exclusively under the control of the institution, consumers of home-based care are subject to many more extrinsic variables that reduce the ability to attribute causation, thereby reducing the accountability of any single provider entity.

In considering the position of the provider in home-based care, Rosalie Kane and her colleagues conclude:

> The nature of home care implies a sharing of power between provider and client. Because home care occurs on the client's turf, providers have much less control over outcomes than for hospital care or nursing home care. . . . Clients and family members have rightful expectations for how and when things are done in their own homes, and professional standards of sanitation, efficiency, and optimal routines are inevitably compromised by the give and take of a household. This shift in the balance of power is, one can argue, highly desirable, but it has made some health care organizations leery of accepting responsibility for outcomes.[7]

Quality assurance is considered particularly challenging and critical in home-based care because, by definition, such care is provided in a more private and secluded manner than other health care; therefore, there is potentially more opportunity for abuse and neglect than in health care settings where others are available to monitor services.[8] Despite this necessity to assure quality care, quality assurance in the area of home care is still at an early stage of development, and lags behind quality assurance in nursing home care by about 15 years.[9]

THE MARKET VS. REGULATION

Throughout this book, the recipient of long-term care services has been described as the consumer. Implicitly, an analogy has been drawn to consumers in a wide array of markets for other services and goods. In a market-based economy, we as a society believe to large extent that consumers will be able to make sound choices among competing providers, and that competition will lead to low prices and high quality.

However, underlying this belief are certain assumptions concerning the consumer, the industry and the market. In particular, consumers are assumed to be autonomous individuals capable of assessing various options and choosing among them. The market is assumed to adhere more or less to the characteristics of a competitive market: many sellers, none of whom unduly control price; many consumers who have access to good information; no significant barriers to entry into the market; and no significant externalities (i.e., costs or benefits of private health care transactions that have a broader impact on society).

To the extent that a particular market deviates from these competitive conditions, we may question the ability of competition to achieve the goals of reasonable price and quality, and we are justified in intervening in the market in some way for the benefit of the public. The health care industry and the market for health care services generally are regarded as deviating substantially from the ideal of a perfectly competitive industry and market.[10]

The Market and the Medical Model

In the acute care context, patients rarely have the information they need to make fully informed decisions, and such decisions are often made under significant stress. There are substantial regulatory barriers to entry, such as licensing and certification requirements; consequently, providers and practitioners often have significant market power. Also, there are significant externalities such as issues concerning iatrogenic medicine in which the conditions of one individual's care may affect other consumers. The market for long-term care services under the medical model similarly deviates from the competitive model for the same reasons. Moreover, informed decision-making in the long-term care market is further impeded, particularly to the extent that consumers are not capable of self-direction and do not have surrogates who are willing and able to make sound decisions on their behalf.[11]

Therefore, we cannot rely entirely on the market to ensure optimal long-term care outcomes. On the other hand, resorting to the other extreme—a laissez-faire "hands-off" approach in which the government does not intervene—is a recipe for disaster in long-term care. We have seen enough of how the less scrupulous components of the long-term care industry behaves when not subject to sufficient public scrutiny.[12] Even the most scrupulous components are likely to cut corners when subject to substantial cost pressures. Some mechanism for ensuring quality is necessary in long-term care. The question is not whether regulation is necessary, but rather what is the optimal form of regulation to ensure quality in an efficient and equitable manner.

Traditionally, quality assurance efforts in the long-term care area have focused on command-and-control government regulation. In other words, federal and state government agencies mandate that providers comply with certain requirements purported to assure quality. Despite being the first industry targeted for deregulation by the Reagan Administration, the federal government quickly withdrew from a strict market approach to ensuring quality.[13] The issue was then studied by the Institute of Medicine, which released its 1986 report, entitled *Improving the Quality of Care in Nursing Homes*.[14] That pivotal report led to the renewed commitment to a command-and-control approach, codified in the Omnibus Budget Reconciliation Act of 1987 with strong bipartisan support in Congress and strong support of the industry and its various stakeholders. The result was a highly-regulated system of standards, inspection processes and enforcement mechanisms.

Some experts defend this system as the alternative to laissez-faire, contending that the real issue is adequate enforcement of the regulatory regime.[15] Others concluded that this approach does not ensure quality, and may actually impose substantial costs on consumers both financially and in terms of lost opportunities resulting from wasted resources, claim that:

> The majority of the regulations are based not on empirical evidence of what activities are associated with better outcomes but on professional judgments, which quickly approach 'dogma'. . . . Strict statements about what should be done for whom become rapidly restrictive at a time when long-term care dearly needs innovation and creativity. Especially because so little has been proven about how to deliver the best care (and there is every likelihood that more than one way is available to achieve this end), it is premature to ossify the process.[16]

Even those committed to a command-and-control regulatory approach recognize that the industry has such an enormous advantage in organizing and lobbying that any regulatory legislation is likely to be written primarily with industry interests in mind.[17] Moreover, even a strong regulatory mandate will not implement itself, and the nursing home and home health industries have demonstrated an ability to undermine implementation and enforcement.[18] One study of enforcement in New York state found that nursing homes were fined at a relatively low rate; while surveyors identified between 1,500 and 2,500 deficiencies annually, there were only 78 enforcement actions. For over 650 facilities in 1992, the year with the most such actions, the average fine was only $7,500.[19] It is clear that fines are only imposed in the most egregious cases, and are unlikely to have a strong deterrent effect.

Therefore, complete reliance on either regulation or the market to ensure quality is misguided.[20] Instead, the better approach is to analyze the market carefully to determine the extent to which competitive market forces are likely to achieve desired quality outcomes, and then to supplement such forces with intelligent market-oriented regulation designed to bolster the capacity of the market to achieve the outcomes desired. This approach, called managed competition, has been applied extensively to acute care but has received little attention in long-term care.[21] Command-and-control regulation simply for the sake of regulating will not achieve quality goals and will ultimately prove counterproductive. Too often, such regulation serves as a pretense to create a public perception of quality assurance, which may cause a false sense of security that quality care is being provided.

The Market and the Independent Living Model

Interestingly, the market for consumer-directed personal assistance services under the independent living model conforms much more closely to the model of perfect competition than care provided under the medical model. Under the independent living model, there are many consumers seeking assistance and many prospective personal assistants seeking employment. Although the knowledge held by both consumers and personal assistants is far from perfect, the nature of the work is not so technically difficult (as compared with medicine or nursing) that this is a problem. There are virtually no barriers to entry to be a personal assistant, and there are no significant external costs or benefits imposed outside the personal assistance relationship. Therefore, theoretically we can rely to large extent on the private market.

This discussion is not meant to suggest that quality assurance measures are unnecessary under the independent living model. Abuse, neglect and incompetence are as likely to occur under this model as they are under the medical model; some approach to assuring quality is useful to help consumers protect themselves. However, the nature of the quality measures used must be compatible philosophically and logistically with the independent living model.

DEFINING AND MEASURING QUALITY LONG-TERM CARE

Traditionally, quality has been assessed in the health care field through measures of the structure, process and outcomes of a provider of services.[22] Each of these types of measures must be examined to determine its applicability and usefulness in assuring the quality of long-term care services.

Structure refers to such variables as accreditation, facility, equipment, staff credentials, and provider-patient ratios that pertain to the entire program of the provider being assessed. An advantage of structural data is that they are typically relatively easy and inexpensive to collect. Most analysts agree that structural measures are not ideal mechanisms for assessing quality, because they rely upon inferences that the structure will translate into positive patient outcomes. Such inferences often are not justified. Examples of structure-oriented quality assurance activities are licensing, standards, and criminal background checks. Structural criteria appear to have limited applicability to home-based care, the quality of which depends largely on the nature of the one-to-one relationship between the provider and the consumer, and much less on the structural characteristics of the home health agency or any other organization involved. The applicability of structural criteria to care provided under the independent living model is particularly limited, in that the model does not use licensed providers or formal organizations.

Process refers to precisely what happens to the consumer over the course of long-term care. Specifically, it considers every interaction with a provider of services and what occurred during that interaction. Process has two major components:

- A technical component involving the specific intervention involved (e.g., insertion of an internal urinary catheter) and
- An interpersonal component involving the nature of the personal interaction between the consumer and the provider.

The technical quality of a health care process consists of appropriateness (whether an intervention is needed) and skill (whether the intervention was conducted competently).[23] The interpersonal quality of a process includes consumer perceptions on whether providers care about them, relate to them in a respectful manner, and provide the physical and emotional comfort they need.[24]

Examples of process-oriented quality assurance activities are provider audits and peer review activities. Although process measures tend to be better assessors of quality than structural measures, a good process still does not guarantee positive outcomes. Moreover, due to the nature of home-based care, which involves many different providers and interventions, any positive or negative outcome cannot necessarily be attributed to any particular provider or intervention. Again, this concern applies in particular to care provided under the medical model and the independent living model, in which a single consumer may receive care from several different providers with different levels of skill and commitment.

Outcomes refer to the ultimate impact of long-term care on the consumer (e.g., functional status, ability to live independently, ability to achieve gainful employment). Outcomes are the ideal quality measure, in that they offer the most direct assessment of quality. Unfortunately, data for outcome measures are often difficult and expensive to obtain, and raise questions of causation and risk selection concerning whether there was adequate consideration of the severity of the patient's condition. Obviously, consumers with the greatest health and functional problems are most likely to have the worst outcomes, all other factors held constant.

The ability to attribute causation of outcomes to the services provided is severely limited in long-term care. Examples of outcome-oriented quality assurance activities include implementation of performance measures and satisfaction surveys. Compared with acute care, in which there are specific interventions targeted at the ideal outcome, i.e., cure of a specific disease, long-term care interventions are not cure-oriented. Also, long-term care outcomes such as the ability to live independently may be attributable to other factors in the consumer's life than care received (e.g., level of functional limitation, accessible environment, financial resources, family support, etc.).

In addition to the traditional quality assessment criteria of structure, process and outcome, some researchers have suggested a fourth category labeled "enabling criteria."[25] These criteria include non-technical pre-conditions for a result that is satisfactory to the consumer, such as courtesy, punctuality, reliability, honesty, and compatibility. Studies indicate that these enabling criteria tend to be extremely important to consumers. Under the independent living model, these criteria are particularly important. If the personal assistant is not reliable, the consumer may not be able to get out of bed in any particular day. If the assistant is not punctual, the consumer may become overcome with anxiety over whether the assistant will show up. Unlike home-based care under the medical model, in which an agency will presumably send an alternative aide if the primary aide fails to show, the consumer under the independent living model is more likely to be without assistance altogether. Under either the independent living or medical model, consumers obviously would not want to welcome into their homes assistants who are not courteous, honest and compatible.

DOMAINS OF QUALITY CARE

Twelve quality indicator domains of care have been identified in the context of assessing nursing home care:
- Accidents
- Behavioral and emotional patterns
- Clinical management
- Cognitive functioning
- Elimination and continence
- Infection control
- Nutrition and eating
- Physical functioning
- Psychotropic drug use
- Quality of life
- Sensory function and communication
- Skin care.[26]

Although these domains were developed to address quality of institutional care, they have applicability to other areas of long-term care, including home-based personal assistance services to some extent. Each of these domains has been assessed through process and outcome measures of quality under the medical model. Future research should apply them to the independent living model.

Quality under the Independent Living Model

Due to the importance of the inter-personal relationship between the consumer and the personal assistant under the independent living model, quality of care is closely related to the quality of their relationship and the personal characteristics of the personal assistant. One study of the quality assurance mechanisms of three states that cover personal assistance services under their programs found that:

. . . hiring the right worker was consistently identified as
the key element in delivering quality care on a consistent

basis. Agencies routinely conduct criminal background checks, require physical exams, tuberculosis screening, and references. Management staff in many of the agencies stressed the importance of supporting their workers and highlighting their value to the organization. Informants in all three states identified complaints as an important but limited quality assurance tool. State administrators, case managers, supervisors, and provider agencies indicated that most clients are reluctant to complain about their workers or case managers. Provider agencies in Washington are required to have a dispute resolution process and to inform clients that it is available. The state agency also operates a complaint hotline.[27]

This study identified several practice issues that affect quality under three general categories: those dealing with wages and workers, those dealing with consumer choice, and those dealing with independent providers of care. Under the first category, low wages resulting from low state reimbursement rates was consistently considered a problem, thus limiting the ability of consumers to hire the workers of their choice.

Advocates of the independent living model contend that the control consumers exercise under the model is itself a form of quality assurance.[28] By giving consumers control over hiring, retaining and firing their assistants, they are empowered to assure that their services satisfy their personal standards of quality. Unlike other areas of health care, in which patients often do not have the technical knowledge to assess the quality of their services, the quality of long-term care services is typically transparent to the consumer.[29] Consumers are uniquely qualified to assess the quality of such services, and the independent living model is uniquely designed to allow consumers to do so.

Independent living advocates further argue that consumers can be used under the model to provide feedback on an ongoing basis.[30] The quality of this mechanism will depend largely on the sophistication of instruments used to measure such quality. Blunt measures of overall satisfaction, asking general questions that do not delve deeply into the real concerns of consumers and payors, are not productive. Well-designed instruments are needed to examine both objective and subjective components of quality in an efficient manner that does not impose an undue burden on consumers. Generally, outcome-based approaches rely heavily on data, and there is very little outcome data available.

PERSPECTIVES OF STAKEHOLDERS

Defining quality of long-term care depends in part on which specific medical, psychological and/or social goals are considered the highest priorities for a particular consumer. In acute care, we can label success or failure somewhat objectively across the board based upon whether medical interventions resulted in a cure or at least resolution of symptoms. Quality in long-term care, however, is subject to the personal perceptions of the consumer and others to much greater degree.

Different participants in the long-term care process have different perspectives on what are the most important goals for a consumer and what constitutes quality care for that particular individual.[31] Although there is some overlap in their perceptions of quality, it is often alarming to realize the disparity of their thoughts and feelings about this often-emotionally-charged issue. An example is where a therapist allocates a substantial amount of time and effort to allow the individual to feed himself or herself using therapeutic equipment, but realizes later that the patient has concluded that this activity is not justified in terms of the amount of time required to set up the equipment or the amount of energy required to use it. In some cases, consumers may justifiably decide that it is simply more efficient for them to be fed by a personal assistant.

Some evidence suggests that stakeholders in home-based care such as providers, payors, government officials and consumers tend to rank outcome indicators of quality as the most important, followed by process, enabling and structural indicators (consumers considered enabling indicators as the most compelling).[32] Among different specific outcome indicators, there is broad agreement that affordability, consumer satisfaction and freedom from exploitation are important outcomes.[33]

Providers

Health care providers traditionally have tended to view quality in terms of structure and process. Because these were the primary types of criteria on which they were assessed by licensors and accrediting agencies, their focus has been on these aspects of quality. Of course, they also have always been concerned about outcomes, but the primary focus was on avoiding negative outcomes that might result in malpractice suits or professional disciplinary actions. Although they have always valued positive outcomes in the form of medical and functional progress in their long-term care consumers, such outcomes were always virtually impossible to measure scientifically and, therefore, were not a major component of their quality reviews. Only in recent years, with payors and accrediting bodies focusing on outcomes have providers adopted this priority. Still, the short-term positive outcomes that are the current focus of providers is not necessarily the highest priority quality issue for consumers.

With respect to structural aspects of quality, home health agencies and nursing homes are subject to state licensure. Similarly, health care professionals who work for or at these nursing homes and home health agencies must also be licensed. Licensing offers a minimalist approach to ensuring quality. While it provides some minimum assurances that the provider has not been guilty of abuse, negligence or other malpractice, and that the provider has at least some minimal level of technical competence, it does not ensure the excellence we would all like to experience from our health care providers. Voluntary accreditation initiatives from organizations such as the Joint Commission on Accreditation of Health care Organizations and the Community Health Accreditation Program (CHAP) of the National League of Nursing, which have focused more on process and outcome approaches in recent years, are more likely to achieve real quality.

With respect to interpersonal process aspects of long-term care quality, providers under the medical model have developed standards indicating that workers should not develop friendships with consumers. The idea that there should be an emotional detachment between the provider and the patient is deeply entrenched in the underlying philosophy of the medical model. Certainly, providers are supposed to treat their patients with respect. However, traditionally this has been the paternalistic respect of a person in control to a person being controlled. This asymmetry in the provider-patient relationship has been moderated in recent years as a result of increasing emphasis on patient autonomy, but the admonition against close personal relationships with patients has not.

Payors

Payors of long-term care, including federal government, state governments, employers, and insurance companies, have always placed a high emphasis on accountability, both with respect to costs and quality. Payors are often thought to represent the interests of their enrollees; the people on whose behalf they are paying. In fact, they have a fiduciary duty of care and loyalty to such individuals. However, they often serve other constituencies as well. For example, the various government programs must satisfy the needs of members of Congress, particularly those who are on the oversight committees for their programs. They in turn must serve other constituencies, some of which are not concerned primarily with quality care. Similarly, in the private sector, insurance companies and managed care organizations often must serve the interests of board members and shareholders who may have different commitments to quality care.

In assessing quality, payors like providers traditionally have focused on structure and process issues, largely by default because of the lack of adequate outcome measures in long-term care care. As discussed earlier, structure and process are not necessarily good indicators of quality, and payors traditionally have had little grasp of quality issues. In times of expansion of the health care sector, it was generally assumed that more care equated with higher quality care. Issues concerning iatrogenic medicine were seldom considered. The focus on quality, particularly on outcome indicators of quality, began in the late 1970s and early 1980s as substantial brakes were placed on health care spending. This focus on quality occurred through the managed care revolution and through government efforts such as the implementation of the Medicare Prospective Payment System in 1983.

Payors can be expected to continue to push for accountability in the manner called for by their constituents. The form of such accountability in implementing programs under the independent living model will depend upon the relative power of consumers as compared with other constituents of these programs.

Consumers

Differences in perceptions of quality between consumers and providers are sometimes subtle and sometimes dramatic. Consumers of long-term care tend to focus primarily on ultimate outcomes, such as the ability to live independently, and on interpersonal process issues, such as whether they were treated with respect and kindness. Technical process issues are of less interest to consumers, except to the extent that procedures are done negligently or otherwise incompetently and result in harm.

Issues concerning interpersonal process are particularly interesting from the perspective of consumers. Many consumers equate control with a favorable interpersonal process. If they cannot control the nature of the services they receive and that affect them fundamentally, they are likely to be dissatisfied with the process, even if the worker is technically competent and the outcomes are excellent.[34] In stark contrast with professional standards discussed above, many consumers judge the quality of their services in part by the personality of the worker and whether there is a comfortable and friendly relationship between the consumer and the worker.

This finding should not be surprising. As discussed in Chapter 1, long-term care becomes a large part of a consumer's life, to the extent that it is impossible to compartmentalize long-term care and treat it separately from the rest of the consumer's life. From the consumer's perspective, quality of care is therefore closely related to quality of life. A consumer's quality of life would be considerably diminished if the consumer was forced to interact with a worker who has an abrasive personality or who is unfriendly. Consumer assessments of quality are based in part on such factors as whether the consumer likes the worker or on how long the worker has been working with the consumer.[35]

The primary mechanism of assessing quality of care from consumers is to conduct satisfaction surveys. However, it is widely agreed among researchers and other experts that there are major methodological problems with most satisfaction surveys. For example, it has been reported that one of the worst ways to assess satisfaction among older consumers of long-term care is simply to ask whether they are satisfied with their care.[36] They respond positively to that question, while in-depth interviews demonstrate much lower levels of satisfaction. Of course, this knowledge has affected the way in which nursing homes, home health agencies and other long-term care providers have inquired about consumer satisfaction. There is now a general consensus that consumers should be involved in the development of satisfaction surveys. One such consumer input is the Home Care Satisfaction Measure.[37]

With respect to outcomes, substantial research conducted over an extensive period of time has demonstrated that consumers who have greater control of their activities express greater satisfaction and achieve better outcomes than consumers who do not have such control.[38] These relationships clearly apply to the satisfaction and outcomes of consumers with respect to long-term care.[39] There has been an enormous growth in research on outcomes over the past 15 years. Among the other outcomes that have been examined are physical functioning, psychological and emotional well-being, independent living and caregiver satisfaction.

Observers have recommended that consumers should be allowed to define quality for non-medical home care if they have the capacity and desire to do so.[40] This recommendation is based on the notion that these are the services consumers know best and are best able to assess. Others have commented that allowing this to occur will require changes in public opinion, politics and the law.[41] Such changes have previously been proven to be controversial and difficult to achieve.[42]

Family Members

The role of the family in long-term care has generated some confusion in the literature. Some analysts view family members as providers of services, based upon the large amount of informal (i.e., uncompensated) care they provide as well as the care some provide under the independent living model. Other analysts view family members primarily as consumers of long-term care services, because of their receipt of respite care and to the extent that the goals of home care include goals relating to the family. The views of family members tend to be similar to those of consumers, as expected. However, family members have additional concerns, such as concerns about having to sacrifice their goals in order to achieve the consumer's goals.

THE NATURE OF LONG-TERM CARE REGULATION

There is a general tendency in this era of smaller government to characterize regulation in derogatory terms. Much of this criticism is justified, in that much of the regulation of the health care industry has been short-sighted, inflexible and even counter-productive. Much regulation of the command-and-control variety has simply served to increase "busy work," those administrative and paperwork burdens and associated costs without providing a concomitant benefit in terms of the quality of care. This criticism appears particularly applicable in the context of long-term care. Some analysts have gone as far as concluding that, "Regulation is part of the problem," with respect to long-term care.[43]

However, the term "regulation" should not be inherently derogatory. Regulations are simply rules of general application formalized in a manner that gives them legal authority. Conceivably, a regulation can be efficient, productive and supportive of autonomy, depending upon its purpose and the manner by which it achieves its purpose. The theory of managed competition recognizes that some pro-competitive regulation is necessary to make imperfect health care markets work competitively. For example, regulations that require information for consumers can improve the functioning of the market.

All aspects of long-term care have been subject to regulatory scrutiny using structural, process and outcome measures. Yet, different types and settings of care may be amenable to one type of measure or another. The following sub-sections consider the means by which the quality of long-term care providers has been measured, assessed and scrutinized.

Regulation of Institutional Care, Including Nursing Homes

Much of the effort to ensure quality in institutional long-term care has focused on structural variables, such as licensing and accreditation, and on process variables, such as sanitary procedures. This approach has been subject to extensive criticism.[44] In summarizing the overall approach to nursing home regulation, Kane has noted:

> After decades of scandal, nursing home care is currently one of the most heavily regulated industries in the United States. This checkered history has established a tradition of regulation designed to avoid catastrophes rather than to encourage good care. Despite major regulatory reform legislation that raised national standards for such care and shifted emphasis toward the outcomes of care, passed in 1987 and implemented in 1990, good care is still effectively defined as the absence of bad events.[45]

One of the primary means of quality assurance is through surveys in which providers are subject to checklists of dozens of technical violations of certain structural and procedural standards. Although this approach ensures that workers will be busy making certain that such technical violations do not exist on the day of an inspection, it does little to ensure that the consumer is actually receiving competent care and achieving desirable outcomes.

Regulation of Home Health Care

Over 41 states require the licensure of home health agencies as a prerequisite to providing services.[46] Moreover, every state requires the licensing of many of the health care professionals who work for or under contracts with home health agencies, including physicians, nurses, psychologists, social workers and therapists.

The federal government also regulates home health care agencies and providers to the extent that they participate in the Medicare and Medicaid programs. Home health agencies that wish to participate in Medicare must satisfy the Medicare Conditions of Participation. Federal regulations require that home health agencies that wish to participate in Medicaid must also satisfy the Medicare Conditions of Participation.

In addition, home health agencies and individual providers are subject to a broad array of federal and state health care laws and regulations designed to deter fraud, anti-competitive conduct and other activities that can adversely affect consumers. Finally, they are also potentially vulnerable to law suits for intentional or negligent tortious conduct or for breaches of contract or fiduciary duties. Despite the claims of consumer protection through supervision, there is evidence in California that approximately 37% of agency workers have very little or no supervision.[47]

Regulation of Personal Assistance Services

Due to the nature of the independent living model, many of the structural and process-related quality assurance mechanisms that apply to long-term care providers under the medical model are not available. Mechanisms such as accreditation, licensing, external supervision and training are inconsistent with the independent living model. To require the use of such mechanisms would effectively eviscerate the model and convert the care provided to something resembling the medical model. Inappropriate regulation of consumer-directed personal assistance services in a manner that is inconsistent with the independent living model can be particularly counter pro-ductive.

Yet, this leaves us with a void in attempting to deal with the essen-tial issue of quality of consumer-directed personal assistance services. Thus far, primary focus has been on implementing quantitative stud-ies of consumer satisfaction. While satisfaction is a key outcome of interest, it is only one of several such outcomes. Ideally, we need to be able to assess other outcomes such as functional improvement or decline, avoidable hospitalizations, ability to maintain independent lifestyle, and ability to maintain major life activity (e.g., work or school).

According to a study of stakeholders, most government officials who address long-term care issues, and most consumers and their representatives, appear to believe that the independent living model offers more control, satisfaction and a higher quality of life.[48] Consumers and their representatives were unanimous in their belief that the independent living model provides a higher quality of care than agency services under the medical model.[49] Representatives of home care agencies and unions that represent their workers indicated that the two models offer a similar quality of care.[50]

Ultimately, the final quality mechanism under the independent living model is consumer control and choice in the market. Tilly, Wiener and Cuellar observe:

> In place of formal quality assurance mechanisms, con-sumer-directed programs rely on the ability of clients to fire unsatisfactory workers and to hire replacements to assure quality—in other words, the market. The current labor short-age in the United States, which makes recruitment difficult for all long-term care services, may threaten the quality of these services by undermining the willingness of clients to fire poor-quality workers, perhaps increasing the need for more formal quality assurance mechanisms.[51]

As indicated earlier, whether in a good or bad labor market, the market has very limited ability to ensure quality. This statement is true with respect to all consumers, but particularly consumers with cognitive deficits. Virtually everyone in the stakeholder study agreed that consumers with cognitive disabilities raise major concerns about quality.[52] Despite such concerns, in all four countries that use the independent living model, consumers with such deficits are still held responsible for the quality of their care under the independent living model.[53]

One observer states:

> Perhaps the ultimate quality riddle is that consumers sometimes seem to choose a lesser standard of care, according to professional or 'objective' standards of quality, but still seem quite pleased with their choices—indeed, often more pleased than consumers who are assured of receiving care from a provider with more professional credentials. Understanding the apparent willingness of consumers to select 'substandard' care is one of the keys to assuring the quality of care of these services.[54]

TOTAL QUALITY MANAGEMENT (TQM) AND CONTINUOUS QUALITY IMPROVEMENT (CQI)

In the past two decades, the concepts of total quality management and continuous quality assurance have been embraced in board rooms and business schools throughout the country. The basic idea underlying these concepts is that those who actually produce a product or service have valuable things to say about defining the quality of the product or service and how to improve such quality over time. These approaches consequently take a bottom-up approach in which work groups are encouraged to define quality and develop strategies to improve quality. In the long-term care context, TQM and CQI have been applied in conjunction with different measures of structure, process, and outcome to improve quality of care.

These concepts were developed to address issues of quality in large bureaucratic organizations. Interestingly, a version of these concepts appears to be inherent in the independent living model, at least to the extent that the model is working well. Consumers often discuss with each other ways in which they take care of their personal assistance needs. Often, new personal assistants who have not gotten into the consumer's routine suggest fresh new ways in which to do things more effectively or efficiently.

Because the independent living model inherently involves decisions by those who are involved directly in receiving and providing care, any new innovation or improvement can be adopted and implemented immediately. There is no need for committee meetings, corporate authorization or approval of legal counsel. New technologies may be effective in enhancing safety and ensuring quality, including monitoring technologies and emergency call systems. This approach may reduce the conflict between autonomy and security, but may increase the conflict between autonomy and privacy.[55]

SUMMARY

Issues concerning quality of care are challenging in virtually all areas of medical and health care. Such are particularly challenging in long-term care because of issues concerning measurement and attribution of causation. Assuring the quality of consumer-directed personal assistance services under the independent living model presents similar challenges. Independent living advocates claim that the control exercised by the consumer provides a significant assurance of quality. These advocates also claim that consumer assessment should be the primary mechanism for measuring quality under this model. This approach may suffice for purposes of services provided to consumers who pay for their own personal assistance, but policymakers typically also demand other "objective" measures and mechanisms to assure technical quality. For this reason, professional standards of quality are still needed to some extent, particularly when the consumer does not have adequate decisional capacity to assess quality.

──11──

Integration and Managed Care

One of the primary criticisms of long-term care in this country is that such services are extremely poorly coordinated with other services needed by consumers. Actually, this lack of integration is a valid criticism of our health care system generally. It is particularly problematic in the long-term care context because consumers typically have substantial physical, mental and sometimes multiple disabilities that make navigation through a complex, fragmented and often inaccessible system extremely difficult. Moreover, while acute care services have been coordinated more extensively in recent years because of the managed care revolution, long-term care has been less influenced and coordinated by managed care. This chapter focuses on the concerns of many people with disabilities and chronic conditions who are highly skeptical that the managed care industry is interested in addressing their challenging and costly health problems, particularly in long-term care which involves the ongoing management of chronic care issues.

A FRAGMENTED HEALTH CARE "SYSTEM"

The ideal health care system would be structured in a manner that would be sufficiently flexible to meet the needs of all consumers, i.e., people of a variety of impairments, disabilities, acute conditions, family situations, ages and ethnicities, in the most efficient way. The unique needs of the consumer should drive the system, not the other way around. Consumers do not come with a standardized set of needs that can be accommodated by a rigid delivery system.

Although there are some commonalities among different consumers, particularly those with similar impairments, disabilities and personal backgrounds, no two consumers are identical; their distinct needs cannot be addressed adequately through a "cookie-cutter" assembly line approach.

Unfortunately, this is largely the approach offered by our fragmented health care system. Services provided are determined more by the rules of the funding agencies and the orientations of specialists than the needs of consumers. Funding agencies often attempt to evade financial responsibility by shifting costs over to other payors or the consumer as much as possible. Only when a single funding entity has full responsibility for the consumer's care is there a fair likelihood that a coordinated effort will be developed. This is one of the primary reasons for the popularity of managed care as an approach to integrate and coordinate services.[1] However, managed care also has strong incentives to contain costs that can be harmful to people with disabilities who require long-term care.

In the actual provision of care, the focus should shift to the consumer as an integrated being with interconnected biological systems that cannot be viewed in isolation. Providers typically segment consumers by their various organ systems and treat them as if each organ were a separate organism. If a consumer with several significant health problems is admitted to the hospital for one problem, it is unusual that requests to address the other problems would be granted. Such special treatment is likely to occur only after aggressive advocacy by the patient or family members, and only if some physician is willing to take charge of the needed coordination. Because physicians are not compensated directly for such efforts, they rarely do so. Seldom is there substantial communication among different providers of health care services for consumers of long-term care services.

One of the leading authorities on long-term care, Joshua Wiener, has concluded:

> For reasons of both quality of care and cost, there is increasing interest in approaches that integrate acute-care and long-term-care services. Almost all of these initiatives depend on extending managed care beyond traditional acute-care services to include long-term care. These approaches face numerous technical, political, and attitudinal barriers. To a large extent, policy makers and providers are just beginning to learn how to create a seamless financ-

ing and delivery system for people with disabilities. Data from evaluations of demonstrations suggest both problems and opportunities. How to meet the needs of the 'whole' person is something we do not understand very well, but with the rising number of people with disabilities, society will have to learn.[2]

DEFINING MANAGED CARE

The mass media, such as television, newspapers and magazines, typically use the term "managed care" in a generic manner, suggesting that it comprises one specific type of health care organization. In fact, managed care is a generic, but very nebulous concept that encompasses a broad array of different types of organizations. Each managed care organization is to some extent unique in the way it finances, organizes and provides services.

The fundamental characteristic distinguishing managed care organizations from other "non-managed" care providers is that managed care integrates the financing and delivery of health care services. Prior to the emergence of managed care as a major force in health care, insurance organizations collected premiums and paid for care on behalf of their enrollees, and provider organizations provided care and collected payments. Except for the few early health maintenance organizations, such as Kaiser Permanente, which had a small market share before the 1980s, financing and delivery of services were segregated functions conducted by separate organizations. Remarkably, there was very little attempt to integrate health care financing and delivery.

The problem with this system is that the provider organizations had a strong incentive to provide as much care as they can be paid for, even unnecessary care, subjecting the patient to risks. The insurance organizations had little control in such situations over the costs incurred by the providers. This process proved to be a recipe for health care inflation. Providers provided services and payors paid for the services, leading providers to provide ever more services, and the cost spiral continued. Ultimately, the consumer/ patient had to pay the bill in the form of higher premiums and higher copayments. The employee paid the bill in the form of lower wages than they would otherwise have earned, and the taxpayer paid the bill in the form of higher taxes for government health care programs.

Managed care was largely a market response to the growing costs of health care. The ultimate payors—employers, employees, consumers and taxpayers—finally reacted to the rapid growth of health care costs being passed on to them. In addition to the integration of financing and delivery of care, managed care organizations tend to use a variety of cost containment mechanisms such as gatekeepers (usually primary care physicians who determine access to specialty care or durable medical equipment), case management (coordinating care throughout the system), and utilization review (determining which care is medically necessary and therefore should be provided).

MODELS OF MANAGED CARE

To greatly oversimplify an extremely complex health care market, there are basically two models of managed care: the health maintenance organization (HMO) and the preferred provider organization (PPO). Each of these models has several sub-models, thousands of variations on the themes, and many types of support organizations that assist managed care organizations to achieve their goals. The following is a rudimentary overview of managed care. A comprehensive treatment of this subject would address the remarkable diversity of managed care plans, the mechanisms they use, and the ways in which they operate.

HMOs are organizations that provide a set of covered services in exchange for a predetermined amount of money per enrollee, known as a capitation payment. There are several sub-models of HMOs. The staff model HMO employs its physicians, in contrast with the more typical arrangement in which physicians are independent contractors on staff. The group model relies upon group practices for the provision of care. The independent practice association (IPA) allows individual physicians to practice in their own offices while participating in the HMO plan. All HMOs use some variation of capitation payment and cost control mechanisms such as gatekeepers and utilization review. Although enrollees are generally required to receive all services from plan providers, some HMOs have a point-of-service option whereby enrollees may receive services from outside providers at higher out-of-pocket costs.

PPOs, which are sometimes more accurately described as preferred provider arrangements (PPAs), involve a contractual relationship between an insurer organization and individual providers who agree to serve on the panel of preferred providers for the PPO. The providers agree to provide their services for the deeply discounted fees negotiated with the PPO. The PPO, in turn, provides a strong financial incentive for its enrollees to receive care from the plan's preferred providers. Enrollees who receive care from providers outside the preferred provider network must pay substantially more money out-of-pocket.

Whether managed care meets the needs of people with disabilities is the subject of an ongoing debate. Some contend that managed care organizations encourage the coordination of care, which should benefit people with disabilities and chronic conditions.[3] Others contend that the financial mechanisms of managed care, particularly capitation payment, create strong incentives to contain costs and deny needed care.[4] One problematic way cost containment is achieved by some managed care organizations is by engaging in preferred risk selection, also known as skimming, i.e., encouraging the most healthy individuals to enroll and discouraging high-cost individuals from enrolling.[5] Depending upon their structures and rules, different managed care plans are likely to be more or less responsive to the needs of people with disabilities.

MANAGED CARE AND LONG-TERM CARE

Over the past 20 years, health care has become more systematized as a result of the managed care revolution and the resulting establishment of integrated delivery systems throughout the country. Managed care organizations have purchased or otherwise consolidated existing facilities, particularly where there has been wasteful excess capacity; they have converted this excess capacity so as to satisfy market demand in other areas of health care.

At this stage of history, our acute health care system is dominated by managed care organizations. With the exception of the traditional Medicare program and the veterans' health care system, virtually the entire acute care system is under some form of managed care. Even the Medicare program is becoming dominated by managed care organizations as more and more beneficiaries sign up with Medicare HMOs. In the private sector, health care organizations that are not organized under managed care principles are not able to contain costs and remain competitive. Therefore, in considering acute health care at the beginning of the 21st century, primarily we are really considering managed care.

The same cannot be said of our long-term care "system." Long-term care in this country remains a highly fragmented set of component parts, including nursing homes, home health agencies, physicians, nurses, therapists, clinics and social service agencies. Although managed care is having an impact on the structure of the long-term care industry, primarily through the development of vertically integrated delivery systems that contain these components, the long-term care industry has not been impacted as substantially as the acute care industry. The likelihood that any individual requiring long-term care would receive such care in a well-integrated manner remains remote.

The primary, direct impact of the managed care revolution has been on primary care, acute care, and medical rehabilitation, because these are the services typically covered by managed care organizations. However, there has also been an important indirect impact on long-term care. In particular, the incentives of managed care to keep patients out of the hospital and reduce length of stay have had two major effects. First, it has increased the need for sub-acute care, requiring somewhat less intensive services than acute care, much of which has been provided by nursing homes, home health agencies and other long-term care providers. Second, it has created the necessity to restructure the health care system to accommodate changes in the balance between the demand and supply of different types of health care services.

Social Health Maintenance Organizations

Some specialized managed care organizations known as "social health maintenance organizations" (Social HMOs or SHMOs) have been established specifically to address the needs of people with disabilities and chronic conditions; many of these organizations have proven effective in doing so.[6] They often are financed through one or more agencies of the federal and/or state governments, and typically receive relatively high levels of payment for their enrollees reflecting the high average costs of their target population.[7] No single model exists for these SHMOs; several have proven capable of providing high quality services to people with disabilities.[8]

Many social HMOs have focused primarily on the frail elderly population. One program in New York state called the Independent Care System (ICS) was designed to enable the broad range of people with disabilities to live at home in the least restrictive setting possible by integrating the full range of health care services, including home- and community-based long-term care.[9] Its goal is to coordinate the var- ious benefits available to these individuals and provide such services in a seamless manner blending needed medical and support services.[10] This system actually contracts with a home health agency for the pro- vision of services by home health aides, and therefore, technically it is under the medical model. However, because of consumer participation on its board of directors, a consumer advisory council, and an ombudsman program, it is considered to offer substantial consumer direction.

ICS offers a full range of supports including an option for consumer- directed para-professional care, respite care for family caregivers, con- sumer peer training, care management, and social day care for those who want it.[11] A full range of medical and other health care services are offered, including durable medical equipment, rehabilitation and nurs- ing home care. To some independent living advocates, this approach is not acceptable because they believe its medical model aspects will inevitably overshadow its independent living aspects. To others, the key component is that consumers may choose this program, which has elements of consumer direction, and therefore it is an acceptable option.

CASE MANAGEMENT

Closely related to managed care and the coordination of services is the concept of case management. Case management has been defined as "a mixture of functions directed at coordinating and negotiating existing resources to assure needed, appropriate, and continuous care for individuals on a case-by-case basis."[12] Case managers come from a variety of professional backgrounds and perform a variety of functions including the following:

- Assessment of consumer need and eligibility;
- Care planning and allocation;
- Arranging and coordinating service delivery;
- Monitoring the quality, appropriateness and outcomes of services;
- Assessment and review of the plan; and
- Discharge or termination from services.[13]

Although the functions of case managers may appear quite innocuous, case management is somewhat controversial within the disability community. Good case management services are appreciated by many people with disabilities, particularly elderly people and people with cognitive disabilities. Some researchers and administrators contend that case management can be a successful component of a program implementing the independent living model.[14] For example, Gilson and and Casebolt argue that, "By focusing case management on doing what the individual directs, the case manager can enhance independence, autonomy, and accommodation."[15] This approach has been adopted by the Paralyzed Veterans of America (PVA) in developing a comprehensive PAS training program using a case management model that supports the principles of consumer empowerment and self-determination.[16]

However, many other people with disabilities, particularly younger and working-age people, express the sentiment that, "I do not want to be managed." Many view case managers as instruments of health care programs designed to reduce their use of resources. These critics have suggested that case managers cannot fully meet the needs of people with disabilities because their commitment to consumers is compromised by inherent conflicts in their goals.[17] A primary function of the case manager is to help manage limited resources. Consequently, their rationing function is always potentially in conflict with the consumer's need and demand for such limited resources. This rationing function could be eliminated by allocating a set amount of money directly to the consumer under the independent living model, allowing consumers to thereby ration their own services.[18] This approach illustrates the transformation from a top-down rationing system, with the case manager representing the management at the top, to a bottom-up rationing system with consumers making decisions at the bottom.

Case managers also have a strong tendency to focus on the needs of the consumer from the perspective of the health care professional.[19] This approach, based upon the ethical principle of beneficence, often is expressed as paternalism. Paternalism is the antithesis of the philosophy behind the independent living movement; the movement was established largely in response to the paternalistic treatment of people with disabilities by health care professionals.[20] This paternalistic tendency is probably inherent in the selection and training of health care professionals generally; it is reinforced by professional practice norms and reactions to the risk of tort liability (e.g., medical malpractice). Even when the actions of case managers are intended to be entirely in the best interests of consumers, perceptions of such interests are likely to diverge; the case manager is likely to interfere with consumer control and choice.

Still, to the extent that case managers expedite the coordination of services, they can benefit consumers. Navigating our health care system is a challenge for experts, and is particularly difficult for people with disabilities who have substantial health care needs. Therefore, an approach to case management that assists consumers in navigating through the system without imposing control over the consumer may be well-received by consumers generally. Case management per se is not necessarily incompatible with the independent living model of long-term care, as long as the consumer has control over whether to use such services.

One study attempted to develop a profile of potential consumer-directed clients in a countywide home care program by having telephone case managers and in-home assessors make independent decisions about the appropriate level of case management for a consumer.[21] Of the 278 clients assessed, only 16.5% were identified by both professionals as candidates for consumer-directed care, and 42.1%, were identified by both professionals as requiring a more intense level of long-term care. The professionals disagreed on the remaining 41.4% of clients. This study suggests the potential arbitrariness of decisions by professional case managers. Professional biases appear to play as large a role as objective analysis in making such determinations. Among the factors indicated by case members as increasing the likelihood of a client's being selected for consumer direction were perceptions that the client had stable health, a good support system, an understanding of the service system and a willingness to make contacts in case of problems. In addition, case managers were more likely to identify clients as candidates for consumer-directed care if they were female, had fewer impairments, received fewer services, had low incomes, and lived alone.

Some analysts, including some independent living advocates, believe that case management can be compatible with the independent living model.[22] They argue that the key to compatibility is the extent to which consumers can choose and control their case manager.[23] The United Kingdom's 5-year demonstration of providing payments directly to consumers for purchasing personal assistance services, discussed in Chapter 12, relies heavily on case managers to determine the amount of assistance needed.[24]

THE INDEPENDENT LIVING MODEL AND INTEGRATED LONG-TERM CARE

Clearly, integration of long-term care with the consumer's other health care and social service needs is important. Any of the three models of long-term care can potentially be coordinated with other services. Again, choice of a model depends largely upon the values, goals and capacities of the consumer. Some consumers simply do not want their care, or any aspect of their lives to be managed by health care professionals or others. For these consumers, the independent living model is likely to be particularly attractive.

In Chapter 7, we concluded that one of the characteristics of the independent living model is that it is challenging to manage. Coordination and integration of services are among the more challenging management tasks for consumers under this model. Unlike the medical model of long-term care, in which the same health care professionals who provide services can assist in integrating and coordinating care, the independent living model does not offer such assistance. However, the consumer under this model can still receive assistance in navigating through the system by becoming a member of a managed care organization that is responsive to the needs of people with disabilities.

Even without such assistance, many consumers operating under the independent living model become sophisticated consumers of health care services. By necessity, they must learn to obtain the services they need in order to survive. Many of these individuals learn through their errors. However, errors can be very harmful or even lethal, and ideally consumers should have assistance available to them to reduce such risks of harm. Ultimately, as discussed at length throughout this book, consumers should be allowed to determine the level of risk to which they are subject.

SUMMARY

Although the traditional long-term care system in this country has always been highly fragmented, there have been some attempts recently at developing a more integrated system. The economic shakeout resulting from government austerity measures and the managed care revolution, have resulted in enormous consolidations throughout the health care sector. In some cases, this consolidation has further resulted in the development of integrated delivery systems that include long-term care providers. However, overall, the system remains largely disjointed. Under any of the long-term care models, there is a need to develop mechanisms of coordination. The extent to which such mechanisms are successful will depend in large part on the consumer's ability to navigate through the system. Some consumers have better navigation skills than others. Obviously, consumers with cognitive disabilities will have great difficulty attempting to navigate the system and require surrogates to do so on their behalf.

——12——

International Perspectives

$\mathbf{S}$ome critics of the independent living model of long-term care contend that this model could never be implemented on a national scale or claim that consumers could never be trusted to direct their own care in a national program. They must respond to the fact that several countries have adopted and successfully implemented long-term care systems that use the independent living model of long-term care.[1] These countries include Austria, Germany, France, and the Netherlands. All of these countries also provide long-term care services through home health agencies under the medical model, with the exception of Austria, which only has an independent living model consumer-directed care program. In Germany and France, the consumer-directed program dominates over the agency-directed program. In the Netherlands, the agency-directed program dominates; the consumer-directed program is limited to only 5% of total expenditures. This chapter examines different approaches these other countries have adopted in implementing variations of the independent living model.

EUROPEAN APPROACHES TO INDEPENDENT LIVING

The following sections describe the independent living model programs of each of the countries, including eligibility criteria, number of beneficiaries, services covered, amounts of benefits, sources of funding, and quality assurance mechanisms (from the work of Jane Tilly, Joshua Wiener and Allison Cuellar).[2] For the benefit of readers from other countries, the native language sources cited and other information sources are included in end notes.

Austria

In Austria, any person over 3 years of age who requires the use of a wheelchair or otherwise requires over 50 hours of care per month meets the functional requirements for eligibility.[3] There is no financial test of eligibility; therefore, all functionally eligible individuals may receive services irrespective of income and resources. Altogether, about 310,000 individuals receive services under the program.

The Austrian program covers any service the consumer desires. The cash benefit received depends upon the number of hours of care the consumer needs. There are seven benefit levels in all. The cash benefit is unencumbered; consumers may use it any way they wish, such as hiring anyone they choose, including family members. The program is funded through general tax revenues and is administered through a sub-national public insurance fund.

In Austria, consumers are provided some assistance with respect to managing their home care. However, this assistance is mostly limited to providing lists of prospective workers and the operation of consumer hotlines to supply needed information. The government agents make random visits to beneficiaries to ensure that they are receiving adequate care. Austria's personal assistance allowance, which was adopted in 1993, has been proposed as a model of consumer-directed care for the United States.[4]

Germany

In Germany, anyone who requires assistance with at least two ADLs and some IADLs is functionally eligible to receive benefits.[5] As implemented, this approach has been criticized for not taking into account the supervisory needs of people with cognitive impairments. Like Austria, there is no means testing; any functionally eligible individual may participate irrespective of income or resources. About 1.28 million home care beneficiaries actually receive benefits.

The German program covers any service the consumer desires. There are three benefit levels based on the consumer's functional deficits. If the beneficiary chooses to receive a cash benefit, the amount of cash is equivalent to about half the value of service benefits the consumer could otherwise receive. The cash benefit is unencumbered. Consumers may use it in any way they wish, such as hiring anyone, including family members. The program is funded by mandatory public insurance premiums paid through a tax of 1.7% of salaries and pensions, which is shared by employers, employees, retirees and pension funds. It is administered through a sub-national public insurance fund.

Like Austria, the German program provides some management assistance in the form of provider lists and hotline information. The primary quality mechanism for this program is periodic visits to determine whether cash beneficiaries are receiving adequate care.

France

In France, functional eligibility depends upon the need for assistance in going to the bathroom and dressing.[6] The assessment instrument used in implementing this approach has been criticized as being too medically oriented. This program is means-tested to the extent that there are income-related reductions in benefits. Also, there are mechanisms to recover expenses from a consumer's estate. Some 86,000 individuals receive benefits under this program.[7]

The French program is not as generous in its benefits as the previous two countries' programs. It primarily covers assistance with ADLs and IADLs. It also provides a small benefit set-aside for flexible use by the consumer. There is a national maximum benefit. The consumer's benefit is calculated using a payment rate formula. The consumer may hire anyone except a spouse, live-in partner, or person receiving retirement income. The program is funded through general tax revenues, and administered through local government.

Fiscal agents pay home care workers and taxes. Otherwise, the program does not provide assistance in recruiting, selecting, or training assistants. Quality is assured through annual visits to ensure beneficiaries are receiving adequate services.

The Netherlands

In the Netherlands, functional eligibility for the program is based on the need for assistance with ADLs or IADLs.[8] However, the need for nursing care cannot exceed three hours per day. Individuals who require more than three hours of nursing care must use the home care program under the medical model. The consumer-directed program is not means-tested. Anyone who qualifies on the basis of the functional criteria may receive benefits irrespective of income or resources. Approximately 7,260 individuals receive such benefits. This number is much smaller than the number of participants in the other countries' consumer-directed care programs because, as mentioned earlier, this program is secondary to the Dutch medical model home care program.

The Dutch independent living model program primarily provides assistance with ADLs and IADLs, as well as a small benefit setaside for the flexible use of beneficiaries. Consumers receive vouchers and may hire anyone they wish, including family members. Workers are paid by fiscal intermediaries. Consumers with substantial cognitive deficits may use the program, but they are required to have surrogates to help them with decision-making. The program is funded through mandatory premiums paid by workers based on salary; it is administered through a sub-national public insurance fund.

The program in the Netherlands provides some informal assistance to the consumer in management tasks such as recruiting and training, as well as payment services by the fiscal agent. In particular, a consumer advocacy group provides telephone assistance to consumers, including information on bureaucratic requirements. The primary quality assurance mechanism involves a legal obligation that consumers obtain good quality care and visits by social insurance banks to ensure that the money is spent appropriately.

Consumer Direction in Other Nations

Several other countries have experimented with consumer-directed long-term care.[9] For example, the United Kingdom implemented a 5-year initiative in which adults with substantial disabilities or chronic conditions were given cash to pay for in-home care which they themselves arrange.[10] In this program, case managers play a primary role in determining the amount of assistance needed by clients in the program. Norway also provides personal assistance services to its citizens with disabilities.[11] These are just some of the countries that have been exploring the concept of consumer-directed personal assistance services as a means by which to satisfy the long-term care needs of their populations.

SUMMARY

A comprehensive treatment of approaches to the provision of consumer-directed personal assistance and long-term care taken by other
countries would require another book. Ideally, that book should be
written in another decade or so, after these programs have been evaluated more extensively. This chapter simply provides a very brief
overview of some of the structural and procedural aspects of several
key programs that have been established and appear to be implemented successfully.

All four of the well-established European personal assistance services programs discussed above have demonstrated that it is possible
to implement a large-scale national program of consumer-directed
personal assistance services under the independent living model.
These programs have some features in common. Although all have
been implemented on a nationwide basis, none is administered at the
national level. There is an apparent consensus that, because of the
very personal nature of personal assistance services, local administration is more appropriate.

All four programs provide some support to consumers in addressing the complex management tasks associated with the independent
living model. All have been criticized to some extent for not providing enough support services. The demand for consumer-directed personal assistance services is substantial in all of these countries, and the
ability to satisfy this large and growing demand under any model is
challenging. The majority of consumers under these programs are
people with physical and/or developmental disabilities. However, all
four programs cover people with cognitive disabilities and either
allow or require them to use surrogate decision-makers.

In the United States, we pride ourselves in having the most state-
of-the-art health care system in the world. Such self-congratulation
may be justified with respect to trauma care and medical rehabilitation. However, in considering long-term care, we lag behind at least
four other countries. This may be a bit of an overstatement, in that
some of our states have been implementing consumer-directed personal assistance programs for many years. It is probably more accurate to say that there is enormous variation among the states in their
long-term care systems, and some states lag seriously behind the
more progressive states and several progressive countries.

—13—

Conclusions: Which Model Will Prevail?

Americans of all ages, ethnicities and functional capacities appreciate, expect and demand their freedom and independence in all aspects of their lives. Until recently, those who could afford long-term care have grudgingly accepted the restrictions on their freedom associated with the medical model, assuming that this surrender of their cherished autonomy was inevitable. Even today, many Americans assume that nursing home care will be their only option in the event that they develop a major disability necessitating long-term care and if there are no family members to take care of them.

However, some significant changes have occurred in the long-term care context over the past 40 years, and most dramatically in the past decade. A major trend toward de-institutionalization has occurred since the 1960s. Although this trend primarily has affected the mentally retarded and mentally ill populations in large state institutions, it has also had a profound effect on the general long-term care policy environment. In conjunction with the general trend toward consumer direction and choice in the health care system, and the normalization and disability rights movements, long-term care policymakers have developed a new emphasis on consumers' rights to control their lives. This emphasis has impacted the rhetoric of even the most restrictive nursing homes and other institutions, if not necessarily their practice.

Since the 1970s, advocates of the independent living movement have been committed to giving people with disabilities living in institutions the option to live independently in their communities. Through their efforts, the independent living model of long-term care—consumer-directed personal assistance services—has grown dramatically since the 1980s. Yet, the majority of individuals who received such services have been young and working-age individuals. The general population, including most elderly people, know very little or nothing at all about the independent living model.

In the past decade, the prospects for greater recognition of the independent living model have increased dramatically. Legislators at the federal and state levels have become familiar with this model as a result of the strong lobbying efforts of disability rights advocates and organizations such as ADAPT. Among other advocacy efforts, they have lobbied for several prominent pieces of legislation supporting expansion of consumer-directed personal assistance services.[1] Evaluations of programs under the independent living model, including variants of the model in which the consumer is simply given a cash payment to purchase personal assistance services, have demonstrated that the model is viable as a basis for major long-term care programs.

EVALUATION OF THE THREE MODELS

The assessment of the three models indicates that each has strengths and weaknesses that may be addressed to some extent through program development. No model is perfect, and no model is appropriate for everyone. However, some models may be better than other models in certain respects and with respect to certain consumers. The foregoing analysis suggests that consumers who insist on maintaining control over their lives will be more satisfied with the independent living model. Consumers who do not wish to deal with the complexities of managing a personal assistance relationship, and those with cognitive impairments who do not have a surrogate willing and able to address these issues on their behalf, will be better off under some version of the medical model.

Any of the models has a potential range of consumer direction associated with it. However, the independent living model, which is based fundamentally on a philosophy of consumer-directed care, is most compatible with consumer autonomy and control. The success of attempts to achieve consumer direction under the other models will depend largely upon the willingness of administrators and caregivers to yield control and authority to consumers. It is likely that the extent to which this occurs, other than when it is legally imposed and

enforced (e.g., negative autonomy such as informed consent requirements), will vary substantially from provider to provider and caregiver to caregiver.

One interesting finding of this analysis is that a large percentage
of consumers in different contexts are receiving care and assistance
under the independent living model from relatives, neighbors and
friends, both in European programs and domestic ones. What is interesting about this trend is that it deviates somewhat from the traditional independent living model. Although there is nothing in that
model that necessarily precludes the use of family members, friends
and close acquaintances as caregivers, the original concept was for
consumer-directed personal assistance services to offer a means for
consumers to escape the dependence inherent in both the medical and
informal support models. It is certainly understandable that consumers would want to hire people they know and trust personally,
such as family members, rather than strangers who could possibly do
them harm.

However, the question must be asked whether this simply substitutes one form of dependence for another. As one consumer
expressed, it is very difficult to fire one's relative. By allowing consumers to hire relatives, programs have in effect authorized a hybrid
informal support/independent living model, which in some cases
more closely resembles a family supplement to other disability cash
benefits than a personal assistance program. This situation is not necessarily a bad thing, but it is different from the original conception of
the independent living model. It may be beneficial to consumers in
the short run, but harmful in the long run, particularly when family
caregivers die or are no longer physically or emotionally capable of
providing care.

On balance, allowing consumers to hire family members is probably justified. It reduces the financial burdens on families and
increases the supply of caregivers needed by our country. This issue
concerning the development of an adequate long-term care work
force will be critical in the coming decades as the population continues to age. However, public policy should also recognize that many
people with disabilities do not have family members or friends willing and able to provide care. Moreover, it would be useful from a
public policy perspective to provide incentives for consumers to
enhance their long-term independence by hiring people outside their
personal circles.

Overall, although the data available are limited, there is clearly sufficient evidence to conclude that the independent living model has enough redeeming features to warrant offering it as an alternative to the medical model. Indeed, there is considerable evidence that the independent living model is superior to the medical model with respect to several key criteria including affordability, autonomy and quality (consumer satisfaction). Professor Benjamin has concluded:

Although health professionals have expressed concerns about the capacity of consumer direction to assure quality, particularly with respect to safety, meeting unmet needs, and technical quality, our findings suggest that the consumer-directed service [independent living] model is a viable alternative to the agency [medical] model. Because public programs are under growing pressure to address the long-term care needs of low-income people of all ages with disabilities, the Medicaid personal assistance benefit needs to be reassessed in light of these findings. Consumer-directed models may offer a less elaborate and possibly less costly option for organizing supportive services at home.[2]

PROSPECTS FOR THE INDEPENDENT LIVING MODEL

Based on the above conclusions, it seems likely that the independent living model will continue to grow rapidly in the next few decades. Yet, the growth of this model is far from a certainty. Due to the substantial control of long-term care by the states through their Medicaid programs and other programs, much will depend upon the political response of state legislators to the growing demand for the independent living model. Unfortunately, most people do not seriously consider the need for long-term care services until they or their family members actually need such services. Consequently, the political pressure for the independent living model is not nearly as great as it would be if people were constantly confronted with this issue and thereby motivated to lobby for long-term care options.

On the other hand, long-term care providers and practitioners who provide services under the medical model have a strong concentrated interest in attempting to maintain as much of their market power as possible.[3] Consequently, they are highly organized politically and likely to continue to oppose encroachments on their market by a model of care that does not rely upon health care professionals.

The bottom line is that the prospects for the independent living model will depend largely upon the relative political clout of those who support the model versus those who oppose it. While the nursing home and home health industries may have a political advantage in this regard, they should not discount the political skills of the independent living advocates. Such disability rights activists have demonstrated repeatedly their ability to attract the attention of the press and political leaders concerning issues that are important to them, such as the enactment and successful implementation of the ADA. There is no issue of greater importance to these independent living advocates than access to consumer-directed personal assistance services under the independent living model.

Perhaps the strongest reason that the independent living model of personal assistance services has not grown as rapidly as feasible is that health care providers who benefit from the status quo have vigorously opposed it.[4] Their primary argument has always been that people with disabilities will be harmed under the independent living model, and that providers who are either professionally trained or supervised by health care professionals are necessary to ensure quality and avoid negligence or abuse. This argument has lost much of its strength in recent years as evidence has mounted concerning negligence, abuse, and rampant fraud in the nursing home and home health industries. Policymakers have realized that the appropriate comparison is not between one model that is subject to problems and another model that provides perfect patient care, but rather between two models that are potentially subject to quality and abuse problems. The policy challenge is to provide services under the model preferred by the consumer in a manner that reduces the likelihood of problems.

The problems identified in the nursing home and home health industries have compromised their public image, adversely affecting their political clout at both the federal and state levels. When providers dominated the health care system, prior to the 1980s, industry trade associations were highly effective in their lobbying efforts to eliminate potential competition. As the health care field has become more and more payor-dominated, and to some degree consumer-oriented, the lobbying effectiveness of provider groups has been diminished relative to other interests. Components of the industry that have been under attack for reasons concerning fraud and/or quality of care issues, such as nursing homes and home health agencies, have been particularly weakened.

This is certainly not to suggest that these long-term care providers have lost their political power altogether. In fact, some nursing facilities and home health agencies have probably gained power through consolidating with large health care systems with significant resources for advocacy and lobbying. However, as an industry, overall these providers have lost power relative to competing political interests such as people with disabilities who have become more organized politically in the past two decades. This relative increase in the political clout of people with disabilities as a potential voting block may accrue to the benefit of the independent living model and programs organized under it.

POLICY OPTIONS

The purpose of this book is not to demonstrate the superiority of the independent living model. A strong argument for such superiority can be made, at least from the perspective of people with disabilities who insist upon maintaining control over their lives and living as independently as possible. However, the burden of proving superiority of any model should be justifiably substantial; satisfying that burden is unnecessary in this case. Instead, my objective was simply to demonstrate that the independent living model is one of several models of long-term care that has the potential to offer high quality care and assistance. I believe this has been adequately demonstrated.

The Need for Balance—the Jungle and the Zoo Revisited

In addition to the need for choice and control, there is a need for balance in our long-term care policy. Currently, the policy remains strongly biased in favor of institutional care and the medical model generally. Those who contend that the long-term care system should remain biased in favor of institutional care and home care supervised by health care professionals must bear the burden of defending the status quo. This book demonstrates that their burden cannot be sustained. In light of the substantial flaws of the medical model, the independent living model should be available to consumers on an equal basis.

We can design our long-term care system in a manner that minimizes the likelihood that anything bad will happen to the recipient, much as animals are fed, protected and cared for in a zoo. However,

in protecting them from risks, we would also be limiting their freedom to do what they want to do. Freedom always entails risks, such
as the possibility that the individuals will be harmed by themselves
or others. Alternatively, we can design the system to maximize freedom, simulating the jungle, which may result in harm to the individual. Most of us would probably agree that the appropriate policy goal is to achieve a reasonable balance between freedom and
security.

Not everyone in the long-term care field accepts the jungle vs. zoo
analogy and a trade-off in risks contemplated by it. For example, Dr.
Pamela Doty prefers an automobile analogy, indicating that like car
transportation, any provision of long-term care services has certain
risks associated with it.[5] She says that receiving care under the independent living model is like driving one's own car rather than driving a rental car or being driven in a taxi, which is more analogous to
the medical model. She concludes that simply because one drives
one's own car does not subject the individual to greater risks, and
that in fact the risk may be less due to the control that one can exercise driving one's own car or receiving care under the independent
living model.

Determining which analogy better describes reality depends in
part upon how each model operates in the real world. To the extent
that consumers hire strangers under the independent living model,
the jungle-zoo analogy is probably better. To the extent that consumers are permitted to hire family members under the independent
living model, and to the extent that they have family members willing and able to provide their care for compensation, the automobile
analogy may be better. Certainly, the empirical data presented indicate that there can be substantial insecurity for many consumers
receiving care through nursing homes and home health agencies;
conversely, there can be a lack of freedom for consumers in a bad personal assistance relationship. Much depends upon the quality of the
provider and working relationship. Choosing the better analogy to
understand long-term care, like many others discussed in this book,
is subject to debate, and reasonable people can agree to disagree.

Overall, the jungle-zoo analogy provides a good general description of the circumstances of consumers who do not have family
members available to provide all or most of their care. Even if one
adopts the automobile analogy, this does not mean that there are no
trade-offs necessary for consumers and no need to consider balance.

Consumers must still be concerned about becoming unduly depend-ent upon their family caregivers and the possibility of losing their family caregivers over time.

The Need for Choices

One way to achieve a balance is to provide a variety of options for long-term care, offering a range of different levels of freedom and security. Clearly, the results of this analysis suggest that the enor-mous range of different types of consumers requires a variety of choices concerning the financing and delivery of long-term care.[6] Ideally, a competitive long-term care system can be devised with choices that can be made from the bottom up by consumers rather than imposed from the top down from government officials.[7] One way to achieve this is simply by trusting consumers with direct cash payments, which they may use flexibly to achieve their goals.[8] This approach has been implemented successfully in several European countries, and is being tested in the Cash and Counseling Demonstration.[9] The amount of cash allocated may be determined according to a variety of formulas, ranging from an unsophisticated per capita payment to a highly complex risk-adjusted approach based upon factors that determine the costs of personal assistance for people with disabilities.

The independent living model is not for everyone. It is probably not for someone who has very limited capacities for self-direction (although a modified version of the model that uses surrogacy may be applicable to such individuals). It may not be for someone who has a limited desire for self-direction. It is also probably not for someone who is unable or unwilling to cope with risks, because there are definitely risks associated with bringing strangers into one's home and receiving care from a person who is not adequately familiar with disability-related problems. Under the independent living model, the individual with a disability is responsible for screening, training and monitoring personal assistants; a mistake in any step of the process can be fatal. However, nursing homes and home health agencies are also far from perfect in screening, training, and monitoring their employees, and therefore present similar risks. *See* Chapter 7.

The independent living model, at least in its pure form, imposes a large administrative burden on the individual with a disability.

The government treats people with disabilities who employ personal assistants just like any other employer, including requiring the filing of quarterly tax and unemployment insurance forms. These
responsibilities can be extremely onerous, and are clearly a downside of the strict independent living model. A modified version of
the independent living model could use independent living centers,
fiscal intermediate service organizations, or other nonprofit entities
to alleviate this burden for people with disabilities.[10]

The Need for Consumer Direction

The independent living model is for the majority of people with
disabilities who want to control their lives and are willing to bear
the responsibilities and risks for doing so. These individuals
should have consumer-directed personal assistance services available to them in their homes and communities. Therefore, in establishing a national personal assistance services program or policy,
the independent living model should be included as a primary
option for people with disabilities. Beyond that, the government
should adopt a neutral posture, neither favoring nor disfavoring
any particular model. The person with the disability should be
allowed to choose the model under which he or she receives services. All bias in favor of institutional providers, such as nursing
homes and home health agencies, should be eliminated. Any
model of long-term care can be modified to ensure greater or lesser degrees of autonomy and independence.

As Professor Kapp concludes:

> As part of their broader health reform agenda, Congress
> and the state legislatures have a historic opportunity to
> move the paradigm of home and community-based LTC
> from the traditional, structured dependency medical
> model toward the more assertive IL [independent living]
> model. Legislation should express a clear (although rebut-
> table) presumption for the latter model in matters pertain-
> ing to client control over service design and delivery.
> Emphasizing the positive autonomy dimension favors
> services that are structured to maximize the client's choice
> and control, rather than services that rely on a client's neg-
> ative right to refuse (i.e., to 'take or leave') proffered items
> selected by professionals from a highly restricted menu.[11]

IN CLOSING

Access to personal assistance services often means the difference between a free life in the community and a severely restricted life in an institutional setting. Even in the best institution, an individual with a major disability cannot choose exactly when to get out of bed, to bathe, to dress, to eat, to pursue his or her interests, and to return to bed. Individuals who require full-time personal assistance (e.g., attendant care) and who cannot obtain those services are not able to live in their communities. If people with disabilities who are recipients of Supplemental Security Income, Medicaid, and other government benefits will eventually lose their personal assistance as a result of accepting employment, it is not in their interest to accept a job that does not provide long-term assurance of at least comparable benefits, or their cash equivalent.[12]

Many people with disabilities indicate that they would strongly prefer to receive their personal assistance services under the independent living model. However, the best way to determine the actual preferences of people with disabilities is through the choices they make under a neutral program that allows them to choose among a broad array of long-term care/personal assistance options. The prospects for establishing a national program that offers such choice appear to have increased in recent years. Specifically, the political acceptability of a national program has grown with the increasing public acceptance of the goals of the independent living movement, increasing acceptance of the independent living model by older people with and without disabilities, specific proposals that have been advanced, insights obtained through Medicaid waiver programs for home and community-based personal assistance services, and decreasing clout of the health care interests opposed to the independent living model.[13]

This does not mean that enactment of a personal assistance services program is inevitable. Nothing in the political arena is inevitable; the establishment of any new national program, particularly at a time of conservative retrenchment from large national programs, is a longshot. Certainly, there is almost no chance of establishing a new open-ended entitlement program. However, the odds in favor of enacting a fiscally responsible program, with substantial controls against fraud and abuse, are now better than they have ever been. Whether such a program will be enacted will depend largely on whether the economy expands and whether disability rights activists will be successful in getting their message through in a manner that is consistent with the goals of policymakers.[14]

Opponents will argue that independent living advocates are just proposing another wasteful big government program. Politicians and other policymakers should be informed that the goal is not to establish a massive new program from nothing. Rather, the goal is to replace an array of poorly coordinated programs currently costing the taxpayers tens of billions of dollars that are not adequately meeting the needs of people with disabilities with a well-coordinated program that meets their needs based on their preferences. It will be essential to design this program well from the outset. As Sabatino and Litvak have concluded:

> ... consumer choice and control can become a reality only if the structure and process of delivery systems are built from the ground up on this premise. Imposing a right of consumer choice on a system after the fact will ultimately not succeed, for the controlling parameters will already be entrenched in a traditional provider-controlled mode.[15]

WHICH MODEL WILL PREVAIL?

In the United States, we often like to examine complex and controversial political issues in much the same way that one would analyze a football game, in terms of winners and losers. Therefore, it is natural to ask, "Which model of long-term care will prevail?" In this context, that may be a particularly inappropriate, or at least an unnecessary, question. This is not to suggest that long-term care policy offering the independent living model on an even basis will not have implications for resource allocation and the distribution of wealth. Virtually all public policy has financial winners and losers in the short run. However, the short run is not the appropriate time frame to consider.

In the medium and long run, the demand for long-term care will be so large over the coming decades that no single model will be able to accommodate it. Although some elements of the long-term care industry appear to fear competition with the independent living model and the prospect of lost revenues associated with such competition, it is likely that such competition will ease pressures on the industry in the face of workforce shortages while providing an outlet for its most disgruntled patients. In this unique context, there may be no real losers. The biggest winners are likely to be the consumers: people with disabilities who want to be able to control their long-term care.

Appendix A:
Legal Accountability

The different models of long-term care considered in this book have different implications for the potential legal liability and accountability of their participants. The paradigm shift from the medical model, in which providers of services are legally accountable and heavily regulated, to the independent living model, in which legal responsibility is placed largely on the consumer, represents a fundamental change in our approach to ensure that the broad interests of society are achieved. These interests include the safety of consumers and workers, the fair treatment of workers, the efficient use of resources and the accountability of payees for funds. This appendix, which is not intended to serve as a legal primer, considers some of the more important legal rights and duties of all parties under the independent living model.*

LEGAL STATUS OF PERSONAL ASSISTANTS: EMPLOYEES VS. INDEPENDENT CONTRACTORS

Legally, personal assistants potentially may be characterized as employees or independent contractors. This characterization has important legal implications. If they are independent contractors,

---

* This chapter is not intended to be a technical guide to the law affecting consumers and personal assistants. Such technical materials are available elsewhere. [See, for example, Sabatino, C.P. and Litvak, S. 1996. "Liability Issues Affecting Consumer-Directed Personal Assistance Services—Report and Recommendations." *The Elder Law Journal* 4: 247.] Even these cannot be relied upon entirely, because the law changes over time and legal rights and obligations change with it. In the event that a legal issue is raised, it is important to consult a knowledgeable attorney. The purpose of this chapter is to familiarize the reader generally with the legal issues that affect the independent living model.

they are on their own with respect to the filing of employment taxes, and nobody else is accountable for their conduct. If they are employees, their employers are responsible for filing such taxes and may be held liable vicariously for their conduct during the scope of employment (i.e., during working hours).

Whether personal assistants are considered employees or independent contractors depends upon their agreements with consumers and the circumstances under which they provide services. The legal status of assistants depends less on how the assistant is characterized in the agreement and more on the amount of control exerted over the personal assistant by the consumer; the more control exerted, the more likely the assistant will be considered an employee. The Internal Revenue Service (IRS) has discouraged classification of workers generally as independent contractors, recognizing that a large percentage of independent contractors have attempted to evade paying taxes by failing to file tax returns.[1]

Due to the nature of the independent living model, which inherently involves substantial consumer control, most legal commentators regard personal assistants as employees if they work full-time or a significant number of hours every week. Sabatino and Litvik conclude that:

> ... even given the variations that exist in consumer direction, the operation of PAS [personal assistance services] necessarily concedes a level of consumer or agency control that most certainly establishes an employer-employee relationship under virtually any definition. This is especially true in so-called [consumer-directed personal assistance services] models, for to conclude otherwise is to contradict the very notion of consumer direction.[2]

However, under certain limited circumstances, personal assistants may be regarded as independent contractors. This legal characterization is likely to apply, primarily in situations in which the assistant is retained for only a few hours per week or on an ad hoc basis. For example, an emergency assistant who works only on an intermittent basis may well be found to be an independent contractor, particularly if that is the way in which the relationship is characterized in a written contract.

Assuming a personal assistant is an employee does not conclude the inquiry concerning his or her legal status.[3] The question must be asked: Whose employee is the assistant? Among the possibilities are the consumer, the state under a public personal assistance program, the insurer under a private insurance agreement, or an intermediary service organization used by the consumer, state or insurer for administrative services. Generally, none of these entities would prefer to serve as "employer of record," because that legal distinction carries with it legal obligations to satisfy paperwork requirements, tax filings and payment of taxes. More importantly, the employer may be held liable for the conduct of the assistant. Even where the state is not classified as employer of record, it will want to ensure that all legal requirements are fulfilled.[4]

Several states initially characterized personal assistants as independent contractors in their consumer-directed personal assistance services programs.[5] They have since changed their characterization to that of employee; consumers were given responsibility for all employer-related tasks, such as the filing of all relevant taxes. Experience has demonstrated that many consumers have difficulty complying fully with all applicable laws without assistance. Unlike large businesses that have human resource professionals to satisfy these requirements, consumers typically must do so themselves while satisfying a variety of other needs and obligations simultaneously. Some states have addressed this management issue by using different forms of intermediary service organizations to provide needed support in this area.

Table 2 lists the various employer-related tasks associated with consumer-directed personal assistance services, some of which are strict legal requirements and all of which have legal implications for potential penalties or liability.

A LEGAL FRAMEWORK FOR THE INDEPENDENT LIVING MODEL

Under the medical model, consumers receive care from home health agencies and their workers, who are subject to an enormous amount of regulatory scrutiny. The traditional approach to assuring quality is to impose strict regulatory requirements with the objective of achieving minimally acceptable standards.[6] Among the regulatory requirements impacting home health care under the medical model are state licensure of agencies, licensure of professionals, Medicare and Medicaid Conditions of Participation,[7] and a variety of statutes to deter fraud. Consumers have the right to participate in planning their care, to be able to voice grievances, and to have personal information

Table 2: Employer-Related Tasks Associated with the Independent Living Model

1. Personal assistant recruitment and hiring
develop a job description and written agreement (i.e., contract)**
advertise job description or otherwise identify potential candidates***
develop an interview protocol*
interview potential candidates**
screen and evaluate candidate qualifications (e.g., reference/criminal background checks)**
develop candidate selection criteria*
select assistant and notify other candidates***
determine/negotiate wages and benefits for new assistant***
supervise submittal of employment forms (e.g., verification of alien status)***
arrange for emergency/backup assistants, if possible**
2. Payroll management and disbursement
obtain an employer identification number***
authorize assistant timesheets and/or vouchers**
withold and deposit state and federal taxes, if requested***
withold and deposit Social Security and Medicare taxes (i.e., FICA)***
withold and deposit federal and state unemployment taxes (i.e., FICA, SUTA)***
purchase and manage witholding for mandatory benefits, if applicable***
purchase and manage witholding for non-mandatory benefits, if applicable***
comply with all federal and state labor laws (e.g., minimum wage)
generate and issue paychecks***
issue IRS W-2 forms annually***
inform assistant about Earned Income Credit provision*
issue pay increases and/or bonuses when appropriate and possible*

Table 2 (continued)

3. Personal assistant supervision
ensure that assistant receives any state-required training if applicable***
develop and discuss with assistant a list of tasks and issues (e.g., no smoking)*
develop and discuss with assistant specific work schedules*
orient and train personal assistant*
evaluate assistant's performance and provide regular, periodic feedback to assistant*

4. Termination of general assistant relationship
assess and discuss problems*
determine whether problems require resolution, notice or immediate termination**
if resolution is indicated, attempt to negotiate solution**
if notice is indicated, provide according to contract or otherwise reasonable notice***
if immediate termination is indicated (e.g., neglect, abuse, theft, etc.) include rationale***

***mandatory task under federal or state law or otherwise necessary task

**highly suggested task, may be mandatory under some state laws and programs

*suggested task, advisable to avoid problems

Much of the information in this table was provided in Flanagan, S. A. & Green, P. S. (1997). Consumer-directed personal assisted services: Key operational issues for state CD-PAS programs using fiscal intermediatry service organizations. Cambridge, Massachusetts, MED-SATA, Inc, at 10-11.

remain confidential. In addition, consumers may sue providers for intentional or negligent infliction of harm under the tort law system.

Under the independent living model, consumers exchange the rights they would have under the medical model for the right to control their care. According to Professor Marshall Kapp, one of the foremost experts on legal issues affecting home care:

> Under consumer-choice models, consumers who purchase services from providers other than Medicare-certified home health agencies effectively forego the protection of these regulatory requirements. In their stead, consumers are entitled to services delivered in accordance with the conditions for which they negotiate and contract—expressly or implicitly—with the providers they hire. Consumers are not forced to depend on the vagaries of a system of government surveys of providers for regulatory compliance and the imposition of sanctions for noncompliance, accompanied by the delay and unpredictability introduced when providers exercise their entitlements to due process. Rather, enforcement of rights in consumer-choice models becomes a matter of consumer responsibility exercised through the power to fire a worker whose performance fails to satisfy the consumer's personal expectations.[8]

The extent to which consumers can exercise control over their care under the independent living model depends upon their capacities for self-direction and their ability to negotiate a contract for services. This model raises a multitude of potential legal issues, some of which are fairly well understood and some of which are subject to debate.

Still, states have imposed protective regulations on their personal assistance services programs. For example, some states require criminal background checks to be performed, and some prohibit consumers from hiring convicted felons. One study by the Medstat Group revealed that Idaho and Washington conducted criminal background checks on all prospective assistants; New Hampshire conducted such checks upon the request of consumers; and other states assist consumers in conducting their own background checks.[9] Conducting such checks does not violate the precepts of the independent living model, particularly when it is the consumer who initiates the background check or requests it. The Medstat study found that consumers are often uncomfortable with initiating background checks themselves because they do not know how to do so or because they are concerned that it will "poison" the relationship from the outset.[10]

Other regulatory requirements do conflict with the basic philosophy of the independent living model. The Medstat study found that 5 of the 23 state personal assistance services programs (22%) require some type of formal training or certification for personal assistance services.[11] As discussed in Chapter 9 on work force issues, most independent living advocates oppose mandatory training and certification. The state of Maine offers consumers the choice of training or determinations of personal assistant competency by a registered nurse.[12] This approach appears to be more in keeping with the independent living philosophy because consumers determine whether they want such supportive services.

Other regulations in conflict with the independent living model include requirements of periodic supervision by registered nurses, and the requirements of Nurse Practice Acts that prohibit personal assistants from engaging in certain activities.

DUTIES UNDER CONTRACT LAW

Due to the private (i.e., non-regulatory) nature of the personal assistance arrangement, the rights and obligations of the parties are defined largely under contract law. A contract is an agreement that may be enforced in a court of law. Although most contracts, including most employment contracts, do not need to be in writing, using written contracts is advisable for the obvious reason that it reduces evidentiary problems concerning the specifics of the agreement in the event of a dispute. Generally, the duties of parties to a contract are defined by the agreement of the parties; courts will generally enforce any and all provisions of a contract if they were entered into voluntarily, and if they are not illegal or otherwise contrary to public policy.

Therefore, consumers and personal assistants may contractually structure their working relationship and any legal risks associated with it, in basically any way they wish that is consistent with law and public policy. Consumers should ideally develop a fair and well-balanced written contract in setting forth the rights and duties of the consumer and the assistant. Research indicates that the process of expressing rights, duties, responsibilities and expectations on paper itself is beneficial to the parties.[13] Both parties should be fully familiar with every provision of the contract. Ideally, the contract should be reviewed by an attorney before being finalized; the personal assistant should be given an opportunity to have his or her attorney review it. However, as a practical manner, neither the consumer nor the assistant typically has the disposable income to hire an attorney for these purposes. The consumer should attempt to develop a well-balanced standard agreement in plain language and discuss it at length with prospective assistants before hiring them.

The contract should be signed by the two parties, the consumer and the personal assistant, but may contain provisions relating to the responsibilities of other parties, such as intermediary service organizations. Although these third parties may not be obligated legally by provisions of a contract that they did not enter into, their services may serve as conditions relating to the obligations of the parties. For example, intermediaries may have obligations to conduct background checks, convey paychecks, and report to tax authorities that may affect the duties of the principal parties.

Competency to Contract

The general rule in our legal system is that people who have reached the age of majority may enter into contractual agreements unless the individual is otherwise legally incompetent (e.g., prisoners or people with mental illnesses that compromise decisional capacity). In the long-term care context, the legal competency issue that is raised most frequently relates to lack of decisional capacity because of a cognitive impairment. This issue is sufficiently important, with implications well beyond the issue of contracting, that Appendix C is dedicated entirely to decisional capacity.

False Representations

As a general matter, consumers and assistants will be held accountable for any representations they make to each other. Some jurisdictions have consumer protection laws requiring honesty in representations. However, even without such laws, courts will typically render a contract void or voidable if one or both of the parties made material misrepresentations of factual issues. For example, if a consumer requires prospective assistants to respond to a set of questions, including whether the job applicant has ever been convicted of a felony, and the assistant lies, this would constitute grounds for immediate dismissal (particularly if the contract lists such misrepresentation as a cause for termination).

DUTIES UNDER TORT LAW

Tort law deals with civil harm caused to people or property. Torts are categorized according to intentional torts, such as assault, battery and trespass, and unintentional torts, such as negligence. Both intentional and unintentional torts have a major impact on long-term care. Consumers may bring tort actions in response to elder abuse and the abuse of people with disabilities generally. Such actions may allege battery, which is an intentional tort in which the abuser acts with substantial certainty that the intended harm of such action will occur. Although such intentional abuse is a big problem in long-term care, it is dwarfed by the even greater prevalence of unintentional harms caused by negligent or reckless actions.

Negligence is defined as the failure to conform to a standard of reasonable care based on what conduct is considered reasonable by the community. Therefore, the most important thing both consumers and personal assistants need to know in this area is that they are expected under the law to act as reasonable consumers and assistants would act under the circumstances. This means, for example, that consumers must maintain a safe work environment for their assistants. Assistants must exercise the level of care that a reasonable assistant would exercise in providing services to the consumer.

DUTIES CONCERNING TAXES

Both consumers and personal assistants have legal obligations with respect to the filing and payment of taxes to the federal and state governments. Failure to comply with such tax obligations can result in an order to pay the required taxes plus interest, as well as the imposition of substantial penalties.[14] The penalties may be particularly severe if the non-compliance is found to be intentional, constituting tax fraud.[15]

Federal and State Income Tax

The federal government and most states impose an annual income tax.[16] Whether a personal assistant is considered an employee or independent contractor, he or she is responsible for filing and paying these income taxes. The consumer-employer must file and provide the assistant with IRS form W-2, the wage and tax statement. Even in the unusual occurrence that the assistant is considered an independent contractor, the consumer still must issue IRS Form 1099 to the assistant.

Although employers generally must withhold and submit part of the assistant's earnings for purposes of income taxation, employers of domestic employees have the option of whether to do so.[17] This option results from a specific exemption from the withholding requirement in the law for "domestic service in a private home," which is defined as "services of a household nature performed by an employee in or about a private home of the person by whom he is employed. . . ."[18] The regulations provide a long list of domestic services that explicitly includes the services of "caretakers" and would encompass personal assistance services.[19]

Personal assistants often request consumers not to withhold income taxes from their paychecks, and consumers typically comply with such requests. Whether or not the consumer withholds some earnings for taxes, the assistant as employee is responsible for filing a federal tax return as well as a state tax return (unless, of course, his or her state has no state income tax). Failure of the assistant to file the appropriate returns is likely to result in penalties if he or she owes the government money.

Finally, it is not clear whether funds paid by some level of government to a consumer for purposes of obtaining personal assistance services constitute taxable income for the consumer. At least one analyst has concluded that it does not have to be reported as income because it is "legislatively provided social benefit program for promotion of general welfare objectives."[20] The more important issue for many consumers is whether such payments constitute income for determining eligibility for other social programs, such as Supplemental Security Income. Much depends upon how the payments are structured.[21] In developing their personal assistance services programs, public officials should attempt to structure payments to allow consumers to maintain program eligibility.

Social Security and Medicare Taxes

Assuming the personal assistant is an employee of the consumer or some other entity, the employer has an obligation to file and pay taxes under the Federal Insurance Contributions Act (FICA).[22] These taxes, which are fully applicable to domestic employees such as personal assistants, include Social Security and Medicare taxes. The Social Security tax is payable by both the consumer-employer and the assistant-employee in equal amounts of 7.65% of earnings each up to a stated limit.[23] Consumers may withhold the employee's share of the taxes from wages. Alternately, consumers may choose to pay the employee's share with their own funds, but if they use their own funds the amount paid on behalf of the employee is considered part of the employee's wages for purposes of calculating income taxes. The Medicare tax is payable by the consumer-employer in the amount of 3% of earnings.

In 1994, Congress made the employer responsibilities for these employment taxes less burdensome for employers of domestic employees.[24] Although the new law was popularly known as the "nanny tax reform bill" because it resulted from exposure of public officials who failed to satisfy their obligations pertaining to their child care employees, it also benefited long-term care consumers who employ personal assistants. The law raised the threshold for withholding and paying Social Security taxes so that employees who receive very little money in a particular year are not subject to the tax.[25] This provision benefits consumers who occasionally hire emergency or supplemental assistants by not subjecting them to excessive paperwork requirements.

The law also provided that employers of only domestic workers are no longer required to file quarterly forms and payments for FICA, federal unemployment taxes, and any other federal income tax withholding, but must instead include them in their own annual personal income tax returns (Form 1040). Again, this reduces the paperwork burden on consumers.

Federal and State Unemployment Tax

The federal-state unemployment insurance system pays cash benefits for a stated period of unemployment to workers who lose their jobs through no fault of their own.[26] The federal unemployment tax

(FUTA) is assessed against the employer on a stated amount of the employee's cash wages. Similarly, states impose the state unemployment tax (SUTA), which must be filed and paid by employers, including consumers who employ personal assistants. Recent changes in the law allow employers of domestic employees to pay this tax in conjunction with filing their federal income tax returns. Consumers must withhold and pay both federal and state unemployment taxes.

DUTIES CONCERNING LABOR LAWS

A broad array of different labor laws at the federal and state levels defines legally acceptable behavior between employers and employees (and even job applicants in certain cases). Some of the major ones are discussed below.

The Fair Labor Standards Act

The Fair Labor Standards Act imposes rules concerning minimum wage, overtime hours and child labor.[27] Employers generally must pay at least the higher of the federal minimum wage or the applicable state minimum wage in their states. Also, any hours worked beyond a 40-hour week must be paid at one and a half times the typical wage. However, under this key federal labor law, personal assistants arguably could be classified as providing "companionship services," a special category involving care and assistance for which an exception applies.[28] The exception does not apply to "trained personnel," referring to people with specific formal training such as nurses, but may apply to personal assistants.[29] Whether personal assistants fit within the exception is not clear.[30] Given the legal ambiguity, the legally prudent and risk-adverse consumer should attempt to comply with the wage and hour regulations to the fullest extent possible.

This advice is often easier said than done. There are many people with disabilities who do not receive any government assistance and require extensive personal assistance services. Many of these individuals have very limited income, and simply cannot afford to pay the required wages for the required number of hours. In other words, they earn too much to be eligible for program assistance, but not enough to pay for their various needs, including personal assistance services. Even consumers with substantial incomes often find their personal assistance costs highly burdensome. Policy makers should recognize that, to the extent that the minimum wage and hours laws apply to these consumers, they create real dilemmas for them.

Perhaps the most complex situation for consumers to analyze is how to pay live-in personal assistants. Some consumers employ assistants who live in their homes. They do so for a variety of reasons. For example, some consumers have an extra bedroom in their residence, and seek assistants who require a place to live. For these consumers, the room and board may apply as part of the assistant's salary for purposes of determining the amount that must be paid to satisfy the minimum wage because it is provided for the convenience of the employee. Other consumers hire live-in assistants primarily for their own convenience because they require extensive care and assistance, sometimes including night assistance.

The general rule concerning live-in assistance is that the employer must pay for the hours that the assistant is actually "on duty."[31] Therefore, the consumer and assistant should carefully agree to the hours in which the assistant is on duty and off duty.

Anti-Discrimination Laws

Other federal laws are intended to prohibit inappropriate discrimination by employers against employees or potential employees. Most of these laws apply only to employers with some minimum number of employees. Although these anti-discrimination laws have limited or no application to small domestic employers, such as consumers of personal assistance services, it is wise for all employers to treat their employees and job applicants with respect and not discriminate against them. Those who wish to be particularly diligent in this regard might establish specific anti-discrimination policies and protocols.

It should also be noted that making determinations based on certain characteristics of job applicants does not necessarily constitute discrimination, even if the anti-discrimination laws applied to consumer-employers. For example, consumers with mobility impairments may choose not to hire a person with back problems if lifting is a job requirement, even though the job applicant would probably qualify as a person with a disability under the ADA. Also, many consumers prefer their assistants to be of a specified gender, due to the intimate nature of the required assistance, and choosing only male or female assistants is permissible.

State Labor Laws

In addition to the federal statutes and regulations, it is necessary to understand state labor laws. To the extent that there is conflict or inconsistency between federal and state laws, federal law applies except to the extent that state law is more stringent. For instance, a state minimum wage that is higher than the federal minimum wage would prevail; employers in that state would have to pay the higher wage.

OTHER REGULATORY REQUIREMENTS

Although the independent living model functions best when it is not extensively regulated, states continue to subject the model to varying levels of regulation. The following are a few key areas involving such regulatory intervention.

Nurse Practice Acts

State laws that regulate the nursing profession were written before the independent living model had become a serious option for most people with disabilities. It has been observed that such nursing "policy and regulations did not anticipate the possibility that a large number of individuals unrelated to the consumer, and not licensed as nurses, might have a role in providing routine nursing services."[32] Some of the duties of personal assistants under the independent living model fall within the definitions of "nursing" or "nursing practice" under the various state Nurse Practice Acts. The Medstat study concluded that, "Unless specifically modified to take into account the desire of consumers to use unlicensed personnel at home or work to assist them in a variety of tasks, Nurse Practice Acts may therefore conflict, or appear to conflict, with CD-PAS [consumer-directed personal assistance services] program design, goals and philosophy.

The 1990 WID survey found that personal assistance services were offered in the following proportions: bowel and bladder care (73%), prosthesis assistance (66%), range of motion (63%), menstrual assistance (63%), foot care (63%), assistance with medications (57%), assistance with respiration (48%), assistance with catheterization (38%), and assistance with injections (33%).[33] These highly intimate tasks are often conducted by nurses. The question raised by Nurse Practice

Acts is whether they can only be provided by nurses. If so, this would effectively eviscerate the independent living model, which is premised on the belief that the consumer should be allowed to decide which services will be provided and by whom.

Two options are available for state personal assistance services programs in which there is a conflict with provisions of a Nurse Practice Act:[34]

• To seek a legislative, regulatory, or administrative exemption to the application of the conflicting provisions, such as the traditional exemptions for care provided by friends and family,[35] care provided by domestic servants,[36] domestic administration of family remedies, care provided by an employee of an institution, and care under the order of a licensed physician; and

• To achieve delegation of authority to conduct the duty.[37]

In the current context, delegation is ". . . the process whereby licensed nursing professionals delegate their authority to perform specific tasks to other personnel serving an individual."[38] If there are no applicable exemptions, delegation may be practically necessary in situations involving tasks that are clearly within the province of nurse professionals. Typically, nurses themselves do not like delegation, because it requires a substantial amount of paperwork documentation; the nurse can also be held liable for problems caused by the assistant who received delegated authority. Moreover, the very notion of delegation is somewhat offensive to the underlying philosophy of the independent living movement, which holds that the consumer's body belongs to the consumer; therefore, any delegation of authority (irrespective of what is contained in Nurse Practice Acts) must derive from the consumer.

Disability rights advocates believe that, if consumers wish for their personal assistants to conduct "nursing practices" without the delegation of authority from nurses, they should be allowed to do so. The preferable way to address limitations imposed by Nurse Practice Acts is by developing specific exemptions for consumer-directed personal assistance services under the independent living model. This approach is most consistent with the independent living philosophy. New York state has established such a specific personal assistance services exemption.[39] Ultimately, the issue of delegation will be resolved on a state-by-state basis through efforts to achieve a reasonable balance among the interests of the home health industry, the nursing profession, payors and independent living advocates in the state.[40]

Verification of Citizen or Legal Alien Status

All employers, including employers of domestic workers such as personal assistants are required to verify and maintain records demonstrating that each of their employees is permitted to work in this country.[41] Specifically, new employees must document that they are U.S. citizens, U.S. nationals, or legal aliens authorized to work in the United States. The employer must ask the employee to complete and sign Immigration and Naturalization Service (INS) Form I-9; the employee must then present the employer with identification and employment eligibility documents. Each reporting violation may result in fines of $100 to $1000 against the employer. If an employer hires an unauthorized alien, the fine can range from $250 to $2000 for a first offense, more for subsequent violations, and even criminal penalties for a "pattern or practice" of hiring illegal aliens.

Many applicants to personal assistant jobs are people who are recent immigrants to this country. Some believe this is a good opportunity to learn both a skill and the language and customs of the United States. Some of these individuals are not authorized to work in this country, and some are not even authorized to be in this country. A study of state personal assistance services programs that use intermediary service organizations found that all states were in full compliance with these laws.[42] The same is probably not true for consumers who are not eligible for government programs. It is likely that most are not familiar with these requirements.

State Worker's Compensation and Disability Insurance Laws

Every state has a worker's compensation statute that insures compensation for injuries and certain illnesses arising out of employment.[43] In exchange for the increased certainty of prompt compensation, workers' rights to have their case heard in a court of law are either limited or foregone. In some states, small employers are exempt from mandatory participation in the program. The Medstat study found that the number of workers' compensation claims filed in personal assistance services programs was "extremely low."[44]

Five states, California, Hawaii, New Jersey, New York and Rhode Island, and Puerto Rico have mandatory disability insurance laws whereby employees and/or employees must purchase private disability insurance or pay into a state fund.[45] These programs are generally coordinated with state workers' compensation or unemployment insurance programs. Such coordination can reduce the paperwork burden on the consumer-employer. However, the financial burden on those consumers whose care is not subsidized by government can be very substantial.

LIABILITY ISSUES

The general legal issues that affect personal assistance services outlined above have implications for the potential legal liability of consumers, personal assistants, states and intermediary service organizations.

Consumer Liability

As indicated above, consumers have many legal duties under the independent living model. Although major liability resulting in substantial monetary damages appears to be rare, the potential exists for this; consumers must be aware of their duties and the risk of liability. Consumers may be held liable for negligent acts resulting in the injury of a personal assistant. To the extent that consumers are able to purchase worker's compensation coverage or other insurance coverage for such risks, they can protect themselves financially. However, they must also maintain a safe environment for the personal assistant to work.

Consumers also can be held liable vicariously for the actions of personal assistants during the scope of employment under the doctrine of respondent superior. Respondent superior applies only if the personal assistant is, in fact, an employee of the consumer, and if the harm caused to another individual or another person's property occurred during the scope of employment. Therefore, if the assistant crashes into another car while driving to work, the consumer typically cannot be held vicariously liable; if the accident occurs during work hours while performing a task on behalf of the consumer, the consumer could be held liable. This situation demonstrates the consumer's need to hire responsible individuals to be personal assistants, and to develop rules to ensure that the assistant acts safely and responsibly.

Consumers can also be held legally responsible for a variety of violations of law, including failure to withhold, file and pay the various taxes discussed above, failure to comply with the various labor laws, and non-compliance with other legal and regulatory requirements. These responsibilities and potential liabilities demonstrate that the independent living model entails a substantial amount of responsibility on the part of the consumer. Not all consumers are capable of bearing such responsibility. Consequently, it is important to make consumers aware of their legal obligations before they agree to receive services under the independent living model. It is also important for supportive services to be available at an affordable cost for consumers who choose the independent living model.

Personal Assistant Liability

Personal assistants are even less likely to be held legally liable than consumers; however, they too can encounter legal problems if they are not aware of their duties. For example, a personal assistant who intentionally or negligently harms a consumer can be subject to both criminal and civil liability. Assistants must recognize further that they cannot simply abandon a consumer when nobody is available to take over the consumer's care. Such abandonment, or other intentional or negligent acts, that harm the consumer may violate specific statutes concerning elder abuse or the abuse of people with disabilities. Intentional abuse may be a battery. The appropriate standard of care for assessing whether a personal assistant did not exercise reasonable care in a negligence action would be what a reasonably prudent personal assistant (i.e., unlicensed worker without formal health care training) would do under the circumstances.

Personal assistants may also defend themselves in negligence cases by demonstrating that the consumer assumed the risk of whatever harm occurred because the consumer agreed to have a worker who is not a trained health care professional. Assistants may also claim that the consumer contributed to his or her own harm by failing to instruct the assistant adequately or failing to satisfy other duties of consumers. Finally, even if a personal assistant is held liable for harm done to the consumer, associated issues concern the collection of damages from personal assistants in that many of these individuals are not people of substantial financial means. If a personal assistant without resources does harm to a consumer, there is likely to be no way to seek compensation. If the personal assistant is an employee and harms another person or another person's property at a time and place within the scope of the individual's employment, the employer may have to pay damages for the harm done by the assistant.

Surrogate Liability

Surrogates of those consumers who do not have decisional capacity generally have very little exposure to liability. However, theoretically they could be held liable for failing to satisfy the requests of the consumer, possibly as expressed in advance directives. Surrogates are typically required to provide substituted judgment, deciding for the consumer in a manner according to the consumer's wishes. In the event that the consumer's wishes cannot be discerned, the surrogate must act in the consumer's best interest. The most likely scenario in which a surrogate may actually be held liable for monetary damages would be when the surrogate makes a decision despite a substantial conflict of interest with the consumer. Surrogates may be considered to have a fiduciary duty to look after the consumer's interests first and foremost above all other interests. This requirement raises questions as to liability when the surrogate follows the consumer's wishes, thereby exposing the consumer to risks.

ISO Liability

Intermediary service organizations retained by individual consumers or by state programs on behalf of their consumers also are subject to potential liability. Such organizations must exercise due care in such responsibilities as filing taxes and other required paperwork or may be required to pay penalties.

State Liability

States that run personal assistance programs also can be brought to court. The risk of being subject to legal liability may be the single largest impediment to expansion of the independent living model. Although states generally have sovereign immunity, and therefore must typically consent to legal actions that can result in monetary damages, simply being brought into court can be very politically damaging. Among the issues identified by experts in the field is potential liability of the state (and other sponsors) for harm done under their programs. One surveyed expert expressed concern that something "awful" might happen to a consumer, and that the following would occur:

> ... some investigative reporter is going to want to make a case about how state officials aren't doing their job. . . . The agency model allows you to shift the blame in a way that consumer-directed services [under the independent living model] don't.[46]

SUMMARY

The potential legal issues affecting consumers and personal assistants are complex and substantial. Fortunately, very few personal assistance relationships ever result in actual legal problems, probably because it is not in the interest of any party to pursue legal action when conflicts arise. However, this absence of legal action is not a good reason for them to ignore or be ignorant of their legal responsibilities and rights. Such awareness is likely to help avoid problems and conflicts in the future by informing each party as to their legitimate expectations under the relationship, and could also help them avoid major legal problems.

Appendix B:
Decisional Capacity

One inevitable reaction to the independent living model of long-term care is "OK, maybe it could work for some younger people with disabilities, but it could never be applied to elderly people, particularly those with cognitive problems and multiple disabilities." As discussed throughout this book, there is substantial evidence that older Americans wish to be able to control their lives, including their long-term care.[1] The question is whether they are capable of controlling their care and whether the independent living model is even applicable to this population. Of course, issues concerning the capacity to make decisions are not limited to elderly people. While a large majority of people with cognitive impairments are elderly, conditions such as Alzheimer's, stroke, and Parkinson's disease can affect individuals before reaching old age; traumatic brain injury is more prevalent among the younger population. Moreover, the individual with the disease or injury is not the only person primarily affected; his or her family is affected in a fundamental manner, often even more so than families of people with other types of disabilities.[2] This chapter considers a broad array of issues concerning decisional capacity.

DECISIONAL CAPACITY IN THE EMERGING CONSUMER MARKET

Autonomy and self-determination are among the most fundamental and cherished values in our society. These are also among the most important values in the areas of health care law and medical ethics, as reflected in the prominence of the doctrine of informed consent, whereby health care services may not be provided without the consent of the patient who has been informed of a procedure's risks and benefits. In considering the general trend toward autonomy in health care, we must also consider the related organizational trend from a health care system in which extensive regulations were developed to protect passive patients toward a system in which active consumers are expected to choose health care financing and delivery packages that meet their needs.[3]

The new consumer market system is manifesting itself in a variety of ways ranging from expanding options for care under Medicare Part C to expanding choices for long-term care under the various Medicaid waiver programs.[4] Even advocates of the market-based approach acknowledge the need to accurately identify those individuals who do not have the capacity to function autonomously as consumers and to determine how to meet the needs of these individuals.[5] The new decisions, such as choosing from among competing health care plans or selecting a personal assistant who must be trained and supervised, are often much more difficult conceptually than the old decisions involving whether to submit to a particular procedure.

Among the questions that are raised by the new decisions are: Who should decide whether an individual has sufficient present capacity to function as an autonomous consumer? Should the courts be involved? Who should be able to initiate judicial involvement? What level of due process is required?[6] It is possible that the rules that have already been devised for assessing decisional capacity in the context of informed consent will prove largely adequate with respect to the new, more complex decision-making. Certainly, we will not have to start from scratch in addressing decisional capacity issues. Yet, we will also not be able to rely entirely on existing approaches.

ASSESSING DECISIONAL CAPACITY

In our society, there is a general presumption that people who have reached the age of majority are legally competent.[7] Adults are presumed to have the capacity to make major decisions that affect their lives, including entering into contracts with substantial financial and other implications. Of course, this presumption may be rebutted that the individual does not have the decisional capacity to make sound decisions. The standards by which to assess legal competence are determined by state law and, therefore, vary from state to state. However, according to Professor Kapp, "[t]here is a broad modern legal and ethical consensus that the question of decisional capacity for any individual ought to be examined and evaluated on a functional, decision-specific basis, rather than as a global, all-or-nothing phenomenon."[8]

This new approach to capacity is based on the idea that an individual's capacity at any point in time is determined by a broad array of specific circumstances, including the nature of the decision being confronted. An individual may have capacity for certain types of decisions while lacking capacity for others. Moreover, capacity is not necessarily a constant over time. Therefore, the ability to engage in the decision-making process in a rational manner may wax and wane from time to time based in part on the individual's disability.

Recognizing this transitory nature of decisional capacity, many state statutes allow or even encourage courts to grant guardianship on a limited or partial basis, taking into consideration the capacities and limitations of the individual in light of the specific decisions that must be made.[9] Even without this statutory authority, courts are generally recognized as having equitable jurisdiction to tailor specific limited guardianship arrangements to meet the needs of a particular individual.[10] Yet, the approaches taken by the different states vary substantially, and there is little systematic analysis of which approaches are best. These approaches include different combinations of guardianship/conservatorship proceedings, advance directives, family consent statutes, and informal approaches; they are complicated, ambiguous, decision-specific, subject to fluctuation over time, and highly ad hoc.[11]

DECISION-MAKING PROCESS

One study of people with cognitive impairments found that individuals with mild to moderate impairments are able to answer questions about their general preferences, provide valid responses to questions about their involvement in everyday care, participate in care decisions, and express values and wishes concerning care with a high degree of reliability and accuracy.[12] Recipients of care were able to choose a person to make decisions on their behalf in the event that they were no longer able to make decisions for themselves.

Care recipients strongly preferred to pass decision-making authority to others. As expected, the person chosen 93% of the time was the family caregiver, who was given decisional authority in six areas: health care, finances, personal care, social activities, living arrangements, and the possibility of living in a nursing home. Care recipients reported that they discussed their daily care wishes with family caregivers, but they also believed that their caregivers understood their wishes for both daily care and nursing home care.[13] Consistently, caregivers also indicated that they had discussed the care recipient's wishes concerning daily care and nursing home care on an equal basis, but that they had a better understanding of the recipient's wishes for daily care.

Some 84% of caregivers reported that they used some paid service provider since the care receiver was diagnosed with cognitive deficits. These services included information about the care recipient's illness, support groups, and assistance with housework, shopping, laundry or cooking. The greater the caregiver's satisfaction with the formal care received, the less likely the caregiver discussed the possibility of nursing home care with the care recipient. The majority of caregivers indicated that they have enough money to pay for the costs of care, but 38% reported that they had "just enough" or "not enough" money. Care recipients who had caregivers under substantial financial strain were more likely to report that their caregivers did not understand their wishes for daily care.

In ranking the top five values concerning their daily lives, care recipients listed:

• To have a comfortable place to live;
• To receive assistance from a particular caregiver;
• To live in their own home;
• To feel safe at home, even if it restricts activities; and
• To allow caregivers not to put their lives on hold.[14]

A substantial majority (78%) of these individuals with cognitive impairments indicated that it is very important to them to remain at home; 73% stated that they do not want to live in a nursing home.[15]

Caregivers were fairly inaccurate concerning the value priorities of their care recipients, although there was general agreement between caregivers and recipients that issues concerning the safety, comfort and social interactions of the care environment are significantly more important than issues of autonomy and self-identity (e.g., allowing the recipient to do things for themselves and to maintain self-dignity). Care recipients preferred to receive assistance from family and friends rather than paid service providers. This rating of values of cognitively-impaired individuals contrasts starkly with the values of younger disabled people without cognitive impairments, who value autonomy and dignity issues highly; many of these younger people prefer using paid providers under the independent living model. The common value among these very different disabled populations is the desire to live at home.

Generally, caregivers chose to use or not use paid assistance consistent with the desires of the care recipient. The greater the disagreement between care recipients and caregivers, the fewer services were actually used.[16]

The researchers who conducted this study conclude:

The findings of this study support the policy direction of utilizing a family systems approach whereby the person with cognitive impairment and the family caregiver are considered legitimate 'consumers' of long-term care. A family systems approach would expand current practice by assessing:1) the care receiver's values and preferences for everyday care, rather than relying solely on information from the 'proxy' or 'surrogate,' who typically, is the family caregiver, and 2) the family caregiver's situation, well-being, and need for targeted support services (e.g., respite, counseling).[17]

SURROGACY ISSUES

Surrogates, who are typically family members, have a variety of difficult decisional issues to address. These issues often involve conflicting factors that must be weighed by the surrogate.[18] Most prominent are conflicts between what the individual would have wanted under the circumstances and what the surrogate or family is able to do. For example, an individual with severe cognitive impairments may have indicated prior to the onset of the disability that he or she did not wish to be taken care of by strangers under any circumstances. However, this desire may conflict with the reality that no family members are physically able or psychologically willing to take care of the individual, or that financial circumstances prevent family members from taking off time from work to assist the individual. Clearly, the needs, preferences and best interests of the family must be taken into consideration in efforts to attempt to satisfy the wishes of the individual with cognitive problems.

The key threshold issue is to determine who would be the ideal surrogate decision-maker on behalf of the consumer. In the context of informed consent decisions, many states have enacted "family consent" statutes indicating which family members have responsibility for making decisions on behalf of the consumer in the event that the consumer does not have adequate capacity to make a decision.[19] If no family members are available, the challenge is to identify other acceptable people who are willing and able to serve as surrogate decision-makers. Typically, efforts are made to identify people who are honest, empathetic and at least somewhat knowledgeable of the values and preferences of the consumer.

Some states have public or volunteer guardianship programs to address the need for surrogates. Guardianship statutes specify the authority of the guardian in acting on behalf of the consumer. Typically, the standard to which surrogates are held is that of "substituted judgment," which means that the surrogate is supposed to do precisely what the consumer would have wanted to do under the circumstances. Obviously, this standard can be strictly met only in circumstances under which the consumer clearly articulated their wishes prior to becoming incapacitated. Otherwise, the surrogate must attempt to discern the consumer's wishes based on an understanding of the consumer's values and preferences generally. When the consumer's likely decision is not discernible, the surrogate is supposed to do what is in the best interests of the consumer as determined by the surrogate.

One key legal issue that is implicated in any surrogacy situation is the emergence of a conflict of interest. Conflicts of interest entail a breach of the surrogate's fiduciary duty of loyalty to the consumer, and may arise in any situation in which the surrogate's loyalties are divided such that the surrogate's interests prevail over those of the consumer. For example, if the surrogate is also an heir to the consumer, and will therefore inherit at least part of the consumer's estate, an effort to limit the consumer's needed services solely to preserve the estate would violate the duty of loyalty.[20] Another potential conflict of interest exists when the surrogate is in a position to hire himself or herself as the consumer's personal assistant even if someone else would be a better provider of services.

Surrogacy through Advance Directives

Another way in which people can make arrangements for decision-making in the event that they develop cognitive impairments is through advance directives, such as living wills, health care proxies and durable medical powers of attorney. Living wills offer an opportunity to specify in detail the types of decisions the individual would wish to make in the event of future decisional incapacity. Health care proxies and powers of attorney allow individuals to designate a trusted individual to serve as a surrogate under such circumstances. Each state has advance directive statutes that permit one or more of these legal mechanisms. These statutes and the case law interpreting them indicate the amount of discretion the surrogate may exercise in that jurisdiction.

An analysis of each jurisdiction's advance directive statutes needs to be analyzed to determine whether it provides adequate legal authority for surrogates to be able to make the range of decisions relevant to the new options available to consumers. Such statutes may need to be amended to provide additional decisional authority for surrogates. However, in so doing, legislatures must be careful to limit such authority to circumstances in which the consumer does not have the capacity or desire to decide. As indicated above, a consumer may have the capacity to make a broad array of lower-level decisions (e.g., scheduling of bathing, choice of clothing) despite being incapable of making higher-level decisions (e.g., choice of long-term care model, selection of assistants).

Decisions While Incapacitated

Another issue is what to do when a consumer expresses a preference while decisionally incapacitated. Although the guardian or other surrogate with full decisional authority does not have a legal obligation to follow the directions of the consumer, and is actually obligated to consider what the consumer would have done under the circumstances when competent, there is a strong tendency to honor their demands unless they are simply irrational. Kapp suggests that, as a matter of policy, there may be some kinds of decisions that are so inherently personal to the consumer that surrogates should not be allowed to make such decisions contrary to the consumer, "in the same sense that we do not permit a surrogate to vote or get married on behalf of even the most incapacitated principal."[21]

If this is the case, policymakers would have to discern what types of decisions fall within this protected category. Perhaps the way in which this would operate would be for the consumer to have an automatic veto power over any surrogate decisions within the protected decision categories, irrespective of how the consumer would have decided when previously competent or if currently rational. An example of this process might be that the consumer could veto the hiring of any personal assistant chosen by the surrogate. This makes sense because the consumer must bear the consequences of the care provided by the assistant. Who is to say that the consumer's intuition concerning a prospective assistant is not as good as the surrogate's presumably rational decision?

Surrogate Conflicts of Interest

In making policy concerning who may serve as a surrogate on behalf of the incapacitated consumer, and how much authority the surrogate should have, there should be a recognition that situations could arise in which there is a conflict of interest between the surrogate and the consumer. Any situation in which the surrogate could receive a payment as a result of a decision could raise such a conflict. For example, a conflict of interest could exist when the surrogate hires himself or herself to serve as the individual's personal assistant when another assistant could do the job better.

Another potential conflict of interest exists whenever the surrogate is expected to inherit money from the consumer. In such circumstances, every dollar spent on the consumer potentially represents one less dollar that the surrogate may inherit. This strong incentive to be conscious of costs could result in refusal to spend money needed by the consumer to maintain health and independence, depending upon the surrogate and his or her relationship with the consumer. Obviously, this type of conflict arises frequently when family members are appointed surrogates; therefore, this conflict is the predominant scenario because most surrogates are chosen from among family members.

Of course, in the vast majority of cases in which family members or other individuals who are likely to inherit are appointed surrogate, the surrogate does not act in a manner contrary to the interests of the consumer. However, the mere potential for such a conflict should be addressed in public policy to ensure that incapacitated consumers are adequately protected. This protection could be achieved by enforcing a strong fiduciary duty of loyalty to the consumer in all surrogacy situations, allowing the consumer to recover from the damages associated with failing to provide adequately for the consumer as a result of an actual conflict of interest. It should be noted that the inheritance conflict of interest could apply to a surrogate who is not a family member or other person intended to inherit money from the consumer. An example might be when the surrogate later attempts to manipulate the consumer to include him or her in the consumer's will.

Decision-Making Standards—Substituted Judgment vs. Objective Analysis

The dominant standard for surrogates to make decisions on behalf of consumers is substituted judgment. The surrogate is expected to discern what the consumer would have chosen to do if the consumer were competent to make the decision. Critics of this standard argue that it is not reasonable to assume that surrogates are capable of discerning the subjective intent of the consumer. They also argue that this standard provides too much discretion on the part of the surrogate who wishes to impose their decisions on consumers. Yet, the purpose of substituted judgment is purportedly to maximize the consumer's autonomy, even when the consumer no longer has decisional capacity. Ultimately, whether the substituted judgment standard will achieve its objective depends upon the commitment of the surrogate to ensure the consumer's will and the surrogate's ability to gain insight into what the consumer's true will would be under the circumstances.

The most important alternative to substituted judgment is an objective analysis by the surrogate of what decision would be in the best interest of the consumer. This supposedly objective best-interest standard requires a careful weighing of burdens, benefits, risks and alternative options. However, this standard is often less objective than it appears, as surrogates may weigh the various criteria and factors in a manner that allows them to impose their preferred options on consumers. Again, whether this standard will achieve its laudable goal—to satisfy the best interest of the consumer—will depend upon the commitment of the surrogate to achieve the goal, and the ability of the surrogate to conduct a rigorous unbiased analysis using appropriate standardized decision criteria. Of course, even the most sincere and committed surrogates do not necessarily have the skills to conduct an objective analysis. Some would argue that no human being has the capacity to be objective.

Recognizing that any standard applied will be subject to the commitment and integrity of the individuals responsible for implementing it, the standard of substituted judgment appears most conceptually consistent with the independent living philosophy. It attempts to honor the autonomy of the consumer by adopting the decision the consumer would have made if decisionally competent. While it is true that some substituted judgments by surrogates would be based largely on speculation with little factual foundation, it is also true that surrogates who knew their consumers well prior to their cognitive disabilities and were aware of the consumers' strongly-held views, values and objectives could make valid and reliable decisions respecting consumer autonomy. Substituted judgment appears to be particularly viable with respect to broad decisions concerning lifestyle and philosophies of life and death. Falling into this broad philosophical category are choices concerning preferred model of long-term care.

Supportive Efforts

The Robert Wood Johnson Foundation has supported research to examine the various issues associated with the provision of consumer-directed care to individuals with cognitive disabilities.[22] The New York City Chapter of the Alzheimer's Association has been implementing a demonstration project that includes the provision of information and counseling to the families of these individuals. The information includes background on financing issues, including the New York Medicaid program and its fiscal intermediary for the payment of services under the medical model. Counseling includes assisting caregivers in making decisions about care options, helping caregivers understand and deal with behavioral problems associated with the disability, serving as a mediator when family members who differ on whether home care is appropriate for the consumer, and on recruiting, training and managing personal assistants.

SUMMARY

Issues concerning lack of adequate decisional capacity are very important in long-term care, because of the substantial number of elderly people and the growing number of younger people with disabilities with major cognitive deficits. Some have used this finding as a rationale for opposing expansion of the independent living model. However, this model can address the needs of people with substantial cognitive disabilities and resulting decisional incapacity with respect to most major decisions that affect them. These people have done so with the assistance of surrogate decision-makers. Issues concerning surrogacy are often complex and need to be addressed and resolved on a case-by-case basis. Several other countries have addressed these issues in their programs based on the independent living model.

Appendix C:
Internet Resources

The internet is an excellent source of information on issues concerning long-term care and personal assistance services. An internet search using any of the major search engines will yield hundreds of web sites that may be useful. Among the search terms that could be used are "long-term care," "personal assistance," home care," and "consumer direction." The following are just a few of those sites:

- ADAPT (Americans Disabled for Attendant Programs Today) at www.adapt.org

- Assistant Secretary for Planning and Evaluation, United States Department of Health and Human Services, at http://aspe.hhs.gov/daltcp/home.htm

- AUTONOMY, Inc. at www.autonomy-now.org

- Cash and Counseling Demonstration and Evaluation, at www.umd.edu/org

- HCBS Resource Network, at www.hcbs.org

- Independent Living Research Utilization, at www.ilru.org

- Liberty Resources at
  www.libertyresources.org

- National Alliance for Caregiving, at
  www.caregiving.org

- National Conference of State Legislatures at
  www.ncsl.org/health

- The National Institute on Disability and Rehabilitation Research at
  www.ed.gov/OSERS/NIDRR/Products

- The Urban Institute at
  www.newfederalism .urban.org

- Vela Microboard Association. "Microboards" at
  www.microboards.org

Glossary

Note: This glossary is adapted in part from several glossaries in the literature, including that from the report of the Blue Ribbon Panel on Personal Assistance Services. Dautel, P.J. and Frieden, L. (August 1999). *Consumer Choice and Control: Personal Attendant Services and Supports in America* (Report of the National Blue Ribbon Panel on Personal Assistance Services). Houston, TX: Independent Living and Research Utilization Program, available on the Internet at www.ilru.org.

Attendant Care Services: A type of personal assistance service typically used by people with mobility disabilities, and by some people with cognitive disabilities, to assist them with activities of daily living (ADLs) and instrumental activities of daily living (IADLs).

Americans with Disabilities Act (ADA): A civil rights statute enacted in 1990 prohibiting discrimination against people with disabilities by employers, certain public entities, and places of public accommodation, and requiring certain reasonable accommodations and modifications to meet the needs of people with disabilities.

Activities of Daily Living (ADLs): The ability to conduct certain basic self-help functions, such as bathing, dressing, eating, using the toilet, and transferring in and out of beds and chairs.

Care Plan: Individualized program of long-term services and supports determined through a needs assessment.

Consumer: Person with a substantial disability who requires some level of personal assistance services and/or other long-term care services.

Consumer Choice: The ability of a consumer to select the specific model, mechanisms and type of program under which long-term services and supports are delivered.

Consumer-Directed Care: An approach to the provision of health care services in which the consumer has a strong role in planning and directing his or her own individualized services. Under the independent living model of long-term care, consumer-direction means that consumers select, train, supervise, and fire their own personal assistants.

Developmental Disabilities: Physical or mental impairments that

239

are manifested before the age of 22 and will continue indefinitely, resulting in substantial disabilities (functional limitations in major life activities).

Disability: A functional limitation in at least one major life activity, which may result in the need for assistance from another person or is otherwise restricted in the conditions, manner, or duration they can perform such activities. This also includes people who can perform an activity only with great difficulty or physical exertion, and people who require supervision, reminding, or the need to have someone nearby.

Home Care: Any kind of health care, personal care, or personal assistance with independent living given to people in their private residences.[1]

Home and Community-Based Services (HCBS): A wide range of long-term care services provided in private residences or other community-based sites that serve as alternatives to institutional care. HCBS services for elderly include home care of various kinds, adult day care, case management, home delivered meals, medical equipment, home modifications, and payment for services in assisted living, small group homes, adult foster care, or other residential settings.

Home and Community-Based Services Waivers: The HCBS waiver permits states to use federally matched Medicaid funds for HCBS services for people who are functionally eligible for nursing homes and other institutional care under the Medicaid program in the state.

Impairment: Any loss or abnormality of psychological, physiological, or anatomical structure or function, which may or may not cause a disability.

Independent Living Model: A general term referring to care and assistance provided to and under the direction of consumers, in which consumers recruit, select, train, manage, and if necessary, fire their personal assistants.

Informal Support Model: A general term referring to care and assistance provided without compensation to consumers by family members and friends.

Independent Provider (IP): A term often used to connote home care workers and personal assistance workers who are "self-employed" as opposed to being employed by home care agencies.

---

[1]Kane, R.A., Kane, R.L., Illston, L.H., and Eustis, N.N. (1994). "Perspectives on home care quality." *Healthcare Financing Review* 16(1): 69-89, at 70.

Institution: In the context of long-term care systems, this term refers primarily to the nursing home, but also includes the larger facilities typically operated by the states to provide residential care and assistance to people with mental retardation, mental illnesses and other disabilities.

Instrumental Activities of Daily Living (IADLs): Tasks necessary for independent living in the community, such as cooking, cleaning, shopping, doing laundry, driving an automobile, using a telephone, reading mail, following instructions, and paying bills.

Long-Term Care: Health care, personal care, personal assistance services, support, training, and related social services provided over a sustained period of time to people who have substantial disabilities and require assistance in caring for themselves.

Managed Care: General term to describe the services of organizations or arrangements that integrate the financing and delivery of health care services, often using such mechanisms as 1) physician gatekeepers who determine access to specialty services; 2) utilization review and case management; 3) provider assumption of financial risk; 4) channeling of patients to providers associated with the plan.

Medicaid: A national program authorized under title 19 of the Social Security Act financed jointly by the federal and state governments according to a matching formula and administered by the states in providing medical benefits for low-income people. States operate their Medicaid programs with substantial policy-setting discretion but under general federal guidelines.

Medicaid Personal Care Option: Since 1975, state Medicaid programs may adopt this policy option, which allows consumers to use consumer-directed personal assistance services under the independent living model.

Medical Model: A general term referring to long-term care provided under the primary control and supervision by physicians, nurses and other health care professionals, in which the recipient of services is considered a patient.

Medicare: A national program authorized under title 18 of the Social Security Act, administered through the federal government, that covers health care services for people 65 and over, for people eligible for social security disability payments for two years or more, and for certain workers and their dependents who need kidney transplantations or renal dialysis. Medicare Part A includes coverage of hospital care and limited nursing home care. Medicare

Part B includes coverage of physician services, home health care, laboratory services, and medical equipment. Consumers contribute to the costs of Medicare through premiums, deductibles, and co-payments.

Mental Retardation: Low intellectual functioning and significant limitation in adaptive skills such as communication, self-care, direction, home and community living, social skills, health and safety, and functional activities, which are present from childhood.

Mental Impairment: Mental or psychological conditions such as mental retardation, organic brain syndrome, emotional or mental illness, and specific learning disabilities.

Most Integrated Setting: The sites and circumstances for the provision of long-term care services that allow consumers the greatest independence, personal responsibility, and ability to participate and community life.

Personal Assistance Services: Any service provided to assist people with substantial disabilities with the ADLs and/or IADLs and thereby help individuals who have deficiencies in their abilities to conduct such activities independently without assistance.

Personal Assistant: Individuals who provide personal assistance services (i.e., assistance with ADLs and/or IADLs) to people with disabilities; typically refers to individuals who provide consumer-directed services under the independent living model.

Physical Impairment: Any of the physiological disorders or medical conditions (e.g., cancer, diabetes), paralysis, disfigurement, or anatomical loss.

Self-Direction: The process of controlling one's own personal assistance services. Self-direction, as manifested under the independent living model of long-term care, involves locating, hiring, training, scheduling, and when necessary, firing one's personal assistants.

Social Security: The federally administered Old-Age, Survivors, and Disability Insurance (OASDI) program, which was established in 1935, is the national pension system in the United States funded through a trust fund funded through a payroll tax.

Surrogate: Typically a family member who assists the person with a disability in directing her/his personal assistance services.

Endnotes

CHAPTER 1

[1]In recent years, this issue has come to the attention of public officials, but it still has not entered into the consciousness of the general public. Senate Committee on Labor and Human Resources. 1991. *Personal Assistance Services and Independence for the Disabled*. United States Senate. Washington, D.C.: 102nd Congress, 1st Session, on examining the need for coverage of personal assistance services to enable Americans with disabilities to achieve more independent living. July 25, 1991.

[2]Stone, R.I. 2000. *Long-Term Care for the Elderly with Disabilities: Current Policy, Emerging Trends, and Implications for the Twenty-First Century*. New York: Milbank Memorial Fund, at 5.

[3]Kane, R.A., Kane, R.L., and Ladd, R.C. 1998. *The Heart of Long-Term Care*. New York; Oxford: Oxford University Press, at 4.

[4]"By and large, the people who literally provide ongoing long-term care services are not and need not be professionals such as nurses, social workers, occupational therapists, physical therapists, or speech therapists. Many of the services are, after all, the same services that people provide for themselves when they can and that family members often provide without any special credentials.

Although many tasks of long-term care are ordinary and well within the abilities of people without formal credentials, nevertheless, professionals do have crucial roles. Professionals may be needed to plan long-term care services, to teach family members or paid providers, or to perform particular specialized tasks (for example, a nurse to do some skin care or catheter insertion, or to teach family members and paid personnel to do so). But, by and large, the labor-intensive tasks that constitute long-term care can be done by nonprofessionals. If regulations require that various long-term care be performed by professionals or be supervised by professionals at frequent, prescribed intervals, the cost of care is likely to soar and perhaps become impractical to be provided in private homes for all but the very wealthy. Paradoxically, informal care of even great complexity can legally be performed by just about anyone, whereas once payment for the service is involved, professional and other regulations often require specific credentials.

... We believe that it is possible, desirable, and necessary to take explicit steps to render long-term care less professional. We also believe such steps can be taken without compromising the quality of long-term care and the competence of those who provide it, or belittling the contributions of professionals." Id. at 16.
[5]Id. at 4.

[6]Personal assistance services have been defined by Pamela Doty and her colleagues as, "A range of human and mechanical assistance provided to people with disabilities of any age who require help with routine activities of daily living." While this definition is appropriate for many purposes, it is overinclusive for purposes of the current analysis. The definition is overinclusive because this book focuses exclusively on human assistance, and therefore does not include assistive technologies and home modifications. Although all these services can be useful in compensating for lost functional capacity, and they may be considered substitutes for each other to some extent under some circumstances, separating them conceptually is helpful analytically. Specifically, because all of the models of long-term care that will be considered focus on human interventions, a definition that includes non-human assistance will obscure the comparison of the models. Doty, P., Kasper, J. and Litvak, S. 1996. "Consumer-Directed Models of Personal Care: Lessons from Medicaid." *The Milbank Quarterly* 74 (3): 377-409, at 378.

[7]DeJong, G., Batavia, A.I. and Griss, R. 1989. "America's Neglected Health Minority: Working-Age Persons with Disabilities." *The Milbank Quarterly* 67 (Supplement 2, Part 2): 311-351.

[8]National Institute on Consumer-Directed Long-Term Services. 1997. *Autonomy or Abandonment: Changing Perspectives on Delegation.* Washington, D.C.: The National Council on the Aging.

[9]Litvak, S., Zukas, H., Heumann, J.E. 1987. *Attending to America: Personal Assistance for Independent Living. A Survey of Attendant Services in the United States for People of All Ages with Disabilities.* Berkeley, CA: World Institute on Disability.

[10]DeJong, G. 1979. "Independent Living: From Social Movement to Analytic Paradigm." *Archives of Physical Medicine and Rehabilitation* 60: 435-446; DeJong, G. and Wenker, T. 1983. "Attendant Care as a Prototype Independent Living Service." *Caring* 2(2): 26-30.

[11]Batavia, A.I., DeJong, G. and McKnew, L. 1991. "Toward a National Personal Assistance Program: The Independent Living Model of Long-Term Care for Persons with Disabilities." *Journal of Health Politics, Policy and Law* 16(3): 525-547; DeJong, G., Batavia, A.I. and McKnew, L. 1992. "The Independent Living Model of Personal Assistance in National Long-Term-Care Policy." *Generations* Winter 1992: 89-95.

[12]Under some state personal assistance services programs, the personal assistants are also referred to as home care workers, private duty homemakers, home health aides, in-home care providers, chore workers, auxiliary workers and/or unlicensed assistive personnel. The important thing to understand is that these are unlicensed workers whose work is directed by consumers. Flanagan, S.A. and Green, P.S. 1997. *Consumer-Directed Personal Assistance Services: Key Operational Issues for State CD-PAS Programs Using Fiscal Intermediary Service Organizations.* Cambridge, MA: MEDSTAT, Inc., at 42.

[13]DeJong, G. and Wenker, T. 1979. "Attendant Care As a Prototype Independent

Living Service." *Archives of Physical Medicine and Rehabilitation* 60(10): 477-82.
[14]Some analysts have used the term "rehabilitation model" to contrast with the "independent living model." It is not clear the extent to which the rehabilitation model overlaps the medical model conceptually. It appears that the rehabilitation model is focused more on functional improvement. The important commonality between these conceptual models is that they are both controlled by professionals in contrast with the independent living model which is controlled by consumers. For purposes of this book, the term "medical model" will be used generally as the counterpoint to the independent living model. Cole, J.A. 1979. "What's New About Independent Living?" *Archives of Physical Medicine and Rehabilitation* 60(10): 458-62.
[15]Flanagan and Green, at 42.
[16]Id.
[17]Even the terms "independent living" and "assisted living" may be misleading to the uninitiated. Independent living is not meant to imply that the consumer is physically independent of other people. In fact, people who receive personal assistance services under the independent living model are often substantially more physically dependent than people who receive the services of assisted living facilities. The term "independent living model" takes its name from the independent living movement in which it was developed (as discussed in Chapter 3). It is meant to imply that the consumer is not dependent on the decisions of other people that affect their lives. People who receive assisted living services are often highly dependent upon the decisions of their assisted living facilities for the services they receive.
[18]Kane, R.A. and Wilson, K.B. 1993. *Assisted Living in the United States: A New Paradigm for Residential Care for Frail Older Persons.* Washington, D.C.: American Association of Retired Persons; Kapp, M.B. and Wilson, K.B. 1995. "Assisted Living and Negotiated Risk: Reconciling Protection and Autonomy." *Journal of Ethics, Law and Aging* 1(1): 5-13.
[19]Professor Marshall Kapp, for instance, identifies five basic models for providing home-based care: 1) the home care providers work directly as employees of the government unit that operates the home care program; 2) the government unit contracts for services with an independent home care agency; 3) the consumer contracts directly with a home care agency for services; 4) the consumer hires and directs an independent home care provider, but the government unit acts as fiscal agent; and 5) the consumer is given cash directly by the government unit and is responsible for all aspects of employing the provider. Kapp, M.B. 1990. "Improving Choices regarding Home Care Services: Legal Impediments and Empowerments." *St. Louis University Public Law Review* 10(2): 441-484, at 445. Kapp's models 1, 2 and 3 may be regarded as variations of the medical model discussed in this book;. models 4 and 5 may be considered variations of the independent living model. Further variations of the models are identified throughout this book.
[20]Batavia, DeJong and Griss. 1991.
[21]Currently, in the Cash and Counseling Demonstration, a version of the independent living model in which consumers actually receive cash to hire their own personal assistants is being tested in Arkansas, Florida and New Jersey. Doty, P. J.

1998. "The Cash and Counseling Demonstration: An Experiment in Consumer-Directed Personal Assistance Services." *American Rehabilitation* 24(3): 27-30. The fact that this "cash and counseling" approach has been funded by the U.S. Department of Health and Human Services and the Robert Wood Johnson Foundation, one of the largest and most prominent health care foundations in the country, demonstrates the credibility of this approach. Doty, P.J. 2000. "The Federal Role in the Move toward Consumer Direction." *Generations* 24(3): 922-27.
[22]Fuchs, V.R. 1975. *Who Shall Live? Health, Economics, and Social Choice.* New York: Basic Books, Inc. , at 26. Reprinted in Fuchs, V.R. 1998. *Who Shall Live? Health, Economics and Choice, Expanded Edition.* Singapore, New Jersey, London: World Scientific Publishing Com. Pte. Ltdd..
[23]Some long-term care experts do not accept the jungle vs. zoo analogy and the associated trade-off between freedom and security. For example, Dr. Pamela Doty prefers an automobile analogy discussed in Chapter 13, suggesting that the independent living model is preferable to the medical model in terms of both freedom and security. Determining which analogy better describes reality depends in part on how the specific models are implemented, particularly whether consumers are allowed to hire family members under the independent living model. The different options for implementation are discussed throughout this book.
[24]There have been some major advances in favor of freedom in recent years, both with regard to human and animal institutionalization. With respect to nursing homes, the general policy is that restraints should only be imposed as a last resort or as a means to protect the patient and others. Although this is a significant advance in terms of consumer freedom, there are limits to the potential amount of flexibility available even in the most progressive institutions.
[25]Kapp, M.B. and Wilson, K.B. 1995. "Assisted Living and Negotiated Risk: Reconciling Protection and Autonomy." *Journal of Ethics, Law and Aging* 1(1): 5-13.

CHAPTER 2

[1]ADLs assess such functions as bathing, toileting, dressing, eating and getting in and out of bed. IADLs assess other functions such as preparing meals, managing finances, doing housework, and using the telephone.
[2]Department of Commerce. 1997. "Disabilities Affect One-Fifth of All Americans: Proportion Could Increase in Coming Decades. *Census Brief* CENBR--97-5 (December, 1997).
[3]Id.
[4]Tilly, J., Goldenson, S. and Kasten, J. 2001. *Long-Term Care: Consumers, Providers and Financing. A Chart Book.* Washington, D.C.: Urban Institute, at 9.
[5]Kaye, S., LaPlante, M.P., Carlson, D., and Wenger, B.L. 1996. *Trends in Disability Rates in the United States, 1970- 1994.* Washington D.C.: U.S. Department of Education, National Institute on Disability and Rehabilitation Research.
[6]Tilly, Goldenson, and Kasten, at 15.
[7]Department of Commerce, 1997.
[8]Kennedy, J. and LaPlante, M.P. 1997. A Profile Of Adults Needing Assistance with Activities of Daily Living, 1991-1992. Disability Statistics Report, (11). Washington DC: U.S. Department of Education, National Institute on Disability and Rehabilitation Research.
[9]Kaye, LaPlante, Carlson, and Wenger. 1996.

[10]U.S. Department of Health and Human Services. 1999. *A Descriptive Analysis of Patterns of Informal and Formal Caregiving among Privately Insured and non-privately Insured Disabled Elders Living in the Community: Final report.* Washington, D.C.: Office of Disability, Aging and Long-term Care Policy, March 1999, at 1.

[11]Tilly, Goldenson, and Kasten, at 18.

[12]Id. at 23.

[13]Id. at 20.

[14]Id. at 21.

[15]Id. at 22.

[16]Id. at 27.

[17]Department of Commerce 1997. "Disabilities Affect One-Fifth of All Americans: Proportion Could Increase in Coming Decades. *Census Brief* CENBR—97-5 (December, 1997).

[18]Tilly, Goldenson, and Kasten, at 10.

[19]Id.

[20]Id.

[21]Id.

[22]Conversely, some individuals who have not reached the age of majority may exhibit the emotional and intellectual maturity to warrant a finding of decisional capacity for purposes of choosing and implementing a model of long-term care.

[23]Kaye, LaPlante, Carlson, and Wenger, 1996; Kennedy and LaPlante, 1997.

[24]Id.

[25]Id.

[26]Tilly, Goldenson, and Kasten, at 24. Based on 1994 NHIS-DS from Spector, W., Fleishman, J., Pezzin, L .Spillman, B. In The Characteristics of Long-term Care Users, Agency for Healthcare Research and Quality, DHHS, 2000. Because the type of caregiver is not known for 17% of these consumers, the actual percentages for unpaid caregivers only, paid and unpaid caregivers, and paid caregivers only may be somewhat higher.

[27]Binstock, at 6.

[28]Tilly, Goldenson, and Kasten, at 18.

[29]Id. at 19.

[30]Id.

[31]U.S. Department of Health and Human Services. 1999, at 1.

[32]Id.

[33]Mack R., Salmoni A., Viverais-Dressler G., Porter E. and Garg R. 1997. "Perceived Risks to Independent Living: The Views of Older, Community-Dwelling Adults." *Gerontologist* 37(6): 729-36.

[34]U.S. Department of Health and Human Services. 1999, at 1.

[35]Tilly, Goldenson, and Kasten, at 25. Based on 1994 NHIS-DS from Spector, W., Fleishman, J., Pezzin, L .Spillman, B. In The Characteristics of Long-term Care Users, Agency for Healthcare Research and Quality, DHHS, 2000.

[36]U.S. Department of Health and Human Services. 1999, at 1.

[37]Cohen, E.S. 1988. "The Elderly Mystique: Constraints on the Autonomy of the Elderly with Disabilities." *The Gerontologist* 28 (Suppl.): 24–31; Cohen, E.S. (1990). "The Elderly Mystique: Impediment to Advocacy and Empowerment." *Generations* 14 (Suppl.): 13–16.

[38]Cohen, at 24.

[39]Doty, P., Kasper, J., Litvak, S. 1996. "Consumer-Directed Models of Personal Care: Lessons from Medicaid," *Milbank Memorial Fund Quarterly* 74 (3): 377-409.

[40]Weiner, J.M. and Hanley, R.J. 1992. "Caring for the Disabled Elderly: There's No Place Like Home." In *Improving Health Policy and Management: Nine Critical Research Issues for the 1990s* (Shortell, S.M. and Reinhardt, U.E., editors), Ann Arbor, MI: Health Administration Press, at 75-110.

[41]Glickman, L.L., Stocker, K.B. and Caro, F.G. 1997. "Self Direction in Home Care for Older People: A Consumer's Perspective," *Home Health Care Services Quarterly* 16(1-2): 41-54. ; Desmond, S.M. et al. 1998. *Comparing Preferences for a Cash Option Versus Traditional Services, Florida Elders and Adults with Physical Disabilities, Telephone Survey Technical Report, Background Research for the Cash and Counseling Demonstration and Evaluation.* Baltimore, MD: University of Maryland Center on Aging.; Simon-Rusinowitz, L., et al. 1998. *Telephone Survey Technical Report: Consumer Preferences for a Cash Option Versus Traditional Services in New Jersey.* Baltimore, MD: University of Maryland Center on Aging.; Mahoney, K.J., et al. 1998. "Determining Consumer Preferences for a Cash Option: New York telephone survey findings." *American Rehabilitation* (winter): 24-36.

[42]Benjamin A.E and Matthias R.E. 2001. "Age, Consumer Direction, and Outcomes of Supportive Services at Home." *Gerontologist* Oct; 41(5): 632-42.

[43]Tilly, Weiner, and Cuellar, 2000.

[44]Id. at 78.

[45]Kelly-Hayes, M., Wolf, P.A., Kannel, W.B, Sytkowski P., D'Agostino, R.B., and Gresham, G.E. 1988. "Factors influencing survival and need for institutionalization Following Stroke: the Framingham Study." *Archives of Physical Medicine and Rehabilitation* 69(6): 415-18.

[46]Department of Commerce. 1997.

[47]Id.

[48]Id.

[49]Tilly, Goldenson, and Kasten, at 16.

[50]Kelly-Hayes, M., Wolf, P.A., Kannel, W.B, Sytkowski P., D'Agostino, R.B., and Gresham, G.E. 1988. "Factors Influencing Survival and Need for Institutionalization Following Stroke: the Framingham Study." *Archives of Physical Medicine and Rehabilitation* 69(6): 415-18.

[51]Id.

[52]Department of Commerce. 1997.

[53]Dwyer, K. 2000. "Culturally Appropriate Consumer-Directed Care: The American Indian Choices Project." Generations, 24(3): 91-93.; Manson, S.M. 1989. "Long-term Care in American Indian Communities: Issues for Planning and Research. *The Gerontologist*, 29(1): 38-44.

[54]Id. at 91.

[55]Id. at 91.

[56]Id. at 91.

[57]Zola, I.K. 1982. "Social And Cultural Disincentives to Independent Living." *Archives of Physical Medicine and Rehabilitation* 63(8): 394-97.

[58]Id. at 394.

[59]U.S. Department of Health and Human Services. 1999, at ii.

[60]Id.

[61]Id.

[62]Id.

[63]Id.

[64]Id. at ii, iv.

[65]Id. at iii.

[66]Id. at iii.

[67]Id. at iii.

[68]Id. at iii.

[69]Id. at iii.

[70]Id. at iii.

[71]Id. at iii.

[72]Tilly, Goldenson, and Kasten, at 29.

[73]American Association of Retired People. 1998. *Medicaid And Long-term Care for Older People*. AARP Policy Institute, Washington, D.C.

[74]Tilly, Goldenson, and Kasten, at 29.

[75]Id. at 30.

[76]Id.

[77]American Association of Retired People. 1997. *Out-of-pocket Health Spending by Medicare Beneficiaries Age 65 and Older*. AARP Policy Institute, Washington, D.C.

[78]Benjamin, A.E., Matthias, R. and Franke, T.M. 1998. *Comparing Consumer-Directed And Agency Models for Providing Supportive Services at Home*. Final Report under HHS Contract #100-94-0022. Los Angeles, California: School of Public Welfare, University of California, Los Angeles.

CHAPTER 3

[1]DeJong, G. 1979. Independent Living: From Social Movement to Analytic Paradigm. *Archives of Physical Medicine and Rehabilitation* 60: 435-446.

[2]Id. at 437.

[3]Id. at 438.

[4]Id. Most people who make reference to the disability rights movement are actually contemplating the independent living movement, sometimes referred to as the modern disability movement. The term "disability rights movement" is typically used broadly to refer to efforts to secure certain fundamental rights for people with disabilities, such as the rights to marry and procreate. The term "independent living movement" is typically used more narrowly to describe efforts to allow people with disabilities to be integrated into their communities, living in their homes often with the help of personal assistants. Clearly, there is substantial overlap in these terms, particularly to the extent that community integration and access to personal assistance are considered fundamental rights for people with disabilities.

[5]Longmore, P.K.and Umansky, L. 2001. *The New Disability History: American Perspectives*. New York, London: New York University Press.

[6]Americans with Disabilities Act of 1990, 42 U.S.C. §§ 12111-12181.

[7]Id.

[8]Relf v. Weinberger, 372 F. Supp. 1196 (D.C. Cir. 1974).

[9]In re Marriage of Carney, 589 P.2d 36 (Cal. 1979).

[10]Individuals with Disabilities Education Act, 20 U.S.C. §1400 et seq. (1991).

[11]Americans with Disabilities Act of 1990, 42 U.S.C. §§ 12111-12181.

[12]DeJong, at 439

[13]Id.

[14]Id.

[15]Levy, C.W. 1988. *A People's History of the Independent Living Movement*. Research and Training Center on Independent Living. The University of Kansas, at 10.

[16]National Council on Disability. 1986. *Toward Independence*. Washington, D.C.: National Council on Disability; National Council on Disability. 1988. *On the Threshold of Independence*. Washington, D.C.: National Council on Disability.

[17]Dautel, P.J. and Frieden, L. 1999. *Consumer Choice and Control: Personal Attendant Services and Supports in America (Report of the National Blue Ribbon Panel on Personal Assistance Services)*. Houston, TX: Independent Living and Research Utilization Program, available on the Internet at www.ilru.org.

[18]Holstein, M. and Cole, T.R. 1996. "The Evolution of Long-Term Care in America." In Binstock, R.H., Cluff, L.E., and von Mering, O. (editors). *The Future of Long-Term Care: Social and Policy Issues*. Baltimore, MD: Johns Hopkins University Press, at 20-22.

[19]Id.

[20]Id.

[21]Haber, C. 1993. "Over the Hill to the Poorhouse: Rhetoric and Reality in the Institutional History Of the Aged." In Schaie, K.W. and Achenbaum, W.A. (editors). 1993. *Societal Impact on Aging: Historical Perspectives*. New York, NY: Springer., at 90-113.

[22]Holstein and Cole, at 21-22.

[23]Id. at 23.

[24]Katz, M. 1984. "Poorhouses and the Origins of Public Old Age Homes." *Milbank Memorial Fund Quarterly/Health and Society* 62 (1): 110-40.

[25]Id.

[26]Id.

[27]Id.

[28]Holstein and Cole,. at 25-26.

[29]Id.

[30]Id.

[31]Id. at 35.

[32]Id. at 36.

[33]Id.

[34]The Medical Retardation Facilities and Community Mental Health Centers Act of 1963, Public Law 88-164, October 31, 1963.

[35]Senate Committee on Finance. 1995. *De-institutionalization, Medical Illness and Medications*. Hearing before the Committee on Finance, United States Senate, 103rd Congress (2nd Session), S. Hrg. 103-1011, May 10, 1994, U.S. Government Printing Office, at 2.

[36]Id. Senator Pete Domenici (R-NM), one on the strongest advocates for people with mental illnesses and disabilities on Capitol Hill, observed in 1994 that: the de-institutionalization has gone full circle. If you want to know where most of the mentally ill are institutionalized, look at the jails, city, county and State. It is now estimated that there are more incarcerated, schizophrenics, manic depressives,

bipolars, and county, city and State jails across this country than go to hospitals for these diseases. Id. at 5.

[37]Id. at 18. The number of mentally ill patients institutionalized in New York, the state with the largest number of such institutionalized patients, dropped from about 100,000 in the 1950s to fewer than 9,000 in the 1990s. Id. at 2.

[38]Hersen, M. 1969. "Independent Living As a Threat to the Institutionalized Mental Patient." *Journal of Clinical Psychology* 25(3): 316-8.

[39]Statement of Karen Greebon, February 3, 1992, available on www.adapt.org, accessed on February 28, 2002.

[40]Tilly, J., Goldenson, S., and Kasten, J. 2001. *Long-Term Care: Consumers, Providers and Financing. A Chart Book.* Washington, D.C.: Urban Institute, at 49. Based on Prouty, R. et al. 1999. *Residential Services for Persons with Developmental Disabilities: Status and Trends Through 1998.* Institute on Community Integration, University of Minnesota, May 1999.

[41]Dunlop, B.D. 1979. *The Growth of Nursing Home Care.* Lexington, MD: Lexington Books.

[42]Holstein and Cole,. at 44.

[43]DeJong, at 442.

[44]Id. at 438.

[45]Id. at 442.

[46]Id. at 439-40; Batavia, A.I. 1999. "Independent Living Centers, Medical Rehabilitation Centers, and Managed Health Care for People with Disabilities." *Archives of Physical Medicine and Rehabilitation* 80: 1357-60.

[47]These include advances in medical rehabilitation, antibiotic drug therapies, durable medical equipment and assistive devices. New antibiotics, for example, allowed individuals to survive severe urinary tract infections that previously would have killed them. New wheelchair cushions prevented decubitus ulcers (i.e., bed sores, pressure sores) that can become infected and life threatening. Medical rehabilitation provided the skills and knowledge needed by newly-disabled people to become independent.

[48]Lifchez R. 1979. "The Environment As a Support System for Independent Living." *Archives of Physical Medicine and Rehabilitation* Oct; 60(10): 467-76.

[49]Pflueger, S.S. 1977. Independent Living: Emerging Issues in Rehabilitation, (unpublished report on file with Independent Living Research Utilization, Houston, Texas), at 1.

[50]Id. at ii.

[51]Batavia, A.I. 2001. "A Right to Personal Assistance Services: 'Most Integrated Setting Appropriate' Requirements and the Independent Living Model of Long-term Care," *American Journal of Law and Medicine* 27(1): 17-43.

[52]Levy, at 5.

[53]During both terms of the Clinton administration, Ms. Heumann held the position of Assistant Secretary for Special Education and Rehabilitation Services of the U.S. Department of Education.

[54]Id. at 6.

[55]Shapiro, J.P. 1993. *No Pity: People with Disabilities Forging a New Civil Rights Movement.* New York, NY: Random House, at 44-53.

[56]Id. at 52-53.

[57]Id. at 41-53.

[58]Gallagher, H.G. 1998. *Black Bird Fly Away: Disabled in an Able-Bodied World.* Arlington, VA: Vandamere Press.

[59]Shapiro, at 53.

[60]Id.

[61]DeJong, at 437.

[62]Id. at 64-70. The history of section 504 and its regulations is documented and analyzed authoritatively by Professor Richard Scotch. Scotch, R.K. 2001. *From Goodwill to Civil Rights: Transforming Federal Disability Policy* (Second edition), Philadelphia, PA: Temple University Press.

[63]National Council on Disability. 1997. *Equality of Opportunity: The Making of the Americans with Disabilities Act.* Washington, D.C.: National Council on Disability.

[64]Batavia, A.I. 2001. "The Ethics of PAS: Morally Relevant Relationships Between Personal Assistance Services and Physician-Assisted Suicide." *Archives of Physical Medicine and Rehabilitation,* 2001;12 Suppl 2:S25-31; Batavia, A.I. 2001. "Are People with Disabilities an Oppressed Minority, and Why Does This Matter?" in (Batavia, AI, guest editor) Special Issue on Oppression and Disability, *Journal of Disability Policy Studies* 12(2): 66-67; Batavia, A.I. 1999. "Independent Living Centers, Medical Rehabilitation Centers, and Managed Health Care for People with Disabilities." *Archives of Physical Medicine and Rehabilitation* 80: 1357-60.

[65]"I'd Rather Go to Jail Than Die in a Nursing Home," by Stephanie Thomas, published in the *Resist* newsletter, available on www.adapt.org, accessed on February 28, 2002.

[66]DeJong, at 435-36.

[67]Mahoney, C., Estes, C., and Heumann, J., Editors. 1986. *Toward a Unified Agenda: Proceedings of A National Conference on Disability and Aging.* San Francisco: University of California and World Institute on Disability.

[68]Eustis, N.N. 2000. "Consumer Directed Long-term Care Services: Evolving Perspectives and Alliances." *Generations,* 24(3): 10-15, at 13.

[69]Simon-Rusinowitz, L., Mahoney, K., Desmond, S.M., et al. 1997. "Determining Consumer Preferences for a Cash Option (AQ1): Arkansas Survey Results." *Health Care Financing Review,* 19(2): 73-96.

[70]Mahoney, Estes, and Heumann, 1986.

[71]DeJong, 1979; DeJong, G. and Wenker, T. 1983. Attendant Care as a Prototype Independent Living Service. Caring 2(2): 26-30; National Council on Disability. 1986. *Toward Independence.* Washington, D.C.: National Council on Disability; National Council on Disability. *On the Threshold of Independence.* Washington, D.C.: National Council on Disability.

[72]Batavia, A.I., DeJong, G. and McKnew, L. 1991. "Toward a National Personal Assistance Program: The Independent Living Model of Long-Term Care for Persons with Disabilities," *Journal of Health Politics,* Policy and Law 16(3): 525-547; DeJong, G., Batavia, A.I. and McKnew, L. 1992. "The Independent Living Model of Personal Assistance in National Long-Term-Care Policy," *Generations* Winter 1992: 89-95. Reprinted in *Aging and Disabilities: Seeking Common Ground* (E.F. Ansello and N.F. Eustis, Eds.), New York: Baywood Publishing Co., 1993.

[73]Batavia, A.I. 2001. "A Right to Personal Assistance Services: 'Most Integrated Setting Appropriate' Requirements and the Independent Living Model of Long-

Term Care," 27 *American Journal of Law and Medicine* 17-43.

[74]See website of ADAPT (Americans Disabled for Attendant Programs Today) at www.adapt.org.

[75]Litvak, S., Zukas, H. and Heumann, J.E. 1987. *Attending to America: Personal Assistance for Independent Living*. Berkeley, CA: World Institute on Disability; Kennedy, J. and Litvak, S. *Case Studies of Six State Personal Assistance Services Funded by the Medicaid Personal Care Option*. Oakland, CA: World Institute on Disability, 1991; Kennedy, J. Policy and Program Issues in Providing Personal Assistance Service. *Journal of Rehabilitation* (July/August/September 1993): 17-22, 1993.

[76]National Health Care Security Act of 1993;

[77]Wiener, J.M., Estes, C.L., Goldenson, S.M., and Goldberg, S.C. 2001. "What Happened to Long-term Care in the Health Reform Debate of 1993-1994? Lessons for the Future." *The Milbank Quarterly* 79(2): 207-252.

[78]Medicaid Community Attendant Services Act of 1997, H.R. 2020, 105th Cong. (1997).

[79]*See* Medicaid Community Attendant Services and Supports Act of 1999, S. 1935, 106th Cong. (1999).

[80]Tommy Olmstead, Commissioner, Georgia Department of Human Resources, et Al., Petitioners v. L. C., by Jonathan Zimring, Guardian Ad Litem and Next Friend, et Al. (No. 98-536), 119 S. Ct. 2176; 1999 U.S. LEXIS 4368; 144 L. Ed. 2d 540; 67 U.S.L.W. 4567; 9 Am. Disabilities Cas. (BNA) 705.

[81]Batavia, 2001.

[82]National Association of Protection and Advocacy Systems. 2000. *Olmstead Progress Report: Disability Advocates Assess State Implementation After One Year*. Washington, D.C.: National Association of Protection and Advocacy Systems, July 25, 2000, www.protectionandadvocacy.com/progressreportfinal.htm.

CHAPTER 4

[1]Benjamin A.E. 2001. "Consumer-Directed Services at Home: A New Model for Persons with Disabilities" *Health Affairs* 20(6): 80-95; Batavia, A.I. 2002 "Consumer Direction, Consumer Choice and the Future of Long-Term Care." *Journal of Disability Policy Studies*. 13(2): 67-73, 86.

[2]Rodin, J. 1986. "Aging and Health: Effects Of the Sense of Control." Science 233: 1271; Winick, B.J. 1992. "On Autonomy: Legal and Psychological Perspectives." *Villanova Law Review* 37: 1705-1777.

[3]Kapp, M.B. 1996. "Enhancing Autonomy and Choice in Selecting and Directing Long-Term Care Services." *The Elder Law Journal* 4 (1): 55-97, at 63; Capitman, J.and Sciegaj, M. 1995. "A Conceptual Approach for Understanding Individual Autonomy in Managed Community Long-Term Care." *Gerontologist* 35 (4): 533-40.

[4]National Institute on Consumer-Directed Long-Term Services. 1996. *Principles of Consumer-Directed Home and Community-Based Services*. Washington, D.C.: The National Council on the Aging.

[5]Nadash, P. 1998. "Independent Choices." *American Rehabilitation* 24(3): 15-20, at 15.

[6]Batavia, 2002.

[7]Stone, R.I. 2000. "Introduction – Consumer Direction in Long-Term Care:

Opportunities, Challenges, and Limitations of This Increasingly Popular Approach." *Generations* 24(3): 5-8, at 5.

[8]DeJong, 1979.

[9]Nosek M.A., Parker, R.M., and Larsen S. 1987. "Psychosocial Independence and Functional Abilities: Their Relationship in Adults with Severe Musculoskeletal Impairments." *Archives of Physical Medicine and Rehabilitation* 68(12): 840-45.

[10]Id.

[11]Id.

[12]Id.

[13]DeJong, 1979.

[14]Batavia, A.I. and Schriner, K. 2001. "The ADA as Engine of Social Change: The Strengths and Limitations of a Civil Rights Approach to Meeting the Needs of People with Disabilities" *Policy Studies Journal* 29(4): 690-702.

[15]DeJong, 1979.

[16]Of course, this is an overstatement, in that many members of the younger disabled population hold more moderate views concerning these models. However, overall, the views of the hardliners continue to be the party line presented by disability rights leaders in public debate.

[17]Desmond, S.M., Shoop, D.M., Simon-Rusinowitz, L., Mahoney, K.J., Squillace, M.R. and Fay, R.A. 1998. *Comparing Preferences for a Cash Option Versus Traditional Services, Florida Elders and Adults with Physical Disabilities, Telephone Survey Technical Report, Background Research for the Cash and Counseling Demonstration and Evaluation.* College Park, MD.: University of Maryland Center on Aging; Simon-Rusinowitz, L., Mahoney, K.J., Desmond, S.M., Shoop, D.M., Squillace, M.R., and Fay, R.A. 1997. "Determining Consumer Preferences for a Cash Option: Arkansas Survey Results." *Health Care Financing Review* 19(2), 73-96.

[18]Mahoney, K.J., Desmond, S.M., Simon-Rusinowitz, L., Loughlin, D.M., and Squillace, M.R. 2001. "Comparing Preferences for a Cash Option Versus Traditional Services: Telephone Survey Results from New Jersey Elders and Adults." *Journal of Disability Policy Studies* 13(2): 74-86, at 77.

[19]Weiner, J.M. and Hanley, R.J. 1992. "Caring for the Disabled Elderly: There's No Place Like Home." In *Improving Health Policy and Management: Nine Critical Research Issues for the 1990s* (Shortell, S.M. and Reinhardt, U.E., editors), Ann Arbor, MI: Health Administration Press, at 75-110.

[20]Glickman, L.L., Stocker, K.B. and Caro, F.G. 1997. "Self Direction in Home Care for Older People: A Consumer's Perspective." *Home Health Care Services Quarterly* 16(1-2): 41-54.

[21]Desmond, et al, 1998; Simon-Rusinowitz, et al., at 73-96.

[22]Mahoney, et al., at 77.

[23]Id.

[24]Simon-Rusinowitz, L. and Hofland, B.F. 1993. "Adopting a Disability Approach to Home Care Services for Adults." *The Gerontologist* 33(2): 159-167.

[25]Cohen, E.S. 1988. "The Elderly Mystique: Constraints on the Autonomy of the Elderly with Disabilities." *The Gerontologist* 28 (Suppl.): 24–31; Cohen, E.S. 1990. "The Elderly Mystique: Impediment to Advocacy and Empowerment." *Generations* 14 (Suppl.): 13–16.

[26]Nadash, at 15.

[27]DeJong, 1979.

[28]Scala, M.A. and Nerney, T. 2000. "People First: The Consumers in Consumer Direction." *Generations* 24(3): 55-59, at 56.

[29]Kapp, M.B. 1999. "Health Care in the Marketplace: Implications for Decisionally Impaired Consumers, Their Surrogates and Advocates." *Southern Illinois University Law Journal* 24 (fall 1999): 1-52; Kapp, M.B. 1999. "From Medical Patients to Health Care Consumers: Decisional Capacity and Choices to Purchase Coverage and Services." *Aging and Mental Health* 3(4): 294-300; Kapp, M.B. 1997. "Who Is Responsible for This? Assigning Rights and Consequences in Elder Care." *Journal of Aging and Social Policy* 9(2): 51-65.

[30]Mayer, R.R., Berson, A. and Marks, J. 2000. "A Consumer-Directed Homecare Program that Works for the Cognitively Impaired." *Generations* 24(3): 98-99.

[31]Vela Micro board Association. 2001. "Microboards" Available at http://www/microboards.org.

[32]Nosek, M.A. 1990. *Personal Assistance Services for People with Mental Disabilities.* Houston, TX: Baylor College of Medicine; Deegan, P. 1992. "The Independent Living Movement and Psychiatric Disabilities: Taking Back Control of Our Lives." *Psychosocial Rehabilitation Journal* 15 (3): 3-19; Dautel, P.J. and Frieden, L. 1999. *Consumer Choice and Control: Personal Attendant Services and Supports in America (Report of the National Blue Ribbon Panel on Personal Assistance Services).* Houston, TX: Independent Living and Research Utilization Program.

[33]Pita, D.D., Ellison, M.L. and Farkas, M. 2001. "Exploring Personal Assistance Services for People with Psychiatric Disabilities." *Journal of Disability Policy Studies* 12(1): 2-9.

[34]Id.

[35]Id., at 7.

[36]An analogy might be drawn to the choices some consumers have in selecting managed care plans. They may choose a health maintenance organization plan that rigidly manages their care, giving them relatively little control of their providers, or they can choose a preferred provider organization plan, which gives them greater control.

[37]Batavia, 2002

[38]Nadash, at 18.

[39]Id.

[40]Administrator awareness of consumer direction was monitored through the Survey of State Administrators on Consumer-Directed Home-and Community-Based Services, National Council on the Aging, which was administered in 1996 and 1999. Velgouse, L. and Dize, V. 2000. "A Review of State Initiatives in Consumer-Directed Long-Term Care." *Generations* 24(3): 28-33.

[41]Id. at 29.

[42]Id.

[43]Id.

[44]Commonwealth Commission on Elderly People Living Alone. 1991. *The Importance of Choice in Medicaid Home Care Programs: Maryland, Michigan, and Texas.* New York: Commonwealth Fund; Doty et al., at 390-92.

[45]Id.; Doty et al., at 391.

[46]Id., at 31.

[47]Vergouse and Dize, at 30-31.

[48]Id., at 32.

[49]Nadash, at 18.

[50]Enthoven, A.C. 1980. *Health Plan: The Only Practical Solution to the Soaring Cost of Medical Care*. Addison-Wesley Publishing Company: Reading, MA.

[51]Leutz, W. 1998. "Home Care Benefits for Persons with Disabilities." *American Rehabilitation* 24(3): 6-14, at 10-12.

[52]Id.

[53]Wong, D. 2000. "Rapid Response: Development of a Home Care Worker Replacement Service." *Generations* 24(3): 88-90.

[54]Mahoney, K.J. and Simon-Rusinowitz L. 1997. "Cash and Counseling Demonstration and Evaluation. Start-Up Activities." *Journal of Case Management*. 6(1): 25-30; Mahoney, K.J., Simone, K. and Simon-Rusinowitz, L. 2000. "Early Lessons from the Cash and Counseling Demonstration And Evaluation." *Generations* 24(3): 41-46.

[55]ADAPT (Americans Disabled for Attendant Programs Today) at www.adapt.org., accessed on February 28, 2002.

[56]Feinberg, L.F. and Ellano, C. 2000. "Promoting Consumer Direction for Family Caregiver Support: an Agency-Driven Model." *Generations* 24(3): 47-54.

[57]Id. at 49.

[58]Id. at 49.

[59]Feinberg, L.F. and Kelly, K.A. 1995. "A Well-deserved Break: Respite Options Offered by California's Statewide System of Caregiver Resource Centers." *Gerontologist* 35: 701-5.

[60]Id.

[61]Feinberg, L.F. and Whitlatch, C.J. 1998. "Family Caregivers and In-Home Respite Options: The Consumer-Directed Versus Agency-Based Experience." *Journal of Gerontological Social Work* 30(3/4): 9-28.

[62]Id.

[63]Id.

[64]Id.

[65]Kane, R.A. and Degenholtz, H. 1997. "Assessing Values and Preferences: Should We, Can We? *Generations* 21(1): 19-24.

[66]Williams G.H. and Wood, P.H. 1988. "Coming to Terms with Chronic Illness: the Negotiation of Autonomy in Rheumatoid Arthritis." *International Disability Studies* 10(3): 128-33.

[67]Id.

CHAPTER 5

[1]Batavia, A.I., DeJong, G. and McKnew, L. "Toward a National Personal Assistance Program: The Independent Living Model of Long-Term Care for Persons with Disabilities," *Journal of Health Politics, Policy and Law* 16(3): 525-547, at 527; DeJong, G., Batavia, A.I. and McKnew, L. 1992. "The Independent Living Model of Personal Assistance in National Long-Term-Care Policy." *Generations* 16: 89-95.

[2]DeJong, G. 1982. "A Legal Perspective on Disability, Home Care, and Relative Responsibility." *Home Health Services Quarterly*, 3 (Fall/Winter) nos. 3/4, 176-187. Abuse and neglect can be prosecuted under state law. Many states have reporting

requirements for certain individuals, including virtually all health care professionals, to report elder abuse.

[3]Kapp, M.B. 1996. "Enhancing Autonomy and Choice in Selecting and Directing Long-Term Care Services." *The Elder Law Journal* 4 (1): 55-97, at 91.

[4]Benjamin, A.E., Matthias, R. and Franke, T.M. 2000. "Comparing Consumer-Directed And Agency Models for Providing Supportive Services at Home." *Health Services Research* 2000 Apr; 35 (1 Pt 2): 351-66.

[5]American Medical Association, Council on Scientific Affairs. 1990. "Home Care in the 1990s." *Journal of the American Medical Association (JAMA)* 263: 1241, at 1243.

[6]*See* National Alliance for Caregiving and American Association of Retired Persons, Family Caregiving in the U.S.: Findings from a National Survey (1997) (visited Feb. 28, 2001) <http://www.caregiving.org/content/repsprods.

[7]Arno P.S., Levine C., and Memmott, M.M. 1999. "The Economic Value of Informal Caregiving; President Clinton's Proposal to Provide Relief to Family Caregivers Opens a Long-Overdue Discussion of This "Invisible" Health Care Sector." *Health Affairs* 18(2): 182-188, at 184, 185.

[8]Senate Committee on Aging, *Long-Term Care for the 21st Century: A Common Sense Proposal to Support Family Caregiver.* 1999. Hearing before the Committee on Aging, United States Senate, 106th Congress (1st Session), S. Hrg. 106-102, March 23, 1999, U.S. Government Printing Office, 1999, at 11.

[9]Tilly, J. , Goldenson, S. and Kasten, J. 2001. *Long-Term Care: Consumers, Providers and Financing.* A Chart Book. Washington, D.C.: Urban Institute, March, 2001, at 26.

[10]Arno, Levine, and Memmott, at 184, 185; Senate Committee on Aging, at 11.

[11]Senate Committee on Aging, at 11.

[12]American Association of Retired People. 1997. *Family Caregiving: From a National Survey.* AARP Policy Institute, Washington, D.C.

[13]Id.

[14]Senate Committee on Aging, at 3.

[15]Kapp, at 90.

[16]Senate Committee on Aging, 1999.

[17]Benjamin, Matthias, and Franke, at 351-66.

[18]Tilly, Weiner, and Cuellar, at 79: citing Baarveld et al. 1998. *Persoonsgebonden Budget Arbeidsmarktpositie van Zorgverleners.* Nijmegen, Netherlands: Instituut voor Toegepaste Sociale Wetenschappen van de Stricting Katholieke Universiteit te Nijmegen.

[19]Id.: citing Simon, M.O. and Martin, P.A. 1996. La Prestation Dependance: Rapport Final du Programme d' Evaluation de l' Experimentation d' une Prestation Dependence. Paris, France: Centre de Recherche pour l'Etude et l'Observation des Conditions de Vie CREDOC.

[20]Id.

[21]Id.

[22]Id.; Badelt, C., et al. 1997. *Analyse der Auswirkungen des Pflegevorsorgesystems.* Vienna, Austria: Bundesministeriums fur Arbeit, Gesundheit un Soziales.

[23]Silverstein, M. and Parrott, T.M. 2001. "Attitudes Toward Government Policies That Assist Informal Caregivers: The Link Between Personal Troubles and Public Issues." *Research on Aging* 23(3): 349-374.

[24]Doty, P., Kasper, J. and Litvak, S. 1996. "Consumer-Directed Models of Personal

Care: Lessons from Medicaid." *Milbank Quarterly* 74 (3): 377-409.

[25]Hanley, R.J., Wiener, J.M. and Harris, K.M. 1991. "Will Paid Home Care Erode Informal Support?" *Journal of Health Politics, Policy, and Law* 16(3): 507-521.

[26]Batavia, DeJong, and McKnew, at 527-28.

[27]Health Care Financing Administration. 1994. "Final Rule: Medicare and Medicaid Programs: Survey, Certification, and Enforcement for Skilled Nursing Facilities and Nursing Facilities." *Federal Register* 59: 56, 116-56, 252. November 10. Washington, D.C.

[28]Pepper Commission. 1990. *A Call for Action (Final report)*. U.S. Bipartisan Commission on Comprehensive Health Care, Washington, D.C.

[29]American Association of Retired People. 1998. *Medicaid and Long-Term Care for Older People*. Washington DC: AARP Policy Institute.

[30]Pepper Commission. 1990.

[31]Benjamin, A.E. and Matthias, R. 2000. "Comparing Consumer-Directed and Agency- Directed Models: California's In-Home Supportive Services Program." *Generations,* 24(3): 85-87, at 86.

[32]Id.

[33]Mahoney, K.J., Desmond, S.M., Simon-Rusinowitz, L., Loughlin, D.M., and Squillace, M.R. "Comparing Preferences for a Cash Option Versus Traditional Services: Telephone Survey Results from New Jersey Elders and Adults." *Journal of Disability Policy Studies* 13(2): 74-86. Mahoney, K.J., et al. 1998. "Determining Consumer Preferences for a Cash Option: New York Telephone Survey Findings." *American Rehabilitation,* (winter): 24-36; Mahoney, K.J. and Simon_Rusinowitz L. 1997. "Cash and Counseling Demonstration and Evaluation. Start-up Activities." *Journal of Case Management.* 6(1): 25-30; Mahoney, K.J., Simone, K. and Simon-Rusinowitz, L. 2000. "Early Lessons from the Cash and Counseling Demonstration and Evaluation." *Generations* 24(3): 41-46.

[34]Collopy, B.J. 1990. "Ethical Dimensions of Autonomy in Long-Term Care." *Generations,* 14 (Supplement): 9-12; Collopy, B.J. 1988. "Autonomy in Long-Term Care: Some Crucial Distinctions." *The Gerontologist,* 28 (Supplement): 10-17.

[35]Id.

[36]Kapp, at 70.

[37]Benjamin, Matthias, and Franke. at 351-66.

[38]Kennedy, J. 1993. "Policy and Program Issues in Providing Personal Assistance Service." *Journal of Rehabilitation* (July/August/September 1993): 17-22.

[39]Kane, Kane and Ladd, at 120-21.

[40]Another conceptual distinction is between therapeutic services, with the goal of improving or preventing the deterioration of the consumer's health and functional capacity, and compensatory services, with the goal of helping consumers pursue their lives. Sometimes, there is a conflict between these objectives. Kane, R.A., Kane, R.L., Ladd, R.C. 1998. *The Heart of Long-Term Care*. New York ; Oxford: Oxford University Press, at 121.

[41]One major reason for the increase in post-hospitalization health care services under Medicare is that patients are being discharged from the hospital "quicker and sicker," largely as a result of strong financial incentives from the Medicare Prospective Payment System and managed care organizations. Kane, Kane and Ladd, at 123-24.

[42]Id.

[43]Id.

[44]General Accounting Office. 1997. *Medicare Home Health Agencies: Certification Process Ineffective in Excluding Problem Agencies* (GAO/HRD-98-29). Washington, D.C.: General Accounting Office.

[45]Due to the financial and time investment in their training, health care workers generally demand more money than is available for personal assistance services, and are likely to be dissatisfied over time with the amount they can earn as personal assistants compared with what they can earn in the health care sector. Moreover, many consumers prefer training their own assistants anyway, claiming that those who have gone through training under the medical model are not as able to adapt to the consumer as employer under the independent living model.

[46]DeJong, G. and Wenker, T. 1983. "Attendant Care as a Prototype Independent Living Service." *Caring* 2(2): 26-30.

[47]Egley, L. 1994. *Program Models Providing Personal Assistance Services (PAS) for Independent Living*, Oakland, CA: World Institute on Disability.

[48]Nosek, M.A. 1991. "Personal Assistance Services: A Review of Literature and Analysis of Policy Implications." *Journal of Disability Policy Studies* 2(2): 1-17.

[49]Coyne, A.C., Reichman, W.E. and Berbig, L.J. 1993. "The Relationship between Dementia and Elder Abuse." *American Journal of Psychiatry* 150: 643-46.

[50]Flanagan, S.A. and Green, P.S. 2000. "Fiscal Intermediaries: Reducing the Burden of Consumer-Directed Support." *Generations*, 24(3): 94-97, at 94.

[51]Id.

[52]Flanagan and Green, at 97; Flanagan, S.A. and Green, P.S. 1997. *Consumer-Directed Personal Assistance services: Key Operational Issues for States Using Fiscal Intermediary Service Organizations.* Cambridge, Mass: MEDSTAT, Inc.

[53]Flanagan and Green, at 12.

[54]Doty, Kasper, and Litvak. 1996.

[55]Beatty, P.W., Richmond, G.W. Tepper, S., and DeJong, G. 1998. "Personal Assistance for People with Physical Disabilities: Consumer-Direction and Satisfaction with Services." *Archives of Physical Medicine and Rehabilitation* 79(6): 674-77; Benjamin, Matthias, and Franke, at 351-66.

[56]Nosek, M.A. 1998. "Personal Assistance: Its Effect on the Long-term Health of a Rehabilitation Hospital Population." *Archives of Physical Medicine and Rehabilitation* 74(2): 127-32.

[57]Verbrugge L.M., Rennert, C., and Madans, J.H. 1997. "The Great Efficacy of Personal and Equipment Assistance in Reducing Disability." *American Journal of Public Health* 1997 Mar; 87 (3): 384-92.

[58]Simon-Rusinowitz, L., Mahoney, K., Desmond, S.M., et al. 1997. "Determining Consumer Preferences for a Cash Option (AQ1): Arkansas Survey Results." *Health Care Financing Review*, 19(2): 73-96; Zacharias, B.L. 1997. *Cash and Counseling Demonstration and Evaluation: A Study to Determine the Preferences of Consumers and Surrogates for a Cash Option.*

[59]Flanagan, S.A., Green, P.S. and Eustis, N. 1998. "You Can Do It: State Initiatives Broaden Access to Consumer-Directed Personal Assistance Services Through the Use of intermediary Service Organizations." *American Rehabilitation* 24(3): 21-26, at 21.

[60]Desmond, S.M., Shoop, D.M., Simon-Rusinowitz, L., Mahoney, K.J., Squillace, M.R. and Fay, R.A. 1998. *Comparing Preferences For a Cash Option Versus Traditional Services, Florida Elders And Adults with Physical Disabilities, Telephone Survey Technical Report, Background Research for the Cash and Counseling Demonstration and Evaluation.* College Park, MD: University of Maryland Center on Aging.

[61]Benjamin and Matthias, at 86.

[62]Id.

[63]Benjamin, A.E., Matthias, R. and Franke, T.M. 2000. "Comparing Consumer-Directed and Agency Models for Providing Supportive Services at Home." *Health Services Research* 2000 Apr; 35 (1 Pt 2): 35-66.

[64]Id.

[65]Tilly, Weiner, and Cuellar, at 80; citing Baarveld et al. 1998. *Persoonsgebonden Budget Arbeidsmarktpositie van Zorgverleners.* Nijmegen, Netherlands: Instituut voor Toegepaste Sociale Wetenschappen van de Stricting Katholieke Universiteit te Nijmegen.

[66]Id. at 87.

[67]Wong, D. 2000. "Rapid Response: Development of a Home Care Worker Replacement Service." *Generations,* 24(3): 88-90.

[68]Mahoney, K.J., et al. 1998. "Determining Consumer Preferences for a Cash Option: New York Telephone Survey Findings." *American Rehabilitation,* (winter): 24-36; Mahoney, K.J., Simone, K. and Simon-Rusinowitz, L. 2000. "Early Lessons from the Cash and Counseling Demonstration and Evaluation." *Generations* 24(3): 41-46.

[69]Batavia, A.I. 1996. "Health Care, Personal Assistance, and Assistive Technology: Are In-Kind Benefits Key to Independence or Dependence for People with Disabilities?," In *Disability, Cash Benefits and Work,* J.L. Mashaw, et al., (eds.), Kalamazoo, MI: W.E. Upjohn Institute for Employment Research.

[70]Litvak, S., H. Zukas, and J.E. Heumann. 1987. *Attending to America: Personal Assistance for Independent Living.* Berkeley, CA: World Institute on Disability; Batavia, DeJong, and McKnew, at 527-28.

[71]Flanagan, Green, and Eustis, at 21.

[72]Id. at 22.

[73]Doty, Kasper and Litvak, 1996.

[74]Cameron and Firman, 1995.

[75]Batavia, A.I. 1998. "The Prospects for a National Personal Assistance Services Program for People With Disabilities." *American Rehabilitation,* 24 (3).

[76]A survey of 20 experts in the field concluded that: *Agencies fear increased business competition.* The most frequently mentioned issue was the increased competition traditional agencies may fear when consumers hire independent providers [11 of the 20 experts made this observation]. According to the experts, agencies' fears of losing business may limit implementation of consumer-directed programs. However, two experts commented that some provider agencies may see consumer direction as an opportunity to expand their services and increase their profits. Simon-Rusinowitz, L., Bochniak, A.M.,. Mahoney, K.J., and Marks, L.N. 2000. "Implementation Issues for Consumer-Directed Programs: A Survey of Policy Experts." *Generations,* 24(3): 34-40, at 36.

[77]The most prevalent issue relating to payors and policy makers was as follows:

Payers and policymakers have concerns about safety, liability, and accountability for cash. The experts most frequently mentioned the concerns of payers and policy makers about accountability for cash payments and the legal liabilities associated with consumer-directed programs [21 of the 22 experts expressed this concern].
Id. at 37.

CHAPTER 6

[1]Health Insurance Association of America. 1998. *Term Care Insurance in 1996: Research Findings*, Washington, D.C; GAO. 1993. *Long-Term Care Insurance: High Percentage of Policy Holders Drop Policies*. (GAO/HRD93-129). Washington, D.C.: General Accounting Office.

[2]Id.

[3]Kane, R.A., Kane, R.L. and Ladd, R.C. 1998. *The Heart of Long-Term Care*. New York; Oxford: Oxford University Press, at 126.

[4]Batavia, A.I., DeJong, G. and McKnew, L.B. 1991. "Toward a National Personal Assistance Program: The Independent Living Model of Long-Term Care for Persons with Disabilities." *Journal of Health Politics, Policy, and Law* 16(3): 523-545.

[5]Benjamin, A.E, Matthias, R., Franke, T., Mills, Hasenfeld, Y., Matras, L., Park, E., Stoddard, S. and Kraus, L. 1998. *Comparing Consumer-Directed and Agency Models for Providing Supportive Services at Home*. Final Report under HHS Contract #100-94-0022. Los Angeles, CA: School of Public Welfare, University of California, Los Angeles; Benjamin, A.E. and Matthias, R. 2000. "Comparing Consumer-Directed and Agency-Directed Models: California's In-Home Supportive Services Program." *Generations* 24(3): 85-87; Benjamin, A.E., Matthias, R. and Franke, T.M. 2000. "Comparing Consumer-Directed and Agency Models for Providing Supportive Services at Home." *Health Services Research* 35(1 Pt 2): 351-66.

[6]Id.

[7]Id.

[8]Kane, Kane and Ladd, at 126.

[9]Benjamin and Matthias, 2000. Benjamin, Matthias, and Franke. 2000.

[10]Doty, P., Kasper, J. and Litvak, S. 1996. "Consumer-Directed Models of Personal Care: Lessons from Medicaid" *Milbank Quarterly* 74 (3): 377-409, at 383.

[11]Id, at 383.

[12]Id, at 383-84.

[13]Id. at 392.

[14]Beatty, P.W., Adams, M. and O' Day, B. 1998. "Virginia's Consumer-Directed Personal Assistance Services Program: A History and Evaluation." *American Rehabilitation* 24(3): 31-35.

[15]Id. at 33-34.

[16]Id. at 34; Beatty, P.W., Richmond, G.W., Tepper, S. and DeJong, G. 1998. "Personal Assistance for People with Physical Disabilities: Consumer-Direction and Satisfaction with Services." *Archives of Physical Medicine and Rehabilitation* 79(6): 674-77.

[17]Bertsch, E.F. 1991. "Barriers to Individualized Community Support Services: The Impact of Some Current Funding and Conceptual Models." *Community Mental Health Journal* 27(5): 337-45.

[18]Mahoney, K.J. and Simon-Rusinowitz L. 1997. "Cash and Counseling

Demonstration and Evaluation. Start-Up Activities." *Journal of Case Management.* 6(1): 25-30; Mahoney, K.J., Simone, K. and Simon-Rusinowitz, L. 2000. "Early Lessons from the Cash and Counseling Demonstration and Evaluation." *Generations* 24(3): 41-46.

[19]Id.

[20]Id.

[21]Id.

[22]Id.

[23]The state of New York, which was originally in the study, dropped out.

[24]Doty, P. 2000. "The Federal Role in the Move toward Consumer Direction." *Generations* 24(3): 922-27.

[25]Doty, at 27.

[26]Desmond, S.M., Shoop, D.M., Simon-Rusinowitz, L., Mahoney, K.J., Squillace, M.R. and Fay, R.A. 1998. *Comparing Preferences for a Cash Option Versus Traditional Services, Florida Elders and Adults with Physical Disabilities, Telephone Survey Technical Report, Background Research for the Cash and Counseling Demonstration and Evaluation.* College Park, Md.: University of Maryland Center on Aging; Zacharias, B.L. 1997. *Cash and Counseling Demonstration and Evaluation: A Study to Determine the Preferences of Consumers and Surrogates for a Cash Option.*

[27]Cameron, K. and Firman, J. *International and Domestic Programs Using "Cash and Counseling" Strategies to Pay for Long-Term Care.* National Council on the Aging, Washington, D.C., 1995; Tilly, J., Weiner, J.M., and Cuellar, A.E. 2000. "Consumer-Directed Home-and Community-based Services Programs In Five Countries: Policy Issues for Older People and Government." *Generations*, 24(3): 74-84.

[28]Leutz, W. 1998. "Home Care Benefits for Persons with Disabilities." *American Rehabilitation* 24(3): 6-14, at 8-10.

[29]Latimer, J. 1997-98. "The Essential Role of Regulation to Assure Quality in Long-term Care." *Generations* 21(4): 10-14.

[30]Id.

[31]Id.

[32]Id.

[33]Stone, R.I. 2001. "Providing Long-Term Care Benefits in Cash: Moving to a Disability Model. The Cause of Patient Autonomy is Well Served by Cash Benefit Programs, Although Challenges Remain." *Health Affairs* 20(6): 96-109.

[34]Id. at 107.

[35]Foster, L., Brown, R., Carlson, B., Phillips, B. and Schore, J. 2000. *Cash and Counseling: Consumer's Early Experiences in Arkansas* (prepared for Office of Disability, Aging, and Long-Term Care Policy, Office of the Assistant Secretary for Planning and Evaluation, DHHS, and The Robert Wood Johnson Foundation). Mathematica Policy Research, Inc.

[36]Id. at 5.

[37]Id.

[38]Id.

[39]Id. at 6 and 15, Table 6.

[40]Id. at 15, Table 6.

[41]Id. at 20, Table 13.

[42]Id. at 6 and 16, Table 7.

[43]Id. at 6 and 17, Table 8.

[44]Id. at 7 and 18, Table 9.

[45]Id. at 8 and 23, Table 16.

[46]Id. at 8 and 23, Table 16.

[47]Id. at 26, Table 18.

[48]Id. at 27, Table 19.

[49]Id. at 25, Table 17.

[50]Simon-Rusinowitz, L., Mahoney, K.J., Desmond, S.M., Shoop, D.M., Squillace, M.R. and Fay, R.A. 1998. *Telephone Survey Technical Report: Consumer Preferences for a Cash Option Versus Traditional Services in New Jersey.* College Park, MD: University of Maryland Center on Aging; Desmond, et al., 1998.

[51]Foster, et al, at 87.

[52]Wong, D. 2000. "Rapid Response: Development of a Home Care Worker Replacement Service." *Generations* 24(3): 88-90.

[53]Id. at 89.

[54]Id.

[55]Id.

[56]Id.

[57]Flanagan, S.A. and Green, P.S. 1997. *Consumer-Directed Personal Assistance Services: Key Operational Issues for State CD-PAS Programs Using Fiscal Intermediary Service Organizations.* Cambridge, MA: MEDSTAT, Inc., at E-1.

[58]Id., at E-2.

[59]Id. at 14.

[60]Vela Microboard Association. 2001. "Microboards" Available at http://www/microboards.org.

CHAPTER 7

[1]Keigher, S.M. 2000. "The Interests of Three Stakeholders in Independent Personal Care For Disabled Elders." *Journal of Health and Human Services Administration* Fall; 23(2): 136-60.

[2]Kane, R.A., Kane, R.L., Ladd, R.C. 1998. *The Heart of Long-Term Care.* New York; Oxford : Oxford University Press.

[3]DeJong, G. 1982. "A Legal Perspective on Disability, Home Care, and Relative Responsibility." *Home Health Services Quarterly* 3(3/4): 176-187.

[4]Nosek M.A., Foley C.C., Hughes R.B., et al. 2001. "Vulnerabilities for Abuse Among Women with Disabilities." *Sex and Disability* 19(3): 177-189; Coyne, A.C., Reichman, W.E. and Berbig, L.J. 1993. "The Relationship Between Dementia and Elder Abuse." *American Journal of Psychiatry* 150: 643-46.

[5]Health Care Financing Administration. 1994. "Final Rule: Medicare and Medicaid Programs: Survey, Certification, and Enforcement for Skilled Nursing Facilities and Nursing Facilities." *Federal Register* 59: 56, 116-56, 252. November 10. Washington, D.C.

[6]GAO. 1997. *Medicare Home Health Agencies: Certification Process Ineffective In Excluding Problem Agencies* (GAO/HRD-98-29). Washington, D.C.: General Accounting Office.

[7]Id.

[8]Goodrich, L.J. 1997. "Medicare Fraud Puts 'Waste Patrols' on Alert: First Comprehensive Report Shows As Much As $23 Billion of Waste and Fraud Each

Year," *The Christian Science Monitor*, July 18, 1997, at 3; "Federal Health Care Fraud Actions Net $1.3 Billion in 2001." *Nursing Home Litigation Reporter* 4(24): 7 (July 26, 2002).

[9]*Medicaid Fraud Report*. 2001. "Home Health Care Agencies: Rhode Island." January 2001, at 19; Eisler, P. 1997. "Health Fraud Hits Home: Fevered Growth Could Turn to Consolidation," USA Today, August 11, 1997, at 1B.

[10]Aronovitz, L. 2001. "Efforts to Control Improper Payments Vary, Medicaid." *GAO Reports*. GAO-01-662 (June 7, 2001).

[11]Pham, A. 1997. "Home Care: A Troubling Diagnosis." *The Boston Globe*, October 5, 1997, at A1.

[12]Aronovitz, 2001.

[13]Id.

[14]General Accounting Office. 1999. *Adults With Severe Disabilities: Federal and State Approaches for Personal Care and Other Services*. (GAO/HEHS-99-101). Washington, D.C.: General Accounting Office; General Accounting Office. 1997. *Medicare Home Health Agencies: Certification Process Ineffective in Excluding Problem Agencies* (GAO/HRD-98-29). Washington, D.C.: General Accounting Office; General Accounting Office. 1994. *Long-Term Care: Status of Quality Assurance and Measurement in Home and Community-Based Services*. (GAO/PEMD-94-19). Washington, D.C.: General Accounting Office, March 1994; General Accounting Office. 1994. *Long-Term Care Reform: States' Views of Key Elements of Well-Designed Programs for the Elderly*. (GAO/HEHS-94-227). Washington, D.C.: General Accounting Office; General Accounting Office. 1994. *Medicaid Long-Term Care: Successful State Efforts to Expand Home Services While Limiting Costs*. (GAO/HEHS-94-167). Washington, D.C.: General Accounting Office.

[15]Batavia, A.I. 1996. "Health Care, Personal Assistance, and Assistive Technology: Are In-Kind Benefits Key to Independence or Dependence for People with Disabilities?," In *Disability, Cash Benefits and Work*. (J.L. Mashaw, et al., eds.), Kalamazoo, MI: W.E. Upjohn Institute for Employment Research.

[16]Stone, R.I. 2000. "Introduction – Consumer Direction in Long-Term Care: Opportunities, Challenges, and Limitations of this Increasingly Popular Approach." *Generations* 24(3): 5-8, at 7.

[17]Arno, P.S., Levine, C., and Memmott, M.M. 1999. "The Economic Value of Informal Caregiving; President Clinton's Proposal to Provide Relief to Family Caregivers Opens a Long-Overdue Discussion of This "Invisible" Health Care Sector." *Health Affairs* March, 1999-April, 1999, at 184-85.

[18]Feinberg, L.F. and Kelly, K.A. 1995. "A Well-Deserved Break: Respite Options Offered by California's Statewide System of Caregiver Resource Centers." *Gerontologist* 35: 701-5; Feinberg, L.F. and Whitlatch, C.J. 1998. "Family Caregivers and In-home Respite Options: The Consumer-Directed Versus Agency-Based Experience." *Journal of Gerontological Social Work* 30(3/4): 9-28.

[19]American Association of Retired People. 1998. *Medicaid and Long-Term Care for Older People*. Washington, D.C.; AARP Policy Institute.

[20]Davis, B.E. 1998. "The Home Health Care Crisis: Medicare's Fastest Growing Program Legalizes Spiraling Costs." *Elder Law Journal* 6: 215-255.

[21]Litvak, S. and Kennedy, J. 1991. *Policy Issues Affecting the Medicaid Personal Care Services Optional Benefit*. Oakland, CA: World Institute on Disability; Doty, P.,

Kasper, J. and Litvak, S. 1996. "Consumer-Directed Models of Personal Care: Lessons from Medicaid," *Milbank Quarterly* 74 (3): 377-409, at 385.

[22]Doty, P., Kasper, J. and Litvak, S. 1996. "Consumer-Directed Models of Personal Care: Lessons from Medicaid," *Milbank Quarterly* 74 (3): 377-409, at 384.

[23]Id.

[24]Litvak and Kennedy; Doty, Kasper and Litvak, at 385.

[25]Id.

[26]Prince, J., Manley, M. and Whiteneck, G. 1995. "Self-Managed Versus Agency-Provided Personal Assistance Care for Individuals with High Level Tetraplegia." *Archives of Physical Medicine and Rehabilitation* 76(10): 919-923; Mattson-Prince J. 1997. "A Rational Approach to Long-Term Care: Comparing the Independent Living Model with Agency-Based Care for Persons with High Spinal Cord Injuries." *Spinal Cord* 35(5): 326-31.

[27]Mattson-Prince, at 326.

[28]Litvak, S., Zukas, H., and Heumann, J.E. 1987. *Attending to America: Personal Assistance for Independent Living. A Survey of Attendant Services in the United States for People of All Ages with Disabilities.* Berkeley, CA: World Institute on Disability; Litvak, S. and Kennedy, J. 1991. *Policy Issues Affecting the Medicaid Personal Care Services Optional Benefit.* Oakland, CA: World Institute on Disability.

[29]Flanagan, S.A. and Green, P.S. 2000. "Fiscal Intermediaries: Reducing the Burden of Consumer-Directed Support." *Generations* 24(3): 94-97; Flanagan, S.A., Green, P.S. and Eustis, N. 1998. "You Can Do It: State Initiatives Broaden Access to Consumer-Directed Personal Assistance Services Through the Use of Intermediary Service Organizations." *American Rehabilitation*, 24(3): 21-26.

[30]Collopy, B.J. 1990. "Ethical Dimensions of Autonomy in Long-Term Care." *Generations*, 14 (Supplement): 9-12.

[31]Kapp, M.B. 1996. "Enhancing Autonomy and Choice in Selecting and Directing Long-term Care Services." *The Elder Law Journal*, 4 (1): 55-97, at 57.

[32]Collopy, B.J. 1988. "Autonomy in Long-Term Care: Some Crucial Distinctions." *The Gerontologist*, 28 (Supplement): 10-17.

[33]Kapp, M.B. 1996, at 63; Capitman, J.and Sciegaj, M. 1995. "A Conceptual Approach For Understanding Individual Autonomy In Managed Community Long-Term Care." *Gerontologist* 35 (4): 533-40; Rodin, J. 1986. "Aging and health: Effects of the Sense of Control." *Science* 233: 1271; Winick, B.J. 1992. "On Autonomy: Legal and Psychological Perspectives." *Villanova Law Review* 37: 1705-1777.

[34]Stone, R.I. 2000. "Introduction – Consumer Direction in Long-Term Care: Opportunities, Challenges, and Limitations of This Increasingly Popular Approach." *Generations*, 24(3): 5-8, at 6.

[35]Doty, et al., at 392.

[36]Id

[37]Id.

[38]Benjamin, A.E., Matthias, R. and Franke, T.M. 2000. "Comparing Consumer-Directed and Agency Models For Providing Supportive Services at Home." *Health Services Research* 2000 Apr; 35 (1 Pt 2): 351-66.; Benjamin, A.E., Matthias, R. and Franke, T.M. 1998. *Comparing Consumer-Directed and Agency Models for Providing Supportive Services at Home.* Final Report under HHS Contract #100-94-0022. Los

Angeles, California: School of Public Welfare, University of California, Los Angeles.

[39]Tilly, J., Weiner, J.M., and Cuellar, A.E. 2000. "Consumer-Directed home-and community-based services Programs in Five Countries: Policy Issues for Older People and Government." *Generations*, 24(3): 74-84, at 78; citing Runde, P. et al. 1996. *Einstellungen und Verhalten zur Pflegeversicherung und zur Hauslichen Pflege.* Hamburg, Germany: Universitat Hamburg.

[40]Id. at 78; citing Miltenburg, T., et al. 1996. *A Personal Budget for Clients: Summary Of an Experiment with Cash Benefits In Home Care in the Netherlands. Institute for Applied Social Sciences.* Nijmegen, Netherlands.; and Woldringh, C. and Ramakers, C. 1998. *Persoonsgebonden Budget Verpleging Verzorging Ervaringen van Budgethouders en Kwaliteit van Zorg.* Nijmegen, Netherlands: Instituut voor Toegepaste Sociale Wetenschappen van de Stricting Katholieke Universiteit te Nijmegen.

[41]Vela Microboard Association. 2001. "Microboards" Available at http://www/microboards.org.

[42]Tilly, Weiner, and Cuellar, at 79.: citing Simon, M.O. and Martin, P.A. 1996. La Prestation Dependance: Rapport Final du Programme d' Evaluation de l' Experimentation d' une Prestation Dependence. Paris, France: Centre de Recherche pour l'Etude et l'Observation des Conditions de Vie CREDOC.

[43]Flanagan, S.A. and Green, P.S. 2000. "Fiscal Intermediaries: Reducing the Burden of Consumer-Directed Support." *Generations* 24(3): 94-97, at 97; citing Flanagan, S.A. and Green, P.S. 1997. *Consumer-Directed Personal Assistance Services: Key Operational Issues for States Using Fiscal Intermediary Service Organizations.* Cambridge, MA: MEDSTAT, Inc.

[44]Three fiscal intermediary models have been identified: 1) the fiscal conduit model, in which the intermediary simply invoices the state and distributes funds to consumers; 2) the IRS employer agent model; and the vendor fiscal intermediary model Id. at 95.

[45]Flanagan and Green, at 95.

[46]Tilly, Weiner, and Cuellar, at 79.

[47]Id. at 79; citing Comite National de Vigilance. 1998. *Le Livre Noir de la P.S.D.* Paris, France.

[48]Id., at 79.

[49]Id.

[50]Id.

[51]Hollnagel, G. 2001. "Reports of Elder Abuse on the Rise." *La Crosse Tribune*, (October 21, 2001).

[52]House Subcommittee on Health and Long-Term Care. 1990. *Elder Abuse: A Decade of Shame and Inaction*, H.R., 101st Cong., 2d Sess. 1.

[53]Id.

[54]Id.

[55]California Assembly Committee on Public Safety. 1998. Committee Analysis of SB 2199, at 3 (June 23, 1998), at 7.

[56]California Assembly Committee on Public Safety. 1998. Committee Analysis of AB 1780, at 2 (Apr. 21, 1998) (claiming that fewer than 44,000 abuse incidents were reported in 1996, though 225,000 incidents of elder abuse occur annually in

California). *See* also California Assembly Committee on Public Safety, Committee Analysis of SB 2199, at 3 (June 23, 1998).

[57]Belkin, D. 1999. "Abuse of Seniors Sometimes Hard to Detect: Fear of Being Sent to Home Cited As Reason for Secret." *The Palm Beach Post* (Florida), at 1B (April 11, 1999).

[58]Nosek, et al., 2001; Coyne, Reichman, and Berbig, 1993.

[59]Saxton M, Curry MA, Powers LE, et al. 2001. "Bring My Scooter So I Can Leave You" - A Study of Disabled Women Handling Abuse by Personal Assistance Providers." *Violence Against Women* 7(4): 393-417.

[60]House Subcommittee on Health and Long-Term Care. 1990.

[61]Health Care Financing Administration, 1994; Health Care Financing Administration. 1993. *Approaches to Quality under Home and Community-Based Services Waivers.* Baltimore, MD: Medicaid Bureau.

[62]Rivlin, A.M. and Wiener, J. 1988. *Caring for the Disabled Elderly: Who Will Pay?* Washington, D.C.: The Brookings Institute.

[63]House Subcommittee on Health and Long-Term Care. 1990.

[64]Washuk, B. 2001. "One-Third Cited for Abuse, Neglect." *Sun Journal* (August 3, 2001).

[65]Benjamin, Matthias, and Franke, 2000.

[66]42 U.S.C. 1395i-3(a)(3).

[67]n4. 1995 Long Term Care Ombudsman Annual Rep. Pt III http://www.aoa.dhhs.gov/napis/95nors/part3.html.

[68]Id. at 2.

[69]Id. at 3.

[70]Id. at 5. In addition, there were 17,780 complaints pertaining to the quality of life, and 25,945 concerning residential care.

[71]Layton, M.J. and Zambito, T. 1999. "The Unlicensed Underground: Tragedy Can Follow Families Seeking Low-Cost Aides." *The Record* (Hackensack, NJ), pA-1 (October 10, 1999); Saxton, et al., 2001.

[72]Ulicny, G.R.,White, G.W., Bradford, B. and Mathews, R.M. 1990. "Consumer Exploitation by Attendants: How Often Does It Happen and Can Anything Be Done about It?" *Rehabilitation Counseling Bulletin* 33: 240-46.

[73]Applebaum, R. and Phillips, P. 1990. "Assuring the Quality of In-Home Care: The 'Other' Challenge for Long-Term Care," *Gerontologist* 30(4): 444-50; Applebaum, R., Mollica, R. and Tilly, J. 1997-8. "Assuring Homecare Quality: A Case Study of State Strategies." *Generations* 21(4): 57-63.

[74]Health Care Financing Administration. 1994. "Final Rule: Medicare and Medicaid Programs: Survey, Certification, and Enforcement for Skilled Nursing Facilities and Nursing Facilities." *Federal Register* 59: 56, 116-56, 252. November 10. Washington, D.C.

[75]Senate Committee on Aging. 1999. *Long-Term Care Hearing before the Special Committee on Aging,* United States Senate, 103rd Congress (2nd Session), Milwaukee, WI, S. Hrg. 103-20, May 9, 1994, U.S. Government Printing Office.

[76]Id.

[77]Mattson, M. 2001. "Nursing Home Quality Declines. Facing a Tide of Lawsuits and Horror Stories, the Industry Says It Is Working to Improve, but Florida Legislature May Not Wait." *The Florida Times-Union*, A-1 (April 1, 2001);. Mattson,

M. 2000. "Nursing Homes in Crisis," *The Florida Times-Union*, A-1 (June 4, 2001); Walters, S. 2001. "Nursing Home Violations Rise: Life-Threatening Problems at Some Long-Term Centers Worry State Officials." *Milwaukee Journal Sentinel*, p01 (April 8, 2001); Boo, K. 1999. "Residents Languish, Profiteers Flourish While Deaths and Abuse Go Unexamined, For-profit Operators Milk a Lax System." *The Washington Post*, A-1 (March 15, 1999); Zambito, T. and Layton, M.J., 1999. "Criminal Caregivers: Home Health Care in Crisis, Lax State Laws Let Danger Enter the Frailest Lives." *The Record*, A-1 (October 3, 1999); Pham, at A-1.

[78]Branstetter, Z and Schafer, S. 2001. "Nearly 1,000 Deaths Were Preventable, Review Shows." *Tulsa World*, p1 (January 14, 2001).

[79]O'Connor, P. 2001. "19 Have Died in 2 Years from Poor Treatment: In Most Cases, When Caregivers Are at Fault, The Penalty Is Minor." *St. Louis Post-Dispatch*, p. A-1 (August 5, 2001).

[80]Harrington, C., Carillo, H. and Wellin, V. 2001. *Nursing Facilities, Staffing, Residents and Facility Deficiencies, 1994-2000*. Department of Social and Behavioral Sciences, University of California at San Francisco, at 80.

[81]Id.

[82]Id., at 82-83.

[83]Id., at 98.

[84]GAO. 1997. *Medicare Home Health Agencies: Certification Process Ineffective in Excluding Problem Agencies* (GAO/HRD-98-29). Washington, D.C.: General Accounting Office.

[85]Benjamin, A.E. and Matthias, R. 2000. "Comparing Consumer-Directed and Agency- Directed Models: California's In-Home Supportive Services Program." *Generations*, 24(3): 85-87, at 86.

[86]Id.

[87]Id.

[88]Mattson-Prince, at 326-31.

[89]Foster, L., Brown, R., Carlson, B., Phillips, B. and Schore, J. 2000. *Cash and Counseling: Consumer's Early Experiences in Arkansas* (prepared for Office of Disability, Aging, and Long-term Care Policy, Office of the Assistant Secretary for Planning and Evaluation, DHHS, and The Robert Wood Johnson Foundation). Mathematica Policy Research, Inc.

[90]Id. at 8 and 23, Table 16.

[91]Id. at 8 and 23, Table 16.

[92]Id. at 26, Table 18.

[93]Id. at 26, Table 18.

[94]Commonwealth Commission on Elderly People Living Alone. 1991. *The Importance of Choice in Medicaid Home Care Programs: Maryland, Michigan, and Texas*. New York: Commonwealth Fund; Doty et al., at 393.

[95]Id. at 396.

[96]The WID case studies found that policies in some states make it more or less likely for consumers to hire people they already know. In Texas, where 75% of surveyed consumers reported that they did not previously know their assistants, the state had a policy requiring all assistants to be employees of home health agencies. In Maryland, where 82% of respondents reported that they did not pre-viously know their assistants, the state had a very restrictive policy prohibiting

almost all relatives from serving as personal assistants. In contrast, about 71% of surveyed consumers in Maryland, which has a much more permissive policy concerning relatives serving as personal assistants, reported that they knew their personal assistant previously. Doty et al., at 393.

[97]Commonwealth Commission on Elderly People Living Alone, Commonwealth Fund; Doty et al., Table 4 at 394.

[98]Id. at 396.

[99]Id. at 396.

[100]Id. at 34; Beatty, P.W., Richmond, G.W., Tepper, S. and DeJong, G. 1998. "Personal Assistance for People with Physical Disabilities: Consumer-Direction and Satisfaction with Services." *Archives of Physical Medicine and Rehabilitation* 79(6): 674-7.

[101]Kane, R.A. and Kane, R.L. 1990. "The Impact of Long-term-Care Financing On Personal Autonomy." *Generations* 14 (Supplement): 86.

CHAPTER 8

[1]U.S. Department of Health and Human Services. 1999. *A Descriptive Analysis of Patterns of Informal and Formal Caregiving Among Privately Insured and Non-Privately Insured Disabled Elders Living in the Community: Final report.* Washington, D.C.: Office of Disability, Aging and Long-term Care Policy, March 1999, at i.

[2]Leutz, W. 1998. "Home Care Benefits for Persons With Disabilities." *American Rehabilitation,* 24(3): 6-14; Tilly, J., Goldenson, S. and Kasten, J. 2001. *Long-Term Care: Consumers, Providers and Financing. A Chart Book.* Washington, D.C.: Urban Institute, March, 2001, at 31 and 41. Based on Office of the Actuary, National Health Statistics Group, Personal Health Care Expenditures, HCFA, DHHS, 2000.

[3]Tilly, Goldenson, and Kasten, at 31 and 34. Based on Office of the Actuary, National Health Statistics Group, Personal Health Care Expenditures, HCFA, DHHS, 2000.

[4]Id. at 35. Based on Office of the Actuary, National Health Statistics Group, Personal Health Care Expenditures, HCFA, DHHS, 2000.

[5]Leutz, at 6-14.

[6]Dautel, P.J. and Frieden, L. August 1999. *Consumer Choice and Control: Personal Attendant Services and Supports in America (Report of the National Blue Ribbon Panel on Personal Assistance Services).* Houston, TX: Independent Living and Research Utilization Program, available on the Internet at www.ilru.org.; Litvak, S., Zukas, H., Heumann, J.E. 1987. *Attending to America: Personal Assistance for Independent Living. A Survey of Attendant Services in the United States For People of All Ages with disabilities.* Berkeley, CA: World Institute on Disability; Litvak, S. and Kennedy, J. 1991. *Policy Issues Affecting the Medicaid Personal Care Services Optional Benefit.* Oakland, CA: World Institute on Disability.

[7]Benjamin A.E 2001. "Consumer-Directed Services at Home: A New Model for Persons with Disabilities" *Health Affairs* 20(6): 80-95.

[8]Tilly, Goldenson, and Kasten, at 31.

[9]U.S. Department of Health and Human Services. 1999. *A Descriptive Analysis of Patterns of Informal and Formal Caregiving Among privately insured and Non-Privately Insured Disabled Elders Living in the Community: Final report.* Washington, D.C.: Office of Disability, Aging and Long-Term Care Policy, March 1999, at 1.

[10]Batavia, A.I. 1998. "The Prospects for a National Personal Assistance Services

Program for People With Disabilities." *American Rehabilitation* 24 (3), Winter.
[11]There has been substantial fraud and abuse by recipients of the earned income tax credit, which is a refundable tax credit for low income individuals.
[12]Arno, Levine, and Memmott, 1999; Tilly, Goldenson, and Kasten, at 34.
[13]Department of Commerce. 1997. "Disabilities Affect One-Fifth of All Americans: Proportion Could Increase in Coming Decades. *Census Brief* CENBR--97-5 (December, 1997).
[14]Tilly, Goldenson, and Kasten, at 26.
[15]Id. at 5l. Health Insurance Association of America. 1998. *Term Care Insurance in 1996: Research Findings*, Washington, D.C.
[16]Id.
[17]Tilly, Goldenson, and Kasten, at 32.
[18]Id. at 5l. Health Insurance Association of America. 1998. *Term Care Insurance in 1996: Research Findings*, Washington, D.C.
[19]Tilly, Goldenson, and Kasten, at 32.
[20]About 59% of purchasers of private long-term care insurance age 55 and older had at least $50,000 in liquid assets in 1994. Id., at 55. Health Insurance Association of America. 1998. *Term Care Insurance in 1996: Research Findings*, Washington, D.C.
[21]GAO. 1993. *Long-term Care Insurance: High Percentage of Policy Holders Drop Policies*. (GAO/HRD93-129). Washington, D.C.: General Accounting Office.
[22]U.S. Department of Health and Human Services. (1999). *A Descriptive Analysis of Patterns of informal and formal caregiving Among Privately Insured and Non-Privately Insured Disabled Elders living in the community: Final report*. Washington, D.C.: Office of Disability, Aging and Long-term Care Policy, March 1999, at 18.
[23]Id. at 19.
[24]Stone, R.I. 2001. "Providing Long-term Care Benefits in Cash: Moving to a disability model. The Cause of Patient Autonomy Is Well Served by cash benefit programs, Although Challenges Remain" *Health Affairs* 20(6): 96-109, at 102.
[25]Tilly, Goldenson, and Kasten, at 31.
[26]Id., at 41.
[27]Id., at 43.
[28]Egley, L. 1994. *New Federal PC Option PAS Funding Rules: Summary*. Berkeley, CA: World Institute on Disability.; Egley, L. 1994. *Program Models Providing Personal Assistance Services (PAS) for Independent Living*. Berkeley, CA: World Institute on Disability.
[29]Doty, P., Kasper, J. and Litvak, S. 1996. "Consumer-Directed Models of Personal Care: Lessons from Medicaid," *Milbank Quarterly* 74 (3): 377-409, at 379-80.
[30]Litvak, S. and Kennedy, J. 1991. *Policy Issues Affecting the Medicaid Personal Care Services Optional Benefit*. Oakland, CA: World Institute on Disability.
[31]Id.
[32]Kennedy, J. and Litvak, S. 1991. *Case Studies of Six State Personal Assistance Services Funded by the Medicaid Personal Care Option*. Oakland, CA: World Institute on Disability.
[33]Doty, Kasper, and Litvak, at 380.
[34]Tilly, Goldenson, and Kasten, at 45. Based on Harrington, C., Carillo, H., Wellin, V., Norwood, F. and Miller, N. 1999. 1915 (c) *Medicaid Home and Community-Based*

Waiver Participants, Services, and Expenditures, 1992-97. Department of Social and Behavioral Sciences, University of California at San Francisco, November 1999.
[35]Id. at 45.
[36]Id. at 50. Based on Prouty, R. et al. 1999. *Residential Services for Persons with Developmental Disabilities: Status and Trends Through 1998*. Institute on Community Integration, University of Minnesota, May 1999.
[37]Kassner, E. and Williams. 1997. *Taking Care of Their Own: State-Funded Home and Community-Based Care Programs for Older Persons*. Washington, D.C.: AARP Public Policy Institute.
[38]Id.
[39]Id.
[40]Tilly, Goldenson, and Kasten, at 31-32.
[41]Id., at 46. Based on Harrington, C., Carillo, H., Wellin, V., Norwood, F. and Miller, N. 1999. *1915 (c) Medicaid Home and Community-Based Waiver Participants, Services, and Expenditures, 1992-97*. Department of Social and Behavioral Sciences, University of California at San Francisco, November 1999.
[42]Pepper Commission. 1990. *A Call for Action (Final report)*. U.S. Bipartisan Commission on Comprehensive Health Care, Washington, D.C.; American Association of Retired People. 1998. *Medicaid and Long-Term Care for Older People*. Washington, D.C.: AARP Policy Institute.
[43]American Association of Retired People. 1998.
[44]Id.
[45]Leutz, at 7.
[46]Adams, K.E., Meiners, M.R. and Burwell, B.O. "Asset Spend-down in Nursing Homes: Methods and Insights." *Medical Care* 31 (1): 1-23.
[47]Pepper Commission. 1990; American Association of Retired People. 1998.
[48]Leutz, W. 1998. "Home Care Benefits for Persons with Disabilities." *American Rehabilitation*, 24(3): 6-14, at 7; Kassner, E. and Martin, J. 1996. *Decisions, Decisions: Service Allocation in Home and Community-Based Long-Term Care Programs – A Four-State Analysis*. AARP Public Policy Institute; Litvak, S. and Kennedy, J. 1991. *Policy issues Affecting the Medicaid Personal Care Services Optional Benefit*. Berkeley, CA: World Institute on Disability.
[49]Tilly, Goldenson, and Kasten, at 47. Based on Harrington, C., Carillo, H., Wellin, V., Norwood, F. and Miller, N. 1999. *1915 (c) Medicaid Home and Community-Based Waiver Participants, Services, and Expenditures, 1992-97*. Department of Social and Behavioral Sciences, University of California at San Francisco, November 1999.
[50]Tilly, Goldenson, and Kasten, at 31.
[51]Id.
[52]U.S. Department of Health and Human Services. 1999, at 1.
[53]Meiners, M.R. 1996. "The Financing and Organization of Long-term Care," in Binstock, R.H., Cluff, L.E., and von Mering, O. (editors). *The Future of Long-Term Care: Social and Policy Issues*. Baltimore: Johns Hopkins University Press, c1996, at 192.
[54]Welch, H.G., Wennberg, D.E. and Welch, W.P. 1996. "The Use of Medicare Home Health Care Services." *The New England Journal of Medicine* 335 (5): 324-29.
[55]American Medical Association, Council on Scientific Affairs. 1990. "Home Care in the 1990s." *JAMA* 263: 1241, at 1243.

[56]Leutz Id. at 6.

[57]Davis, B.E. 1998. "The Home Health Care Crisis: Medicare's Fastest Growing Program Legalizes Spiraling Costs." *Elder Law Journal* 6: 215-255.

[58]Stone, at 101.

[59]The regulations for this program are contained in 38 U.S.C. Chapter 11 concerning compensation for service-connected disability or death.

[60]42 U.S.C. Section 3001.

[61]42 U.S.C. sections 1397a- 1397e.

[62]Litvak, S., Zukas, H., Heumann, J.E. 1987. *Attending to America: Personal Assistance for Independent Living*. Berkeley, CA: World Institute on Disability.

[63]Batavia, A.I. 1996. "Health Care, Personal Assistance, and Assistive Technology: Are In-Kind Benefits Key to Independence or Dependence for People with Disabilities?," In *Disability, Cash Benefits and Work*, J.L. Mashaw, et al., (eds.), Kalamazoo, MI: W.E. Upjohn Institute for Employment Research.

[64]Id.

[65]Id.

[66]An MSA is a tax-advantaged savings account, similar to an Individual Retirement Account (IRA), which could be used for certain specified purposes (e.g., medical costs, long-term care, personal assistance services) and could accumulate from year to year.

[67]Batavia, A.I. and DeJong, G. 2001. "Disability, Chronic Illness and Risk Selection, *Archives of Physical Medicine and Rehabilitation* 81: 546-52.

[68]Id.

[69]Newcomer, R., Manton, K., Harrington, C., Yordi, C. and Vertrees, J.C. 1995. "Case Mix Controlled Service Use and Expenditures in the Social/Health Maintenance Organization Demonstration." *Journal of Gerontology* 50A(1): M35-44.

[70]Master, R,. Dreyfus, T., Connors, S., Tobias, C., Zhou, Z. and Kronick, R. 1996. "The Community Medical Alliance: An Integrated System of Care in Greater Boston for People with Severe Disability and AIDS." *Managed Care Quarterly* 4(2): 26-37.

CHAPTER 9

[1]Department of Commerce. 1997. "Disabilities Affect One-Fifth of All Americans: Proportion Could Increase in Coming Decades. *Census Brief* CENBR--97-5 (December, 1997); Tilly, J., Goldenson, S. and Kasten, J. 2001. *Long-Term care: Consumers, Providers and Financing. A Chart Book.* Washington, D.C.: Urban Institute, March, 2001, at 9; Kaye, S., M.P. LaPlante, D. Carlson, and B.L. Wenger. 1996. *Trends in Disability Rates in the United States, 1970-1994.* Washington DC: U.S. Department of Education, National Institute on Disability and Rehabilitation Research.

[2]Arno P.S., Levine C., and Memmott M.M. 1999. "The Economic Value of Informal Caregiving; President Clinton's Proposal to Provide Relief to Family Caregivers Opens a Long-Overdue Discussion of This "Invisible" Health Care Sector." *Health Affairs* 18 (2): 182-188, at 184, 185.

[3]Yamada Y. 2001. "Profile of Home Care Aides, Nursing Home Aides, and Hospital Aides." *Gerontologist* 41: 395-395 Sp. Iss. 1.

[4]Shellenbarger, S. 1994. "Home Aide Shortage Upsets Delicate Balance." *Wall*

Street Journal June 1, 1994, at B1.

[5]Davis, H.L. and Herbeck, D. "Staffing Shortage Reaches a Crisis: The Lack of Nurse Aides at Homes for the Elderly Hurts Quality, And Mistakes in Care Are Common, Sometimes with Deadly Results." *The Buffalo News*, December 11, 2001, p A1.

[6]Crown, W.H. 1994. "A National Profile of Home Care, Nursing Home, and Hospital Aides." *Generations* 18(3): 29-33.

[7]Binstock, R.H., Cluff, L.E., and von Mering, O. 1996. "Issues Affecting the Future of Long-Term Care." In Binstock, R.H., Cluff, L.E., and von Mering, O. (editors). *The Future of Long-Term Care: Social and Policy Issues.* Baltimore, MD: Johns Hopkins University Press, at 14.

[8]For example, some people find the job responsibilities of attorneys, whose profession is considered among the most prestigious in our society, boring and distasteful.

[9]Close, L., Estes, C.L., Linkins, K.W. and Binney, E.A. 1994. "A Political-Economy Perspective on Frontline Workers in Long-Term Care." *Generations* 18(3): 23-27.

[10]Holmes D. 2001. "Staffing Issues As They Pertain to Nursing Home Care of Elderly Persons with Dementing Illness." *Gerontologist* 41: 58 Sp. Iss. 1.

[11]Branin J.J. 2001. "Burnout Among Nursing Home Personnel: The Effectiveness of an Education Training Intervention." *Gerontologist* 41: 92 Sp. Iss. 1.

[12]Doty, P., Kasper, J. and Litvak, S. 1996. "Consumer-Directed Models of Personal Care: Lessons from Medicaid." *Milbank Quarterly* 74 (3): 377-409, at 385; Kennedy, J. and S. Litvak. 1991. *Case Studies of Six State Personal Assistance Services Funded by the Medicaid Personal Care Option.* Oakland, CA: World Institute on Disability.

[13]The WID study found that the average number of hours per week per recipient of services was 25 hours for consumers using independent providers and only 16 hours for consumers using agency providers. Id.

[14]Benjamin, A.E., Matthias, R. and Franke, T.M. 2000. "Comparing Consumer-Directed and Agency Models For Providing Supportive Services at Home." *Health Services Research* 35 (1 Pt 2): 351-66.

[15]Tilly, Weiner, and Cuellar, at 80.

[16]Id.

[17]Id. at 80-81.

[18]O'Connor, A., "Study Offers Complex Portrait of Domestic Workers Labor: Many Feel Invisible and Excluded from the Lives of the Families They Serve. Wages in the Richest Areas Aren't Always Highest." *Los Angeles Times*, April 11, 2001, at B-1.

[19]Tilly, Weiner, and Cuellar, at 80; citing Baarveld et al. 1998. *Persoonsgebonden Budget Arbeidsmarktpositie van Zorgverleners.* Nijmegen, Netherlands: Instituut voor Toegepaste Sociale Wetenschappen van de Stricting Katholieke Universiteit te Nijmegen.

[20]Benjamin, Matthias, and Franke, 2000.

[21]Id.

[22]Id.

[23]Id.

[24]Wilner, M.A. 2000. "Toward a Stable and Experienced Caregiving Workforce." *Generations*, 24(3): 60-65, at 62.

[25]Nadash, P. 1998. "Independent Choices." *American Rehabilitation* 24(3): 15-20, at 18.

[26]Id. at 18.

[27]Stone, D.A. 1991. "Commentary: Caring Work in a Liberal Polity." *Journal of Health Politics, Policy and Law* 16(3): 547-552.

[28]Batavia, A.I. 1991. "Caring Through Personal Assistance Policy: A Response," *Journal of Health Politics, Policy and Law* 16(4).

[29]Wilner, at 64.

[30]Leutz, W. 1998. "Home Care Benefits for Persons with Disabilities." *American Rehabilitation*, 24(3): 6-14, at 9.

[31]Pijl, M. 1994. "When Private Care Goes Public: An Analysis of Concepts and Principles Concerning Payments for Care." In Evers, A., Pijl, M., and Ungerson, C. (editors), *Payments for Care*. Brookfield, VT: Ashgate, at 3-18.

[32]Leutz at 9.

[33]Stryckman, J. and Nahmiash, D. 1994. "Payments for care: The Case of Canada." In Evers, A., Pijl, M., and Ungerson, C. (editors), *Payments for Care*. Brookfield, VT: Ashgate, at 307-19.

[34]Pijl, M., Mandmaker, T., Daal, H.J.V., and Schoonman, B. 1994. "Payments for Care: the Case of the Netherlands." In Evers, A., Pijl, M., and Ungerson, C. (editors), *Payments for Care*. Brookfield, VT: Ashgate, at 145-64.

[35]Horowitz, A. and Shindelman, L. 1983. "Social and Economic Incentives For Family Caregivers." *Health Care Financing Review* 5(2): 25-33.

[36]Id. at 12.

[37]Flanagan, S.A., Green, P.S. and Eustis, N. 1998. "You Can Do It: State Initiatives Broaden Access to Consumer-Directed Personal Assistance Services through the Use Of Intermediary Service Organizations." *American Rehabilitation* 24(3): 21-26, at 22.

[38]Id.

[39]Id. at 22-23.

[40]Id. at 23.

[41]Id. at 24.

[42]Id. at 25.

[43]Id. at 24.

[44]Id. at 25.

[45]Id. at 25.

[46]Wong, D. 2000. "Rapid Response: Development of a Home Care Worker Replacement Service." *Generations* 24(3): 88-90, at 89.

CHAPTER 10

[1]Tanenbaum, S.J. and Hurley, R.E. 1995. "Managed Care, Disability and the 1115 Waiver Frenzy: A Cautionary Note. *Health Affairs* 14 (4): 113-19.

[2]Brook, R.H., McGlynn, E.A. and Cleary, P.H. 1996. "Measuring Quality of Care." *The New England Journal of Medicine* 335(13): 966-69.

[3]Verweij M. 2001. "Individual and Collective Considerations in Public Health: Influenza Vaccination in Nursing Homes." *Bioethics* 15 (5-6): 536-546 Sp. Iss. SI.

[4]Bresnitz E, Grant C, Ostrawski S, et al. 2001. "Outbreak of Pneumococcal Pneumonia Among Unvaccinated Residents of a Nursing Home." *Journal of the American Medical Association (JAMA)* 286 (13): 1570-1571; Ghilardi G, Wietlisbach

V, Petignat C, et al. 2001. "The Reciprocal Relationship Between Infections and Functional Impairment in Nursing Home Residents." *Gerontologist* 41: 346 Sp. Iss. 1.

[5]Id.

[6]Kane, R.A., Kane, R.L., Illston, L.H., and Eustis, N.N. 1994. "Perspectives on Home Care Quality." *Healthcare Financing Review* 16(1): 69-89, at 69.

[7]Id. at 74.

[8]Id. at 72.

[9]Id. at 71.

[10]Enthoven, A.C. 1980. *Health Plan: The Only Practical Solution to the Soaring Cost of Medical Care*. Addison-Wesley Publishing Company: Reading, MA.

[11]Latimer, J. 1997-98. "The Essential Role of Regulation To Assure Quality in Long-term Care." *Generations* 21(4): 10-14.

[12]Institute of Medicine. 1986. *Improving the Quality of Care in Nursing Homes*, Washington, D.C., National Academy of Sciences; Mattson, M. 2001. "Nursing Home Quality Declines. Facing a Tide of Lawsuits and Horror Stories, the Industry Says It Is Working to Improve, but Florida Legislature May Not Wait." *The Florida Times-Union*, A-1 (April 1, 2001);. Mattson, M. 2000. "Nursing Homes in Crisis," The Florida Times-Union, A-1 (June 4, 2001); Walters, S. 2001. "Nursing Home Violations Rise: Life-threatening Problems at Some Long-term Centers Worry State Officials." *Milwaukee Journal Sentinel*, at 1 (April 8, 2001); Boo, K. 1999. "Residents Languish, Profiteers flourish While Deaths and Abuse Go Unexamined, For-Profit Operators Milk a Lax System." *The Washington Post*, A-1 (March 15, 1999); Zambito, T. and Layton, M.J. 1999. "Criminal Caregivers: Home Health Care in Crisis, Lax State Laws Let Danger Enter the Frailest Lives." *The Record*, A-1 (October 3, 1999); Pham, A. 1997. "Home Care: A Troubling Diagnosis." *The Boston Globe*, A-1 (October 5, 1997).

[13]Hawes, C. 1997-8. "Regulation and the Politics of Long-Term Care." *Generations* 21(4): 5-9, at 5.

[14]Institute of Medicine. 1986.

[15]Latimer, 1997-98.

[16]Kane, R.A., Kane, R.L., Ladd, R.C. 1998. *The Heart of Long-Term Care*. New York; Oxford : Oxford University Press, at 209-210; quoted in Kapp, M.B. 1999. "Home Health Care Regulation: Is It Good for the Patient?" *Journal of Long-Term Home Health Care* 1(4): 251-57, at 251-52.

[17]Hawes, at 5-9.

[18]Edelman, T.E. 1997-98. "The Politics of Long-Term Care at the Federal Level and Implications for Quality." *Generations* 21(4): 37-41, at 39-40.

[19]Phillips, C.D., Hawes, C., Mor, V., Fries, B.E, and Morris, J.N. 1997-8. "Geriatric Assessment in Nursing Homes in the United States: Impact of a National Program." *Generations* 21(4): 15-24, at 22-24.

[20]Hawes, at 7-8.

[21]Enthoven, A.C. 1980.

[22]Kane, Kane, Illston, and Eustis, at 72.

[23]Kane, R.L. 1995. "Improving the Quality of Long-Term Care." *JAMA* 273(17): 1376-80, at 1377.

[24]Bowers, B.J., Fibich, B. and Jacobson, N. 2001. "Care-As-Service, Care-As-

Relating, Care-As-Comfort: Understanding Nursing Home Residents' Definitions of Quality." *Gerontologist* 41 (4): 539-545.

[25]Kane, Kane, Illston, and Eustis, at 76.

[26]Zimmerman, D.R. 1997-98. "The Power of Information: Using Resident Assessment Data to Assure and Improve Quality of Nursing Home Care." *Generations* 21(4): 52-56, at 53.

[27]Applebaum, R., Mollica, R. and Tilly, J. 1997-8. "Assuring Homecare Quality: A Case Study of State Strategies." *Generations* 21(4): 57-63, at 61.

[28]Nadash, P. 1998. "Independent Choices." *American Rehabilitation* 24(3): 15-20, at 18.

[29]Id.

[30]Id.

[31]Geron, S.M. 2000. "The Quality of Consumer-Directed Long-term Care." *Generations*, 24(3): 66-73, at 68-69.

[32]Id. at 78.

[33]Id. at 80.

[34]Geron, at 69.

[35]Eustis, N.N., Fischer, L.R. and Kane, R.A. 1994. "The Home Care Worker: On the Frontline of Quality." *Generations*, 18: 43-49; Eustis, N.N. and Fischer, L.R. 1992. "Common Needs, Different Solutions? Younger and Older Home Care Clients." *Generations*, 16: 17-22.

[36]Geron, at 70.

[37]Geron, S.M., et al. 2000. "The Home Care Satisfaction Measure: A Client-Centered Approach on Assessing the Satisfaction of Frail Older Adults With Home Health Care services." *Journal of Gerontology: Social Services* 52B(5): 259-70.

[38]Reid, D., Haas, W. and Hawkings, D. 1977. "Locus of Desired Control and Positive Self-concept of the Elderly." *Journal of Gerontology* 32(4): 441-50.; Lefcourt, H.M., editor. 1981. *Research With the Locus of Control Construct.* Volume 1. New York, Academic Press.

[39]Doty, P., Kasper, J. and Litvak, S., 1996. "Consumer-Directed Models of Personal Care: Lessons from Medicaid," *Milbank Memorial Fund Quarterly* 74 (3): 377-409; Doty, P., et al. 1999. *In-home Supportive Services for the Elderly And Disabled: Comparison of Client-Directed and Professional Management Models of Service Delivery.* Non-technical summary report. Washington, D.C.: Office of the Assistant Secretary for Planning and Evaluation, U.S. Department of Health and Human Services.; Geron, S.M., et al. 2000.

[40]Geron, S.M. 2000. "The Quality of Consumer-Directed Long-term Care." *Generations*, 24(3): 66-73, at 69.

[41]Kapp, M.B. 1997. "Who Is Responsible for This? Assigning Rights and Consequences in Elder Care." *Journal of Aging and Social Policy*, 9(2): 51-65; Kapp, M.B. 1999. "From Medical Patients to Health Care Consumers: Decisional Capacity and Choices to Purchase Coverage And Services." *Aging and Mental Health* 3(4): 294-300; Sabatino, C.P. and Litvak, S. 1992. "Consumer-directed homecare: What Makes It Possible?" *Generations* 14 (3): 53-58.

[42]Flanagan, S.A. 1994. *Consumer-Directed Attendant Services: How States Address Tax, Legal, and Quality Assurance Issues.* Cambridge, Massachusetts: SysteMetrics/MEDSTAT, Inc.; Flanagan, S.A. and Green, P.S. (1997). *Consumer-*

Directed Personal Assistance Services: Key Operational Issues for States Using Fiscal Intermediary Service Organizations. Cambridge, MA: MEDSTAT, Inc.

[43]Hofland, B.F. and David, D. 1990. "Autonomy and Long-Term Care Practice: Conclusions and Next Steps." *Generations* 14 (Supplement): at 91; Kapp, M.B. 1996. "Enhancing Autonomy and Choice in Selecting and Directing Long-Term Care Services." *The Elder Law Journal* 4 (1): 55-97, at 70.

[44]Kapp., M.B. 2000. "Quality of Care and Quality of Life in Nursing Facilities: What's Regulation Got to Do with It? 31 *McGeorge Law Review* 707 .

[45]Kane, R.L. 1995. "Improving the Quality of Long-Term Care." *JAMA* 273(17): 1376-80, at 1376.

[46]Kapp, M.B. 1999. "Home Health Care Regulation: Is it Good for the Patient?" *Journal of Long-Term Home Health Care* 1(4): 251-57, at 251.

[47]Benjamin, A.E., Matthias, R. and Franke, T.M. 2000. "Comparing Consumer-Directed and Agency Models for Providing Supportive Services at Home." *Health Services Research* 2000 Apr; 35 (1 Pt 2): 351-66.

[48]Tilly, J., Wiener, J.M., and Cuellar, A.E. 2000. "Consumer-Directed Home-and Community-based Services Programs in Five Countries: Policy Issues for Older People and Government." *Generations,* 24(3): 74-84, at 81.

[49]Id.

[50]Id.

[51]Id. at 82.

[52]Id.

[53]Id. at 81.

[54]Geron, S.M. 2000. "The Quality of Consumer-Directed Long-Term Care." *Generations* 24(3): 66-73, at 68.

[55]Id. at 72.

CHAPTER 11

[1]Wiener, J.M. 1996. "Managed Care and Long-Term Care: The Integration of Financing and Services." *Generations* 20(2): 47-52.

[2]Id. at 51.

[3]DeJong, G. and Sutton, J. 1998. "Managed Care and People with Disabilities: Framing the Issues." *Archives of Physical Medicine and Rehabilitation* 79:1312; DeJong, G. and Sutton, J. 1998. "Managed Care and Catastrophic Injury: The Case of Spinal Cord Injury." *Topics in Spinal Cord Injury Rehabilitation* 1998: 3(4): 1-16.

[4]Frieden, L., Smith, L., Wilkinson, W., Redd, L., and Smith, Q. 1998. "Spinal Cord Injury and Managed Care: A Consumer Viewpoint." *Topics in Spinal Cord Injury Rehabilitation* 1998:3(4): 80-88.

[5]Batavia, A.I. and DeJong, G. 2001. "Disability, Chronic Illness and Risk Selection, *Archives of Physical Medicine and Rehabilitation,* 81: 546-52.

[6]Master R., Dreyfus, T., Connors, S., Tobias, C., Zhou, Z., and Kronick, R. 1996. "The Community Medical Alliance: An Integrated System of Care in Greater Boston for People with Severe Disability and AIDS." *Managed Care Quarterly* 4(2): 26-37; Newcomer, R., Manton, K., Harrington, C., Yordi, C., and Vertrees, J.C. 1995. "Case Mix Controlled Service Use and Expenditures in the Social/Health Maintenance Organization Demonstration." *Journal of Gerontology* 50A(1): M35-44.

[7]Newcomer, et al., 1995.

[8]Criscione, T., Kastner, T.A., O'Brien, D. and Nathanson, R. 1994. "Replication of a

Managed Health Care Initiative for People with Mental Retardation Living in the Community." *Mental Retardation* 32(1): 43-52; Criscione, T., Walsh, K.K. and Kastner, T.A. 1995. "An Evaluation the Care Coordination in Controlling Inpatient Hospital Utilization of People with Developmental Disabilities." *Mental Retardation* 33(6): 364-73.
[9]Wilner, M.A. and Wyatt, A. 1998. "Independent Care System: Managed Care for People with Disabilities." *American Rehabilitation* 24(3): 2-5, at 2.
[10]Id. at 3.
[11]Id. at 4.
[12]Kapp, M.B. 1996. "Enhancing Autonomy and Choice in Selecting and Directing Long-term Care Services." *The Elder Law Journal* 4 (1): 55-97, at 62.
[13]Id. at 62-63.
[14]Gilson, S.F. and Casebolt, G.J. 1997. "Personal Assistance Services and Case Management." *Journal of Case Management* 6(1): 13-17.
[15]Id., at 13.
[16]Id.
[17]Kane, R.A. 1988. "Case Management: Ethical Pitfalls on the Road to High-quality Managed Care." *Quality Review Bulletin* 161.
[18]Kapp, at 73.
[19]Id.
[20]DeJong, G. 1979. "Independent Living: From Social Movement to Analytic Paradigm." *Archives of Physical Medicine and Rehabilitation* 60: 435-446; Shapiro, J.P. 1993. *No Pity: People with Disabilities Forging a New Civil Rights Movement.* New York, NY: Random House.
[21]Scala M.A., Mayberry, P.S. and Kunkel, S.R. 1996. "Consumer-Directed Home Care: Client Profiles and Service Challenges." *Journal of Case Management* 5(3): 91-8.
[22]Kafka, B. 1994. "Perspectives on Personal Assistance Services." *Independent Living* Winter-Spring 1994, at 11.
[23]Kapp at 80.
[24]Phillips V.L. 1996. "The Role of Case Managers in a United Kingdom Experiment with Self-Directed Care." *Journal of Case Management* Winter;5(4): 142-5.

CHAPTER 12

[1]Much of the information in this chapter is derived from the following sources: Tilly, J. and Bechtel, R. 1999. *Consumer-Directed Long-Term Care: Participant's Experiences in Five Countries.* Washington, D.C.: American Association of Retired Persons; Tilly, J., Weiner, J.M., and Cuellar, A.E. 2000. "Consumer-Directed Home-and Community-based Services Programs in Five Countries: Policy Issues for Older People and Government." *Generations*, 24(3): 74-84.
[2]*See* table 1 in Tilly, Weiner, and Cuellar, at 76.
[3]Information on the Austrian program derives from the following: Badelt, C., et al. 1997. *Analyse der Auswirkungen des Pflegevor-sorgesystems.* Vienna, Austria: Bundesministeriums fur Arbeit, Gesundheit un Soziales.
[4]Keigher, S.M. 1997. "Austria's New Attendance Allowance: A Consumer-Choice Model of Care For the Frail and Disabled." *International Journal of Health Services* 27(4): 753-65.
[5]Information on the German program derives from the following: Runde, P. et al. 1996. *Einstellungen und Verhalten zur Pflegeversicherung und zur Hauslichen Pflege.* Hamburg, Germany: Universitat Hamburg.

[6]Information on the French program derives from the following: Comite National de Vigilance. 1998. *Le Livre Noir de la P.S.D.* Paris, France.; Observatoire National de' Action Socialee Decentralisee (OANSD). 1998. *La PSD un An Apres: Premieres Tendances.* Paris, France.; Simon, M.O. and Martin, P.A. 1996. La Prestation Dependance: Rapport Final du Programme d' Evaluation de l' Experimentation d' une Prestation Dependence. Paris, France: Centre de Recherche pour l'Etude et l'Observation des Conditions de Vie CREDOC.

[7]Id.

[8]Information on the Dutch program derives from the following: Baarveld et al. 1998. *Persoonsgebonden Budget Arbeidsmarktpositie van Zorgverleners.* Nijmegen, Netherlands: Instituut voor Toegepaste Sociale Wetenschappen van de Stricting Katholieke Universiteit te Nijmegen.; Miltenburg, T., et al. 1996. *A Personal Budget for Clients: Summary of An Experiment with Cash Benefits in Home Care in the Netherlands. Institute for Applied Social Sciences.* Nijmegen, Netherlands.; Woldringh, C. and Ramakers, C. 1998. *Persoonsgebonden Budget Verpleging Verzorging Ervaringen van Budgethouders en Kwaliteit van Zorg.* Nijmegen, Netherlands: Instituut voor Toegepaste Sociale Wetenschappen van de Stricting Katholieke Universiteit te Nijmegen.

[9]European Social Network (John Halloran, editor). 1998. *Towards a People's Europe: A. Report on the Development of Direct Payments in 10 Member States of the European Union.* East Sussex, United Kingdom: European Social Network.

[10]Phillips V.L. 1996. "The Role of Case Managers in a United Kingdom Experiment with Self-Directed Care." *Journal of Case Management* 5(4): 142-5.

[11]Askheim, O.P. 1999. "Personal Assistance for Disabled People-the Norwegian Experience." *International Journal of Social Welfare* 8(2): 111-119.

CHAPTER 13

[1]Senate Committee on Labor and Human Resources. 1991. *Personal Assistance Services and Independence for the Disabled.* United States Senate. Washington, D.C.: 102nd Congress, 1st Session, on examining the need for coverage of personal assistance services to enable Americans with disabilities to achieve more independent living. July 25, 1991.

[2]Benjamin, A.E., Matthias, R. & Franke, T.M. 2000. "Comparing Consumer-Directed and Agency Models for Providing Supportive Services at Home." *Health Services Research* 2000 Apr; 35 (1 Pt 2): 351-66, at 351.

[3]Feldstein, P.J. 2001. *The Politics of Health Legislation: An Economic Approach,* 3rd ed., Chicago, IL: Health Administration Press.

[4]Batavia, A.I., DeJong, G. & McKnew, L.B. 1991. "Toward a National Personal Assistance Program: The Independent Living Model of Long-Term Care for Persons with Disabilities." *Journal of Health Politics, Policy, and Law* 16(3): 523-545; Batavia, A.I. 1998. "The Prospects for a National Personal Assistance Services Program for People with Disabilities." *American Rehabilitation* 24 (3).

[5]Personal e-mail correspondence, August 2002.

[6]"The rich heterogeneity of attitudes and preferences regarding autonomy among potential LTC clients firmly underscores the need for a national policy that assures the availability of a variety of service financing and delivery models rather than the inflexible bureaucratic imposition of any single model – even one sincerely intended to promote autonomy – on all home and community-based clients. Legislative overgeneralization and oversimplification, even in what most people would consider a socially

desirable direction, must be guarded against." Kapp, M.B. 1996. "Enhancing Autonomy and Choice in Selecting and Directing Long-Term Care Services." *The Elder Law Journal* 4 (1): 55-97, at 68.

[7]Id. at 69.

[8]Batavia, A.I. 1996. "Health Care, Personal Assistance, and Assistive Technology: Are In-Kind Benefits Key to Independence or Dependence for People with Disabilities?," In *Disability, Cash Benefits and Work* (Mashaw, J.L., et al., (eds.), Kalamazoo, MI: W.E. Upjohn Institute for Employment Research.

[9]Doty, P. 2000. "The Federal Role in the Move toward Consumer Direction." *Generations* 24(3): 922-27; Doty, P. J. 1998. "The Cash and Counseling Demonstration: An Experiment in Consumer-Directed Personal Assistance Services." *American Rehabilitation* 24(3): 27-30.

[10]Flanagan, S.A. 1994. *Consumer-Directed Attendant Services: How States Address Tax, Legal, and Quality Assurance Issues.* Cambridge, MA.: SysteMetrics/MEDSTAT, Inc. Flanagan, S.A. and Green, P.S. 1997. Consumer-Directed Personal Assistance Services: Key Operational Issues for State CD-PAS Programs Using Fiscal Intermediary Service Organizations. Cambridge, MA.: MEDSTAT, Inc.

[11]Kapp at 66.

[12]Batavia, 1996.

[13]Batavia, 1998; Batavia, A.I. 2002. "Consumer Direction, Consumer Choice and the Future of Long-Term Care." *Journal of Disability Policy Studies* 13(2): 67-73, 86.

[14]Id.

[15]Sabatino, C.P. & Litvak, S. 1992. "Consumer-Directed Homecare: What Makes It Possible?" *Generations* 14 (3): 53-58, at 57.

APPENDIX A

[1]Flanagan, S.A. 1994. *Consumer-Directed Attendant Services: How States Address Tax, Legal, and Quality Assurance Issues.* Cambridge, MA: SysteMetrics/MEDSTAT, Inc.

[2]Sabatino, C.P. and Litvak, S. 1996. "Liability Issues Affecting Consumer-Directed Personal Assistance Services—Report and Recommendations." *The Elder Law Journal* 4: 247, 259.

[3]Flanagan, S.A. and Green, P.S. 1997. *Consumer-Directed Personal Assistance Services: Key Operational Issues for State CD-PAS Programs Using Fiscal Intermediary Service Organizations.* Cambridge, MA: MEDSTAT, Inc., at 9.

[4]In one case, the state of Missouri was required to pay back taxes that were not a paid by consumers who were the actual employers of record. Id. at 9.

[5]Id. at 19.

[6]Kapp, M.B. 2000. "Consumer Direction in Long-Term Care: ATaxonomy of Legal Issues." *Generations* 24(3): 16-21, at 16.

[7]42 CFR Part 484; 42 CFR Section 440.70 (d).

[8]Kapp, at 18.

[9]Flanagan and Green, at 12.

[10]Id.

[11]Id. at 13.

[12]Id.

[13]Flanagan and Green, at 48.

[14]Sabatino and Litvik, at 265.

[15]I.R.C. 3403, 3509.

[16]26 U.S.C. 3401-3406.

[17]26 U.S.C. 3401(a)(3).

[18]26 C.F.R. 31.3121(a)(7)-1(a)(2).

[19]Domestic services include: "services performed by cooks, waiters, butlers, house-keepers, governesses, maids, valets, baby sitters, janitors, laundresses, furnacemen, caretakers, handymen, gardeners, footmen, grooms, and chauffeurs of automobiles for family use." Id. Sabatino and Litvik, at 265.

[20]Rev. Rul. 74-205, 1974-1 C.B. 21; Sabatino and Litvik, at 267.

[21]Sabatino and Litvik, at 267.

[22]Federal Insurance Contribution Act (FICA), I.R.C. 3101, 3102, 3121 (1994) (regarding tax on employees, tax on employers, and definitions).

[23]I.R.C. 3121(a).

[24]Social Security Domestic Employment Reform Act of 1994, Pub. L. No. 103-387, 108 Stat 4071 (codified as amended in 26 U.S.C.), signed into law on October 22, 1994.

[25]The threshold was set at $1,000 annually for 1994 and is now indexed annually for inflation.

[26]Federal Unemployment Tax Act (FUTA), I.R.C. 33013311.

[27]The Fair Labor Standards Act (FLSA), 29 U.S.C. 201-219.

[28]The companionship services exemption to the minimum wage and maximum hour requirement states that: "Any employee employed on a casual basis in domestic service employment to provide babysitting services or any employee employed in domestic service employment to provide companionship services for individuals who (because of age or infirmity) are unable to care for themselves." 29 U.S.C. 213(a)(15). "Companionship services" are defined as "those services which provide fellowship, care, and protection for a person who, because of advanced age or physical or mental infirmity, cannot care for his or her own needs. Such services may include household work related to the care of the aged or infirm person such as meal preparation, bed making, washing of clothes, and other similar services. They may also include the performance of general household work. Provided, however, That such work is incidental, i.e., does not exceed 20 percent of the total weekly hours worked." 29 C.F.R. 552.6.

[29]The term "companionship services" does not include services relating to the care and protection of the aged or infirm which require and are performed by trained personnel, such as a registered or practical nurse." 29 C.F.R. 552.6.

[30]Sabatino and Litvak, at 277-78.

[31]Id., at 285.

[32]Kane, R., O'Connor, C. and Baker, M. 1995. *Delegation of Nursing Activities: Implications for Patterns of Long-term Care.* AARP Public Policy Institute #9515: Washington, D.C. (November 1995), at 2.

[33]Flanagan. and Green, at 43.

[34]Id. at 44-45.

[35]This exemption for care provided by friends and family provides legal authorization for care provided under the informal support model.

[36]This exemption for care provided by domestic servants also arguably provides legal authorization for care provided under the independent living model, particularly for consumers who are not eligible for care under a state program and who pay for their personal assistance services out-of-pocket. The question raised is whether a more specific exemption is needed for personal assistants under state programs.

[37]National Institute on Consumer-Directed Long-Term Services. 1997. *Autonomy or Abandonment: Changing Perspectives on Delegation.* Washington D.C.: The National Council on the Aging.
[38]Id.
[39]Flanagan and Green, at 45.
[40]Nadash P. 1998. "Delegation. Creating a Balance among Home Care, the Disability Community, Regulators, and Payors." *Caring* 17(7): 20.
[41]Flanagan and Green, at 39-40.
[42]Id. at E-9.
[43]5 U.S.C. 8101 (1994).
[44]Id. at 38.
[45]Id. at 39.
[46]Simon-Rusinowitz, L., Bochniak, A.M.,. Mahoney, K.J., and Marks, L.N. 2000. "Implementation Issues for Consumer-Directed Programs: a Survey of Policy Experts." *Generations* 24(3): 34-40, at 37.

APPENDIX B

[1]Doty, P., Kasper, J., Litvak, S., 1996. "Consumer-Directed Models of Personal Care: Lessons from Medicaid," *Milbank Memorial Fund Quarterly* 74 (3): 377-409.
[2]Feinberg, L.F., Whitlatch, C.J. and Tucke, S. 2000. *Making Hard Choices: Respecting Both Voices—Final Report.* San Francisco: Family Caregiver Alliance.
[3]Kapp, M.B. 1999. "From Medical Patients to Health Care Consumers: Decisional Capacity and Choices to Purchase Coverage and Services." *Aging and Mental Health* 3(4): 294-300, at 300.
[4]Id. at 295.
[5]Id.
[6]Kapp, M.B. 2001. "Consumer Choice in Long-term Care: What the United States Can Teach and Learn From Others about Decisionally Incapacitated Consumers." *International Journal of Law and Psychiatry* 24(3): 199-211, at 205.
[7]Kapp, M.B. 1996. "Enhancing Autonomy and Choice in Selecting and Directing Long-term Care Services." *The Elder Law Journal* 4 (1): 55-97, at 85.
[8]Id. at 295.
[9]Id.
[10]Id.
[11]Kapp, M.B. 1990. "Evaluating Decisionmaking Capacity in the Elderly: A Review of Recent Literature." *Journal of Elder Abuse and Neglect* 2: 15.
[12]Feinberg, Whitlatch, and Tucke, at 3, 6.
[13]Id. at 4.
[14]Id.
[15]Id. at 5.
[16]Id. at 6.
[17]Id. at 9.
[18]Id.
[19]Kapp, at 296.
[20]Id. at 297.
[21]Kapp, at 207.
[22]Mayer, R.R, Mahoney, Berson, A. and Marks, J. 2000. "A Consumer-Directed Home Care Program for the Cognitively Impaired." *Generations* 24(3): 98-99.

Bibliography

Congressional and other Governmental Materials

General Accounting Office. 1999. *Adults With Severe Disabilities: Federal and State Approaches for Personal Care and Other Services.* (GAO/HEHS-99-101). Washington, D.C.: General Accounting Office.

General Accounting Office. 1997. *Medicare Home Health Agencies: Certification Process Ineffective in Excluding Problem Agencies* (GAO/HRD-98-29). Washington, D.C.: General Accounting Office.

General Accounting Office. 1994. *Long-Term Care: Status of Quality Assurance and Measurement in Home and Community-Based Services.* (GAO/PEMD-94-19). Washington, D.C.: General Accounting Office, March 1994.

General Accounting Office. 1994. *Long-Term Care Reform: States' Views of Key Elements of Well-designed Programs for the Elderly.* (GAO/HEHS-94-227). Washington, D.C.: General Accounting Office.

General Accounting Office. 1994. *Medicaid Long-term Care: Successful State Efforts to Expand Home Services While Limiting Costs.* (GAO/HEHS-94-167). Washington, D.C.: General Accounting Office.

General Accounting Office. 1993. *Long-Term Care Insurance: High Percentage of Policy Holders Drop Policies.* (GAO/HRD93-129). Washington, D.C.: General Accounting Office.

General Accounting Office. 1993. *Long-Term Care Case Management: State Experiences and Implications for Federal Policy.* (GAO/HRD93-52). Washington, D.C.: General Accounting Office.

Health Care Financing Administration. 1994. "Final Rule: Medicare and Medicaid Programs: Survey, Certification, and Enforcement for Skilled Nursing Facilities and

Nursing Facilities." *Federal Register* 59: 56, 116-56, 252. November 10. Washington, D.C.

Health Care Financing Administration. 1993. *Approaches to Quality under Home and Community-Based Services Waivers*. Baltimore, MD: Medicaid Bureau.

Senate Committee on Aging. 1994. *Long-Term Care*. Hearing before the Special Committee on Aging, United States Senate, 103rd Congress (2nd Session), Milwaukee, WI, S. Hrg. 103-20, May 9, 1994, U.S. Government Printing Office.

Senate Committee on Aging. 1999. *Long-Term Care for the 21st Century: A Common Sense Proposal to Support Family Caregiver*. Hearing before the Committee on Aging, United States Senate, 106th Congress (1st Session), S. Hrg. 106-102, March 23, 1999, U.S. Government Printing Office.

Senate Committee on Finance. 1995. *Deinstitutionalization, Medical Illness and Medications*. Hearing before the Committee on Finance, United States Senate, 103rd Congress (2nd Session), S. Hrg. 103-1011, May 10, 1994, U.S. Government Printing Office.

Pepper Commission. 1990. *A Call for Action (Final report)*. U.S. Bipartisan Commission on Comprehensive Health Care, Washington, D.C.

Senate Committee on Labor and Public Welfare. 1935. *The Aged and Aging in the United States: A National Problem: Summary and Recommendations*. United States Senate. Washington, D.C.:86th Congress, 2nd Session.

Senate Committee on Labor and Human Resources. 1991. *Personal Assistance Services and Independence for the Disabled*. United States Senate. Washington, D.C.: 102nd Congress, 1st Session, on examining the need for coverage of personal assistance services to enable Americans with disabilities to achieve more independent living. July 25, 1991.

U.S. Department of Health and Human Services. 1999. *A Descriptive Analysis of Patterns of Informal and Formal Caregiving among Privately Insured and Non-Privately Insured Disabled Elders Living in the Community: Final Report*. Washington, D.C.: Office of Disability, Aging and Long-Term Care Policy.

U.S. Department of Health and Human Services. Office of Disability, Aging and Long-Term Care Policy. 1994. *Summary of Long-Term Care Provisions under the Health Security Act*. Washington D.C.: U.S. Government Printing Office.

Books, Chapters, Monographs and Reports

Agosta, J. 1999. Human Services Research Institute, for the New Jersey Personal Preference Cash and Counseling Demonstration Program. *You Can Do It! A Consumer Guide for Managing Your Own Cash Grant for Household Employees*. University of Maryland Center on Aging.

American Association of Retired People. 1998. *Medicaid and Long-Term Care for Older People*. Washington, D.C.: AARP Policy Institute.

American Association of Retired People. 1997. *Out-of-Pocket Health Spending by Medicare Beneficiaries Age 65 and Older*. Washington, D.C.: AARP Policy Institute.

American Association of Retired People. 1995. *Home and Community-Based Long-Term Care* (13R). Washington, D.C.: Center on Elderly People Living Alone.

Baarveld et al. 1998. *Persoonsgebonden Budget Arbeidsmarktpositie van Zorgverleners*. Nijmegen, Netherlands: Instituut voor Toegepaste Sociale Wetenschappen van de Stricting Katholieke Universiteit te Nijmegen.

Badelt, C., et al. 1997. *Analyse der Auswirkungen des Pflegevorsorgesystems*. Vienna, Austria: Bundesministeriums fur Arbeit, Gesundheit un Soziales.

Barresi, C.M. and Stull, D.E. 1993. *Ethnic Elderly and Long-Term Care*. New York: Springer Publishing.

Batavia, A.I. 1996. "Health Care, Personal Assistance, and Assistive Technology: Are In-Kind Benefits Key to Independence or Dependence for People with Disabilities?," *In Disability, Cash Benefits and Work* (Mashaw, J.L., et al., (eds.), Kalamazoo, MI: W.E. Upjohn Institute for Employment Research.

Benjamin, A.E, Matthias, R., Franke, T., Mills, Hasenfeld, Y., Matras, L., Park, E., Stoddard, S. and Kraus, L. 1998. *Comparing Consumer-Directed and Agency Models for Providing Supportive Services at Home*. Final Report under HHS Contract #100-94-0022. Los Angeles, CA: School of Public Welfare, University of California, Los Angeles.

Binstock, R.H., Cluff, L.E., and von Mering, O. (editors). 1996. *The Future of Long-Term Care: Social and Policy Issues*. Baltimore, MD: Johns Hopkins University Press.

Cameron, K. and Firman, J. 1995. *International and Domestic Programs Using "Cash and Counseling" Strategies to Pay for Long-Term Care*. Washington, D.C.: National Council on the Aging.

Coleman, B. 1998. "New Directions for State Long-Term Care Systems." 2nd Edition. Washington D.C.: American Association of Retired Persons.

Commonwealth Fund Commission on Elderly People Living Alone. 1993. *The Importance of Choice in Medicaid Home Care Programs: Maryland, Michigan, and Texas*. (Survey conducted for Commonwealth Fund by Taylor, H., Leitman, R. and Barnett, S.). New York: Louis Harris and Associates.

Comite National de Vigilance. 1998. *Le Livre Noir de la P.S.D*. Paris, France.

Dautel, P.J. and Frieden, L. 1999. *Consumer Choice and Control: Personal Attendant*

Services and Supports in America (Report of the National Blue Ribbon Panel on Personal Assistance Services). Houston, TX: Independent Living and Research Utilization Program, available on the Internet at www.ilru.org.

Department of Commerce. 1997. "Disabilities Affect One-Fifth of All Americans: Proportion Could Increase in Coming Decades. *Census Brief* CENBR--97-5 (December, 1997).

Desmond, S.M., Shoop, D.M., Simon-Rusinowitz, L., Mahoney, K.J., Squillace, M.R. and Fay, R.A. 1998. *Comparing Preferences for a Cash Option Versus Traditional Services, Florida Elders and Adults with Physical Disabilities, Telephone Survey Technical Report, Background Research for the Cash and Counseling Demonstration and Evaluation*. College Park, MD: University of Maryland Center on Aging.

Doty, P., Benjamin, A.E., Matthias, R.E.and Franke, T.M. 1999. *In-Home Supportive Services For the Elderly and Disabled: Comparison of Client-Directed and Professional Management Models of Service Delivery*. Non-technical summary report. Washington, D.C.: Office of the Assistant Secretary for Planning and Evaluation, U.S. Department of Health and Human Services.

Dunlop, B.D. 1979. *The Growth of Nursing Home Care*. Lexington, MA: Lexington Books.

Egley, L. 1994. *Program Models Providing Personal Assistance Services (PAS) for Independent Living*. Berkeley, CA: World Institute on Disability.

Egley, L. 1994. *New Federal PC Option PAS Funding Rules: Summary*. Berkeley, CA: World Institute on Disability.

Ellison, M.L. and Ashbaugh, J. 1990. *The Dollars and Sense of Promoting Self-sufficiency of Persons with Disabilities Through Programs of Independent Living, In-Home and Family Supports*. Cambridge, MA: Human Services Research Institute.

Enthoven, A.C. 1980. *Health Plan: The Only Practical Solution to the Soaring Cost of Medical Care*. Reading, MA: Addison-Wesley Publishing Company.

European Social Network (Halloran, J., editor). 1998. *Towards a People's Europe: A. report on the Development of Direct Payments in 10 Member States of the European Union*. East Sussex, United Kingdom: European Social Network.

Feldstein, P.J. 2001. *The Politics of Health Legislation: An Economic Approach*, 3rd ed., Chicago, IL: Health Administration Press.

Feinberg, L.F., Whitlatch, C.J. and Tucke, S. 2000. *Making Hard Choices: Respecting Both Voices—Final report*. San Francisco, CA: Family Caregiver Alliance.

Flanagan, S.A. 1994. *Consumer-Directed Attendant Services: How States Address Tax,*

Legal, and Quality Assurance Issues. Cambridge, MA.: SysteMetrics/MEDSTAT, Inc.

Flanagan, S.A. and Green, P.S. 1997. *Consumer-Directed Personal Assistance Services: Key Operational Issues for State CD-PAS Programs Using Fiscal Intermediary Service Organizations.* Cambridge, MA.: MEDSTAT, Inc.

Foster, L., Brown, R., Carlson, B., Phillips, B. and Schore, J. 2000. *Cash and Counseling: Consumer's Early Experiences in Arkansas* (prepared for Office of Disability, Aging, and Long-Term Care Policy, Office of the Assistant Secretary for Planning and Evaluation, DHHS, and The Robert Wood Johnson Foundation). Mathematica Policy Research, Inc.

Fuchs, V.R. 1993. *The Future of Health Policy.* Cambridge, MA.: Harvard University Press.

Fuchs, V.R. 1975. *Who Shall Live? Health, Economics, and Social Choice.* New York: Basic Books, Inc. Reprinted in Fuchs, V.R. 1998. *Who Shall Live? Health, Economics and Choice, Expanded Edition.* Singapore, New Jersey, London: World Scientific Publishing Com. Pte. Ltdd.

Gallagher, H.G. 1998. *Black Bird Fly Away: Disabled in an Able-Bodied World.* Arlington, VA: Vandamere Press.

Harrington, C., Carillo, H. and Wellin, V. 2001. *Nursing Facilities, Staffing, Residents and Facility Deficiencies, 1994-2000.* Department of Social and Behavioral Sciences, University of California at San Francisco, June 2001.

Harrington, C., Carillo, H., Wellin, V., Norwood, F. and Miller, N. 1999. *1915 (c) Medicaid Home and Community-Based Waiver Participants, Services, and Expenditures, 1992-97.* San Francisco, CA: Department of Social and Behavioral Sciences, University of California at San Francisco, November 1999.

Health Insurance Association of America. 1998. *Term Care Insurance in 1996: Research Findings.* Washington, D.C.: HIAA.

Institute of Medicine. 1986. *Improving the Quality of Care in Nursing Homes.* Washington, DC: National Academy Press.

Institute of Medicine. 1996. *Nursing Staff in Hospitals and Nursing Homes.* Washington, D.C.: National Academy of Sciences.

Kapp, M.B. 2000. *Consumer Choice in Home and Community-Based Long Term Care: Policy Implications for Decisionally Incapacitated Consumers.* Oxford, OH: Miami University, Scripps Gerontology Center.

Kane, R.A. and Penrod, J.D. 1995. *Family Caregiving in an Aging Society: Policy*

Perspectives. Thousand Oaks, CA: Sage.

Kane, R., O'Connor, C. and Baker, M. 1995. *Delegation of Nursing Activities: Implications for Patterns of Long-Term Care*. Washington, D.C.: AARP Public Policy Institute #9515.

Kane, R.A., Kane, R.L., and Ladd, R.C. 1998. *The Heart of Long-Term Care*. New York; Oxford : Oxford University Press.

Kane, R.A. and Wilson, K.B. 1993. *Assisted Living in the United States: A New Paradigm for Residential Care for Frail Older Persons*. Washington, D.C.: American Association of Retired Persons.

Kassner, E. and Martin, J. 1996. *Decisions, Decisions: Service Allocation in Home and Community-based Long-term Care Programs—a Four-State Analysis*. Washington, D.C.: AARP Public Policy Institute.

Kassner, E. and Williams. 1997. *Taking Care of Their Own: State-Funded Home and Community-Based Care Programs for Older Persons*. Washington, D.C.: AARP Public Policy Institute.

Kaye, S., LaPlante, M.P., Carlson, D. and Wenger, B.L. 1996. *Trends in Disability Rates in the United States, 1970–1994*. Washington, DC: U.S. Department of Education, National Institute on Disability and Rehabilitation Research.

Kennedy, J. and LaPlante, M.P. 1997. A Profile of Adults Needing Assistance with Activities of Daily Living, 1991-1992. Disability Statistics Report, (11). Washington, DC: U.S. Department of Education, National Institute on Disability and Rehabilitation Research.

Kennedy, J. and S. Litvak. 1991. *Case Studies of Six State Personal Assistance Services Funded by the Medicaid Personal Care Option*. Oakland, CA: World Institute on Disability.

Kerkstra, A. and Hutton, J.B.F. 1996. "A Cross-National Comparison on Home Care in Europe--Summary of the Findings." In *Home Care in Europe* (Kerkstra, A. and Hutton, J.B.F. , editors).

Kimmick, M. and Godfrey, T. 1991. *New Models for the Provision of Personal Assistance Services. Final Report*. Cambridge, MA: Human Services Research Institute.

Lefcourt, H.M., editor. 1981. *Research with the Locus of Control Construct*. Volume 1. New York: Academic Press.

Levy, C.W. 1988. *A People's History of the Independent Living Movement*. Research and Training Center on Independent Living. The University of Kansas.

Lerman, P. 1984. *Deinstitutionalization and the Welfare State.* New Brunswick, NJ: Rutgers University Press.

Linsk, N.L., Keigher, S.M., Simon-Rusinowitz, L. and England, S.E. 1992. *Wages for Caring: Compensating Family Care of the Elderly.* New York: Praeger.

Litvak, S., Zukas, H., and Heumann, J.E. 1987. *Attending to America: Personal Assistance for Independent Living. A Survey of Attendant Services in the United States for People of All Ages with Disabilities.* Berkeley, CA: World Institute on Disability.

Litvak, S. and Kennedy, J. 1991. *Policy Issues Affecting the Medicaid Personal Care Services Optional Benefit.* Oakland, CA: World Institute on Disability.

Litvak, S. 1990. *New Models for the Provision of Personal Assistance Service: A Research and Demonstration Project.* Berkeley, CA: World Institute on Disability and Bureau of Economic Research at Rutgers University.

Liu, K. and Manton, K. 1994. *Changes in Home Care Use by Disabled Elderly Persons: 1982-1989,* Congressional Research Service, Library of Congress.

Longmore, P.K. and Umansky, L. 2001. *The New Disability History: American Perspectives.* New York, London: New York University Press.

Mahoney, C., Estes, C.and Heumann, J.,Editors. 1986. *Toward a Unified Agenda: Proceedings of a National Conference on Disability and Aging.* San Francisco: University of California and World Institute on Disability.

Mathematica Policy Research. 1987. *The Evaluation of the National Long-Term Care Demonstration: Final Report.* Princeton, NJ: Mathematica Policy Research.

Miltenburg, T., et al. 1996. *A Personal Budget for Clients: Summary of an Experiment with Cash Benefits in Home Care in the Netherlands.* Institute for Applied Social Sciences. Nijmegen, Netherlands.

National Academy on Aging. 1994. *Advisory Panel Report on the Future of Community-Based Long-Term Care,* New York: The Maxwell School of Citizenship and Public Affairs, Syracuse University, Syracuse.

National Association of Protection and Advocacy Systems. 2000. *Olmstead Progress Report: Disability Advocates Assess State Implementation After One Year.* Washington, D.C.: National Association of Protection and Advocacy Systems, www.protectionandadvocacy.com/progressreportfinal.htm.

National Council on Disability. 1986. *Toward Independence.* Washington, D.C.: National Council on Disability.

National Council on Disability. 1988. *On the Threshold of Independence.*

Washington, D.C.: National Council on Disability.

National Council on Disability. 1997. *Equality of Opportunity: The Making of the Americans with Disabilities Act.* Washington, D.C.: National Council on Disability.

National Conference of State Legislatures. 2001. *The States' Response to the Olmstead decision: A Status Report.* National Conference of State Legislatures, www.ncsl.org/programs/health/forum/olmsreport.htm.

National Institute on Consumer-Directed Long-Term Services. 1998. *State Administrator Knowledge, Practices, and Attitudes Regarding Consumer Direction.* Washington D.C.: The National Council on the Aging.

National Institute on Consumer-Directed Long-Term Services. 1996. *Principles of Consumer-Directed Home and Community-Based Services.* Washington D.C.: The National Council on the Aging.

National Institute on Consumer-Directed Long-Term Services. 1996. *Cash and Counseling Technical Analysis: The Counseling Component.* Washington D.C.: The National Council on the Aging, University of Maryland Center on Aging, World Institute on Disability.

National Institute on Consumer-Directed Long-Term Services and the Independent Choices Grants Program. (1996-Present). *Consumer Choice News.* Washington D.C.: The National Council on the Aging.

National Institute on Consumer-Directed Long-Term Services. 1997. *Autonomy or Abandonment: Changing Perspectives on Delegation.* Washington D.C.: The National Council on the Aging.

Nosek, M.A. 1990. *Personal Assistance: Key to Employability of Persons with Physical Disabilities in the United States.* Report. San Francisco, CA: Disability Rights Advocates.

Nosek, M.A. 1990. *Personal Assistance Services for People with Mental Disabilities.* Houston, TX: Baylor College of Medicine.

Observatoire National de' Action Socialee Decentralisee (OANSD). 1998. *La PSD un An Apres: Premieres Tendances.* Paris, France.

Rivlin, A.M. and Wiener, J. 1988. *Caring for the Disabled Elderly: Who Will Pay?* Washington, D.C.: The Brookings Institute.

Runde, P. et al. 1996. *Einstellungen und Verhalten zur Pflegeversicherung und zur Hauslichen Pflege.* Hamburg, Germany: Universitat Hamburg.

Schaie, K.W. and Achenbaum, W.A. (editors). 1993. *Societal Impact on Aging:*

Historical Perspectives. New York, NY: Springer.

Scotch, R.K. 2001. *From Goodwill to Civil Rights: Transforming Federal Disability Policy* (Second edition), Philadelphia, PA: Temple University Press.

Pflueger, S.S. 1977. Independent Living: Emerging Issues in Rehabilitation, (unpublished report on file with Independent Living Research Utilization, Houston, Texas).

Pijl, M. 1994. "When Private Care Goes Public: an Analysis of Concepts and Principles Concerning Payments for Care." In Evers, A., Pijl, M., and Ungerson, C. (editors), *Payments for Care*. Brookfield, VT: Ashgate, pages 3-18.

Pijl, M., Mandmaker, T., Daal, H.J.V., and Schoonman, B. 1994. "Payments for Care: the Case of the Netherlands." In Evers, A., Pijl, M., and Ungerson, C. (editors), *Payments for Care*. Brookfield, VT: Ashgate, at 145-64.

Sabatino, C.P. 1996. "Competency: Refining Our Legal Fictions." In Smyer, M., Schaie, K.W.and Kapp, M.B. *Older Adults' Decision-Making and the Law*. New York: Springer.

Shapiro, J.P. 1993. *No Pity: People with Disabilities Forging a New Civil Rights Movement*. New York, NY: Random House.

Simon, M.O. and Martin, P.A. 1996. *La Prestation Dependance: Rapport Final du Programme d' Evaluation de l' Experimentation d' une Prestation Dependence*. Paris, France: Centre de Recherche pour l'Etude et l'Observation des Conditions de Vie CREDOC.

Simon-Rusinowitz, L., Mahoney, K.J., Desmond, S.M., Shoop, D.M., Squillace, M.R. and Fay, R.A. 1998. *Telephone Survey Technical Report: Consumer Preferences for a Cash Option Versus Traditional Services in New Jersey*. College Park, MD: University of Maryland Center on Aging.

Spector, W., Fleishman, J., Pezzin, L. and Spillman, B. 2000. *The Characteristics of Long-Term Care Users*, Agency for Healthcare Research and Quality, U.S. Department of Health and Human Services.

Stone, R.I. 2000. *Long-Term Care for the Elderly with Disabilities: Current Policy, Emerging Trends, and Implications for the Twenty-First Century*. New York: Milbank Memorial Fund.

Stryckman, J. and Nahmiash, D. 1994. "Payments for Care: The Case of Canada." In Evers, A., Pijl, M., and Ungerson, C. (editors), *Payments for Care*. Brookfield, VT: Ashgate, 307-19.

Tilly, J. , Goldenson, S. and Kasten, J. 2001. *Long-Term Care: Consumers, Providers and Financing. A Chart Book.* Washington, D.C.: Urban Institute.

Tilly, J. and Bechtel, R. 1999. *Consumer-Directed Long-Term Care: Participant's Experiences in Five Countries.* Washington, D.C.: AARP Public Policy Institute.

Tilly, J, Wiener, J.M. and Cuellar, A.E. 2000. *"Consumer-Directed Home and Community Services Programs in Five Countries: Policy Issues for Older People and Government."* Washington, D.C.: Urban Institute.

Tilly, J. and Wiener, J.M. 2001. *Consumer-Directed Home and Community Services: Policy Issues.* Washington, D.C.: Urban Institute.
http://newfederalism.urban.org/html/op44/occa44.html

Wagner, D., Nadash, P. and Sabatino, C. 1997. *Autonomy or Abandonment: Changing Perspectives on Delegation.* Proceedings of a conference sponsored by the National Institute on Consumer-Directed Services, a partnership of the National Council on Aging (Washington, D.C.) and the World Institute on Aging (Oakland, CA, Washington, D.C.: Office of the Assistant Secretary for Planning and Evaluation, U.S. Department of Health and Human Services.

Weiner, J.M. and Hanley, R.J. 1992. "Caring for the Disabled Elderly: There's No Place Like Home." In *Improving Health Policy and Management: Nine Critical Research Issues for the 1990s* (Shortell, S.M. and Reinhardt, U.E., editors), Ann Arbor, MI: Health Administration Press, at 75-110.

World Institute on Disability. 1990. *The Personal Assistance for Independent Living Act of 1989 – A Draft Bill.* Berkeley, CA: World Institute on Disability.

World Institute on Disability. 1999. *Personal Assistance Services: Political and Personal Insights in Developing a National System.* Report. Oakland, CA: World Institute on Disability.

World Institute on Disability. 1999. *PAS: A New Millennium Conference. Executive Summary.* Berkeley, CA: World Institute on Disability.

Woldringh, C. and Ramakers, C. 1998. *Persoonsgebonden Budget Verpleging Verzorging Ervaringen van Budgethouders en Kwaliteit van Zorg.* Nijmegen, Netherlands: Instituut voor Toegepaste Sociale Wetenschappen van de Stricting Katholieke Universiteit te Nijmegen.

Zacharias, B.L. 1997. *Cash and Counseling Demonstration and Evaluation: A Study to Determine the Preferences of Consumers and Surrogates for a Cash Option.*

Journal Articles

Adams, K.E., Meiners, M.R. and Burwell, B.O. "Asset Spend-Down in Nursing Homes: Methods and insights." *Medical Care* 31 (1): 1-23.

Ansello, E.F. and Eustis, N.N. 1992. "A Common Stake? Investigating the Emerging 'Intersection' of Aging and Disabilities." *Generations* 16: 5-8.

American Medical Association, Council on Scientific Affairs. 1990. "Home Care in the 1990s," *Journal of the American Medical Association (JAMA)* 263: 1241.

Applebaum, R. and Phillips, P. 1990. "Assuring the Quality of In-Home Care: The 'Other' Challenge for Long-Term Care," *Gerontologist* 30(4): 444-50.

Applebaum, R., Mollica, R. and Tilly, J. 1997-8. "Assuring Homecare Quality: A Case Study of State Strategies." *Generations* 21(4): 57-63.

Arno P.S., Levine C., and Memmott M.M. 1999. "The Economic Value of Informal Caregiving; President Clinton's Proposal to Provide Relief to Family Caregivers Opens a Long-Overdue Discussion of This "Invisible" Health Care Sector." *Health Affairs* 18 (2): 182-188.

Askheim O.P. 1999. "Personal Assistance for Disabled People - the Norwegian Experience." *International Journal of Social Welfare* 8(2): 111-119.

Asher, C.C., Asher, M.A., Hobbs, W.E, and Kelley, J.M. 1991. "On Consumer Self-Direction of Attendant Care Services: An Empirical Analysis of Survey Responses," *Evaluation and Program Planning* 14: 131-139.

Baker, D. and Pallett-Hehn, P. 1995. "Care or Control: Barriers to Service Use by Elderly People." *Journal of Applied Gerontology* 14 (3): 261-74.

Barnes, A. 1995. "The Policy and Politics of Community-Based Long-Term Care." *Nova Law Review* 19: 487.

Bass, S. 1996. "Recommended Federal Policy Directions on Personal Assistance Services for Americans with Disabilities' The Consortium for Citizens with Disabilities and Task Force on Personal Assistance Services. Quandaries Persist, But Consumer Choice Calls for Experimentation, Education." *Perspective on Aging* 25(4): 4-7.

Batavia, A.I. 1993. "Health Care Reform and People With Disabilities," *Health Affairs* 12(1): 40-57.

Batavia, A.I. 2003. "The Growing Prominence of Independent Living and Consumer Direction as Principles in Long-Term Care: A Content Analysis." *Elder Law Journal* (In press).

Batavia, A.I. 2002. "Consumer Direction, Consumer Choice and the Future of Long-Term Care." *Journal of Disability Policy Studies* 13(2): 67-73, 86.

Batavia, A.I. 2002. "Even Playing Field for Consumer-Directed Long-Term Care."

Health Affairs 21(1): 271 (Letter to the editor).

Batavia, A.I. 2001. "A Right to Personal Assistance Services: 'Most Integrated Setting Appropriate' Requirements and the Independent Living Model of Long-Term Care," *American Journal of Law and Medicine* 27(1): 17-43.

Batavia, A.I. 2001. "The Ethics of PAS: Morally Relevant Relationships Between Personal Assistance Services and Physician-Assisted Suicide." *Archives of Physical Medicine and Rehabilitation*, 2001; 12 Suppl 2:S25-31.

Batavia, A.I. 2001. "Are People with Disabilities an Oppressed Minority, and Why Does This Matter?" in (Batavia, AI, guest editor) Special Issue on Oppression and Disability, *Journal of Disability Policy Studies*, 12(2): 66-67.

Batavia, A.I. 1999. "Independent Living Centers, Medical Rehabilitation Centers, and Managed Health Care for People with Disabilities." *Archives of Physical Medicine and Rehabilitation*, 80: 1357-60.

Batavia, A.I. 1998. "The Prospects for a National Personal Assistance Services Program for People with Disabilities." *American Rehabilitation* 24 (3).

Batavia, A.I. 1991. "Caring Through Personal Assistance Policy: A Response," *Journal of Health Politics, Policy and Law* 16(4) (Letter to the editor).

Batavia, A.I. and DeJong, G. 2001. "Disability, Chronic Illness and Risk Selection." *Archives of Physical Medicine and Rehabilitation*, 81: 546-52.

Batavia, A.I., DeJong, G. and McKnew, L.B. 1991. "Toward a National Personal Assistance Program: The Independent Living Model of Long-Term Care for Persons with Disabilities." *Journal of Health Politics, Policy, and Law* 16(3): 523-545.

Beatty, P.W., Adams, M. and O' Day, B. 1998. "Virginia's Consumer-Directed Personal Assistance Services Program: A History and Evaluation." *American Rehabilitation* 24(3): 31-35.

Beatty, P.W., Richmond, G.W., Tepper, S. and DeJong, G. 1998. "Personal Assistance for People with Physical Disabilities: Consumer-Direction and Satisfaction with Services." *Archives of Physical Medicine and Rehabilitation* 79(6): 674-77.

Benjamin A.E. 2001. "Consumer-Directed Services at Home: A New Model for Persons with Disabilities" *Health Affairs* 20(6): 80-95.

Benjamin, A.E. 1993. "An Historical Perspective on Home Care Policy." *The Milbank Quarterly* 71: 129.

Benjamin, A.E. and Matthias, R. 2000. "Comparing Consumer-Directed and

Agency-Directed Models: California's In-Home Supportive Services Program." *Generations* 24(3): 85-87.

Benjamin, A.E., Matthias, R. and Franke, T.M. 2000. "Comparing Consumer-Directed and Agency Models for Providing Supportive Services at Home." *Health Services* Research 35(1 Pt 2): 351-66.

Benjamin, A.E. , et al. 1999. "Consumer Direction and In-Home Services: Recipient Perspectives on Family and Non-Family Service Provision." *Journal of Rehabilitation Administration* 22: 233-47.

Benjamin A.E and Matthias R.E. 2001. "Age, Consumer Direction, and Outcomes of Supportive Services at Home." *Gerontologist* Oct; 41(5): 632-42.

Bertsch, E.F.. 1991. "Barriers to Individualized Community Support Services: The Impact of Some Current Funding and Conceptual Models." *Community Mental Health Journal* 27(5): 337-45.

Bowers B.J., Fibich B. and Jacobson N. 2001. "Care-As-Service, Care-As-Relating, Care-As-Comfort: Understanding Nursing Home Residents' Definitions of Quality." *Gerontologist* 41 (4): 539-545.

Branin J.J. 2001. "Burnout Among Nursing Home Personnel: The Effectiveness of an Education Training Intervention." *Gerontologist* 41: 92 Sp. Iss. 1.

Bresnitz E, Grant C, Ostrawski S, et al. 2001. "Outbreak of Pneumococcal Pneumonia Among Unvaccinated Residents of a Nursing Home." *Journal of the American Medical Association (JAMA)* 286 (13): 1570-1571.

Brook, R.H., McGlynn, E.A. and Cleary, P.H. 1996. "Measuring Quality of Care." *New England Journal of Medicine* 335(13): 966-69.

Capitman, J.and Sciegaj, M. 1995. "A Conceptual Approach for Understanding Individual Autonomy in Managed Community Long-term Care." *Gerontologist* 35 (4): 533-40.

Clark, P.G. 1988. "Autonomy, Personal Empowerment, and Quality of Life in Long-Term Care." *Journal of Applied Gerontology*, 7: 279-297.

Clark, P.G. 1987. "Individual Autonomy, Cooperative Empowerment, and Planning for Long-Term Care Decision-Making." *Journal of Aging Studies*, 1: 65-76.

Close, L., Estes, C.L., Linkins, K.W. 1994. "A Political-Economy Perspective on Frontline Workers in Long-Term Care." *Generations* 18(3): 23-27.

Cohen, E.S. 1990. "The Elderly Mystique: Impediment to Advocacy and Empowerment." *Generations* 14 (Supplement): 13-16.

Cohen, E.S. 1992. "What Is Independence?" *Generations* 16: 49-52.

Cohen, E.S. 1998. "The Elderly Mystique: Constraints on the Autonomy of the Elderly with Disabilities." *The Gerontologist* 28(Suppl): 24 -31.

Cole, J.A. 1979. "What's New about Independent Living?" *Archives of Physical Medicine and Rehabilitation* 60(10): 458-62.

Collopy, B.J. 1990. "Ethical Dimensions of Autonomy in Long-Term Care." *Generations*, 14 (Supplement): 9-12.

Collopy, B.J. 1988. "Autonomy in Long-Term Care: Some Crucial Distinctions." *The Gerontologist*, 28 (Supplement): 10-17.

Coyne, A.C., Reichman, W.E. and Berbig, L.J. 1993. "The Relationship between Dementia and Elder Abuse." *American Journal of Psychiatry* 150: 643-46.

Criscione, T., Kastner, T.A., O'Brien, D. and Nathanson, R. 1994. "Replication of a Managed Health Care Initiative for People with Mental Retardation Living in the Community." *Mental Retardation* 32(1): 43-52.

Criscione, T., Walsh, K.K., and Kastner, T.A. 1995. "An Evaluation the Care Coordination in Controlling Inpatient Hospital Utilization of People with Developmental Disabilities." *Mental Retardation* 33(6): 364-73.

Crown, W.H. 1994. "A National Profile of Home Care, Nursing Home, and Hospital Aides." *Generations* 18(3): 29-33.

Davis, B.E. 1998. "The Home Health Care Crisis: Medicare's Fastest Growing Program Legalizes Spiraling Costs." *Elder Law Journal* 6: 215-255.

Deegan, P. 1992. "The Independent Living Movement and Psychiatric Disabilities: Taking Back Control of Our Lives." *Psychosocial Rehabilitation Journal* 15 (3): 3-19.

DeJong, G. 1982. "A Legal Perspective on Disability, Home Care, and Relative Responsibility." *Home Health Services Quarterly*, 3 (Fall/Winter) nos. 3/4, 176-187.

DeJong, G. 1979. "Independent Living: From Social Movement to Analytic Paradigm." *Archives of Physical Medicine and Rehabilitation* 60(10): 435-446.

DeJong, G. and Sutton, J. 1998. "Managed Care and People with Disabilities: Framing the Issues." *Archives of Physical Medicine and Rehabilitation* 79: 1312.

DeJong, G. and Sutton, J. 1998. "Managed Care and Catastrophic Injury: The Case of Spinal Cord Injury." *Topics in Spinal Cord Injury Rehabilitation* 3(4): 1-16.

DeJong, G. and Wenker, T. 1983. "Attendant Care as a Prototype Independent

Living Service." *Caring* 2(2): 26-30.

DeJong G. and Wenker T. 1979. "Attendant Care As a Prototype Independent Living Service." *Archives of Physical Medicine and Rehabilitation* Oct; 60(10): 477-82.

DeJong, G., Batavia, A.I. and Griss, R.. 1989. "America's Neglected Health Minority: Working-Age Persons with Disabilities." *The Milbank Quarterly*, 67 (Supplement 2, Part 2): 311-351.

DeJong, G., Batavia, A.I. and McKnew, L. 1992. "The Independent Living Model of Personal Assistance in National Long-Term-Care Policy." *Generations* 16: 89-95. Reprinted in *Aging and Disabilities: Seeking Common Ground* (E.F. Ansello and N.F. Eustis, Eds.), New York: Baywood Publishing Co., 1993.

Desai, M.M., Lentzner, H.R. and Weeks, J.D. 2001. "Unmet Need for Personal Assistance with Activities of Daily Living Among Older Adults." *Gerontologist* 41(1): 82-88.

Doty, P. 2000. "The Federal Role in the Move Toward Consumer Direction." *Generations*, 24(3): 922-27.

Doty, P. J. 1998. "The Cash and Counseling Demonstration: An Experiment in Consumer-Directed Personal Assistance Services." *American Rehabilitation*, 24(3): 27-30.

Doty, P., Kasper, J., Litvak, S. and Taylor, H. 1994. "Consumer Choice and the Frontline Worker." *Generations* 18(3): 65-70.

Doty, P., Kasper, J. and Litvak, S. 1996. "Consumer-Directed Models of Personal Care: Lessons from Medicaid." *Milbank Quarterly* 74 (3): 377-409.

Dubler, N.N. 1990. "Autonomy and Accommodation: Mediating Individual Choice in the Home Setting." *Generations*, 14 (Supplement), 29-31.

Dwyer, K. 2000. "Culturally Appropriate Consumer-Directed Care: The American Indian Choices project." *Generations*, 24(3): 91-93.

Edelman, T.E. 1997-98. "The Politics of Long-Term Care at the Federal Level and Implications For Quality." *Generations* 21(4): 37-41.

Estes, C.L. and Bodenheimer, T. 1994. "Paying for Long-Term Care." *Western Journal of Medicine* 160: 64.

Eustis, N.N. 2000. "Consumer Directed Long-Term Care Services: Evolving Perspectives and Alliances." *Generations*, 24(3): 10-15.

Eustis, N.N., Fischer, L.R. and Kane, R.A. 1994. "The Home Care Worker: On the

Frontline of Quality." *Generations*, 18: 43-49.

Eustis, N.N., Kane, R.A., and Fischer, L.R. 1993. "Home Care Quality and the Home Care Worker: Beyond Quality Assurance As Usual." *The Gerontologist* 33: 64-73.

Eustis, N.N. and Fischer, L.R. 1992. "Common Needs, Different Solutions? Younger and Older Home Care Clients." *Generations*, 16: 17-22.

Feinberg, L.F. and Kelly, K.A. 1995. "A Well-Deserved Break: Respite Options Offered by California's Statewide System of Caregiver Resource Centers." *Gerontologist* 35: 701-5.

Feinberg, L.F. and Whitlatch, C.J. 1998. "Family Caregivers and In-Home Respite Options: The Consumer-Directed Versus Agency-Based Experience." *Journal of Gerontological Social Work* 30(3/4): 9-28.

Feinberg, L.F. and Ellano, C. 2000. "Promoting Consumer Direction for Family Caregiver Support: an Agency-Driven Model." *Generations*, 24(3): 47-54.

Feldblum, C.R. 1985. "Home Health Care for the Elderly: Programs, Problems and Potentials." *Harvard Journal on Legislation* 22: 193.

Flanagan, S.A. and Green, P.S. 2000. "Fiscal Intermediaries: Reducing the Burden of Consumer-Directed Support." *Generations* 24(3): 94-97.

Flanagan, S.A., Green, P.S. and Eustis, N. 1998. "You Can Do It: State Initiatives Broaden Access to Consumer-Directed Personal Assistance Services Through the Use of Intermediary Service Organizations." *American Rehabilitation*, 24(3): 21-26.

Frieden, L., Smith, L., Wilkinson, W., Redd, L. and Smith, Q. 1998. "Spinal Cord Injury and Managed Care: A Consumer Viewpoint." *Topics in Spinal Cord Injury Rehabilitation* 1998: 3(4): 80-88.

Geron, S.M. 2000. "The Quality of Consumer-Directed Long-Term Care." *Generations*, 24(3): 66-73.

Geron, S.M., et al. 2000. "The Home Care Satisfaction Measure: A Client-Centered Approach on Assessing the Satisfaction of Frail Older Adults with Home Health Care Services." *Journal of Gerontology: Social Services* 52B(5): 259-70.

Geron, S.M. 1998. "Assessing the Satisfaction of Older Adults with Long-Term Care Services: Measurement and Design Challenges." *Research on Social Work Practice* 8(1): 103-19.

Ghilardi G., Wietlisbach V., Petignat C., et al. 2001. "The Reciprocal Relationship Between Infections and Functional Impairment in Nursing Home Residents."

Gerontologist 41: 346-346 Sp. Iss. 1.

Gilson, S.F. and Casebolt, G.J. 1997. "Personal Assistance Services and Case Management." *Journal of Case Management*, 6(1): 13-17.

Glickman, L.L., Stocker, K.B. and Caro, F.G. 1997. "Self Direction in Home Care for Older People: A Consumer's Perspective," *Home Health Care Services Quarterly* 16(1-2): 41-54.

Gomolin, I.H. and Kathpalia, R.K. 2002. "Influenza - How To Prevent and Control Nursing Home Outbreaks." *Geriatrics* 57 (1): 28.

Hanley, R.J., Wiener, J.M. and Harris, K.M. 1991. "Will Paid Home Care Erode Informal Support?" *Journal of Health Politics, Policy, and Law* 16(3): 507-521.

Hawes, C. 1997-8. "Regulation and the Politics of Long-Term Care." *Generations* 21(4): 5-9.

Hennessy, C.H. 1989. "Autonomy and Risk: The Role of Client Wishes In Community-Based Long-Term Care." *The Gerontologist* 29: 633-639.

Hersen M. 1969. "Independent Living As a Threat to the Institutionalized Mental Patient." *Journal of Clinical Psychology* 25(3): 316-18.

Hoenig, H., Taylor, D. and Sloan, F. 2001. "Assistive Technology is Associated with Reduced Use of Personal Assistance Among Disabled Older Persons." *Journal of The American Geriatric Society* 49 (4): A40.

Hofland, B.F. and David, D. 1990. "Autonomy and Long-Term Care Practice: Conclusions and Next Steps." *Generations* 14 (Supplement): 13-16.

Hofland, B.F. 1988. "Autonomy in Long-Term Care: Background Issues and a Programmatic Response." *Gerontologist* 28: 3.

Holmes D. 2001. "Staffing Issues As They Pertain to Nursing Home Care Of Elderly Persons with Dementing Illness." *Gerontologist* 41: 58 Sp. Iss. 1.

Home Care Aide Association of America. 1995. "Guiding Principles Governing the Delivery of Long-Term Care." *Caring*, 14(4): 70-71.

Horowitz, A. and Shindelman, L. 1983. "Social and Economic Incentives for Family Caregivers." *Health Care Financing Review* 5(2): 25-33.

Infeld, D.L 2000. "Personal Assistance: The Future of Home Care." *Inquiry* 37 (1): 111-112.

Jette, A.M., Smith, K.W. and McDermott, S.M. 1996. "Quality of Medicare-

Reimbursed Home Health Care." *Gerontologist* 36(4): 492-501.

Johnson, R.W. and LoSasso, A.T. 2001. "Does Informal Care Reduce Nursing Home Admissions for the Frail Elderly?" *Gerontologist* 41(Sp. Iss. 1): 61.

Kafka, B. 1994. "Perspectives on Personal Assistance Services." *Independent Living* Winter-Spring 1994.

Kapp, M.B. 2001. "Consumer Choice in Long-Term Care: What the United States Can Teach and Learn from Others About Decisionally Incapacitated Consumers." *International Journal of law and Psychiatry* 24(3): 199-211.

Kapp, M.B. 2000. "Consumer Direction in Long-Term Care: ATaxonomy of Legal Issues." *Generations* 24(3): 16-21.

Kapp, M.B. 1999. "Health Care in the Marketplace: Implications for Decisionally Impaired Consumers, Their Surrogates and Advocates." *Southern Illinois University Law Journal* 24 (fall 1999): 1-52.

Kapp, M.B. 1999. "From Medical Patients to Health Care Consumers: Decisional Capacity and Choices to Purchase Coverage and Services." *Aging and Mental Health* 3(4): 294-300.

Kapp, M.B. 1999. "Home Health Care Regulation: Is It Good for the Patient?" *Journal of Long Term Home Health Care* 1(4): 251-57.

Kapp, M.B. 1997. "Who Is Responsible for This? Assigning Rights and Consequences in Elder Care." *Journal of Aging and Social Policy*, 9(2): 51-65.

Kapp, M.B. 1998. " 'A Place like That': Advance Directives and Nursing Home admissions." *Journal of Psychology, Public Policy, and Law* 4(3): 805-28.

Kapp, M.B. 1996. "Enhancing Autonomy and Choice in Selecting and Directing Long-Term Care Services." *The Elder Law Journal*, 4 (1): 55-97.

Kapp, M.B. and Wilson, K.B. 1995. "Assisted Living and Negotiated Risk: Reconciling Protection and Autonomy." *Journal of Ethics, Law and Aging* 1(1): 5-13.

Kapp, M.B. 1990. "Home Care Client-Centered Systems: Consumer Choice vs. Protection." *Generations*, 14 (Supplement): 33-35.

Kapp, M.B. 1990. "Improving Choices Regarding Home Care Services: Legal Impediments and Empowerments." *St. Louis University Public Law Review* 10(2): 441-484.

Kane, R.A. 2001. "Long-Term Care and a Good Quality of Life: Bringing Them Closer Together." *Gerontologist* 41 (3): 293-304.

Kane, R.A. and Degenholtz, H. 1997. "Assessing Values and Preferences: Should We, Can We? *Generations*, 21(1): 19-24.

Kane R.L and Kane, R.A. 2001. "What Older People Want from Long-Term Care, and How They Can Get It." *Health Affairs* 20(6): 114-127.

Kane, R.A. and Kane, R.L. 1990. "The Impact of Long-Term-Care Financing on Personal Autonomy." *Generations* 14 (Supplement): 86.

Kane, R.L. 1995. "Improving the Quality of Long-Term Care." *JAMA* 273(17): 1376-80.

Kane, R.A. 1992. "Case Management in Long-Term Care: It Can Be Ethical and Efficacious." *Journal of Case Management* Fall 1992: 76.

Kane, R.A., Kane, R.L., Illston, L.H., and Eustis, N.N. 1994. "Perspectives on Home Care Quality." *Healthcare Financing Review* 16(1): 69-89.

Kane, R.A. 1988. "Case Management: Ethical Pitfalls on the Road to High-quality Managed Care." *Quality Review Bulletin* 161.

Katz, M. 1984. "Poorhouses and the Origins of Public Old Age Homes." *Milbank Memorial Fund Quarterly/Health and Society* 62 (1): 110-40.

Kelly, C.M. and Liebig, P.S. 2001. "Nursing Home Oversight: Problems in Intergovernmental Regulation." *Gerontologist* 41(Sp. Iss. 1): 13.

Kelly_Hayes, M., Wolf, P.A., Kannel, W.B, Sytkowski P., D'Agostino, R.B., and Gresham, G.E. 1988. "Factors Influencing Survival and Need for Institutionalization Following Stroke: The Framingham Study." *Archives of Physical Medicine and Rehabilitation* 69(6): 415-18.

Kemper, P. 1992. "The Use of Formal and Informal Home Care by the Disabled Elderly." *Health Services Research* 27: 421-51.

Kemper, P. 1988. "The Evaluation of the National Long Term Care Demonstration: Overview of the Findings," *Health Services Research* 23: 161.

Kennedy J. 2001. "Unmet and Undermet Need for Activities of Daily Living and Instrumental Activities of Daily Living Assistance among Adults with Disabilities - Estimates from the 1994 and 1995 Disability Follow-up Surveys." *Medical Care* 39 (12): 1305-1312.

Kennedy J. 1997. "Personal Assistance Benefits and Federal Health Care Reforms: Who Is Eligible on the Basis of ADL Assistance Criteria?" *Journal of Rehabilitation* 63 (3): 40-45.

Kennedy, J. 1993. "Policy and Program Issues in Providing Personal Assistance Service," *Journal of Rehabilitation* (July/August/September 1993): 17-22.

Kramer, A.M., Shaughnessy, P.W., Baumman, M.K., et al. 1990. "Assessing and Assuring the Quality of Home Health Care: A Conceptual Framework." *The Milbank Quarterly* 68(3): 413-43.

Keigher, S.M. 1997. "Austria's New Attendance Allowance: A Consumer-Choice Model of Care for the Frail and Disabled." *International Journal of Health Services* 27(4): 753-65.

Keigher, S.M. 2000. "The Interests of Three Stakeholders in Independent Personal Care for Disabled Elders." *Journal of Health and Human Services Administration* Fall; 23(2): 136-60.

Kingston, B.J. and Wright, C.V. 2002. "Influenza in the Nursing Home." *American Family Physician* 65 (1): 75-78.

Laditka, S.B. and Laditka, J.N. 2001. "Effects of Improved Morbidity Rates on Active Life Expectancy and Eligibility for Long-Term Care Services." *Journal of Applied Gerontology* 20(1): 39-56.

Latimer, J. 1997-98. "The Essential Role of Regulation to Assure Quality in Long-Term Care." *Generations* 21(4): 10-14.

Leutz, W., Sciegaj, M., Capitman, J. 1997. "Client-Centered Case Management: A Survey of State Programs." *Journal of Case Management* 6(1): 18-24.

Leutz, W. 1998. "Home Care Benefits for Persons with Disabilities." *American Rehabilitation*, 24(3): 6-14.

Levine C. 1999. "The Loneliness of the Long-Term Care Giver." *New England Journal of Medicine* 340 (20): 1587-1590.

Levy-Storms L., Gutierrez V.F., Schnelle, J.F., et al. 2001. "Assessing the Quality of Nursing Home Care Processes from Residents' Perspectives." *Gerontologist* 41(Sp. Iss. 1): 54.

Lifchez R. 1979. "The Environment As a Support System For Independent Living." *Archives of Physical Medicine and Rehabilitation* Oct; 60(10): 467-76.

Mahoney, K.J., Desmond, S.M., Simon-Rusinowitz, L., Loughlin, D.M., and Squillace, M.R. "Comparing Preferences for a Cash Option Versus Traditional Services: Telephone Survey Results from New Jersey Elders and Adults." *Journal of Disability Policy Studies* 13(2): 74-86.

Mahoney, K.J., et al. 1998. "Determining Consumer Preferences for a Cash Option:

New York Telephone Survey Findings." *American Rehabilitation*, (winter): 24-36.

Mahoney, K.J. and Simon_Rusinowitz L. 1997. "Cash and Counseling Demonstration and Evaluation. Start-up Activities." *Journal of Case Management*. 6(1): 25-30.

Mahoney, K.J., Simone, K. and Simon-Rusinowitz, L. 2000. "Early Lessons from the Cash and Counseling Demonstration and Evaluation." *Generations* 24(3): 41-46.

Mack R., Salmoni A., Viverais-Dressler G., Porter E. and Garg R. 1997. "Perceived Risks to Independent Living: The Views of Older, Community-Dwelling Adults." *Gerontologist* 37(6): 729-36.

Manton K., Corder L., and Stallard E. 1993. "Changes in the Use of Personal Assistance and Special Equipment from 1982 to 1989 - Results from the 1982 and 1989 NLTCS." *Gerontologist* 33 (2): 168-176.

Manson, S.M. 1989. "Long-Term Care in American Indian Communities: Issues for Planning and Research. *The Gerontologist*, 29(1): 38-44.

Master R., Dreyfus, T., Connors, S., Tobias, C., Zhou, Z., and Kronick, R. 1996. "The Community Medical Alliance: An Integrated System of Care in Greater Boston for People with Severe Disability and AIDS." *Managed Care Quarterly* 4(2): 26-37.

Martin NE and Melichar DY. 2001. "Home Sweet Home: Staffs' Perceptions on Creating Homelike Nursing Home Environments." *Gerontologist* 41 (Sp. Iss. 1): 309.

Mattson-Prince, J. 1997. "A Rational Approach to Long-Term Care: Comparing the Independent Living Model with Agency-Based Care for Persons with High Spinal Cord Injuries." *Spinal Cord* 35(5): 326-31.

Mauser, E. 1997. "Medicare Home Health Initiatives: Current Activities and Future Directions." *Health Care Financing Review* 18(3): 275-91.

Mayer, R.R., Berson, A. and Marks, J. 2000. "A Consumer-Directed Homecare Program that Works for the Cognitively Impaired." *Generations*, 24(3): 98-99.

Micco, A., Hamilton, A.C.S., Martin, M.J., McEwan, K.L. 1995. "Case Manager Attitudes Toward Client-Directed Care." *Journal of Case Management* 4: 95-101.

Miller, N. 1992. "Medicaid Home and Community-based Care Waivers: The First Ten Years." *Health Affairs* 11(4): 162-72.

Miller, N.A., Ramsland, S., and Harrington, C. 1999. "Trends and Issues in the

Medicaid 1915(c) Waiver Program." *Health Care Financing Review* 20 (4): 139-160.

Nadash P. 1998. "Delegation. Creating a Balance Among Home Care, The Disability Community, Regulators, and Payors." *Caring* Jul; 17(7): 20-25.

Nadash, P. 1998. "Independent Choices." *American Rehabilitation*, 24(3): 15-20.

Newcomer, R., Manton, K., Harrington, C., Yordi, C., and Vertrees, J.C. 1995. "Case Mix Controlled Service Use and Expenditures in the Social/Health Maintenance Organization Demonstration." *Journal of Gerontology* 50A(1): M35-44.

Nosek, M.A. 1993. "Personal Assistance: Its Effect on the Long-Term Health of a Rehabilitation Hospital Population." *Archives of Physical Medicine and Rehabilitation* 74(2): 127-32.

Nosek, M.A. and Foley, C.C. 1995. "Personal Assistance: A Key to Employability." *Directions in Rehabilitation Counseling* 6(5): 1-9.

Nosek, M.A. 1991. "Personal Assistance Services: A Review of Literature and Analysis of Policy Implications." *Journal of Disability Policy Studies* 2(2): 1- 17.

Nosek, M.A., Fuhrer, M. and Potter, C. 1995. "Life Satisfaction of People with Physical Disabilities: Relationship to Personal Assistance, Disability Status and Handicap." *Rehabilitation Psychology* 40(3): 191-202.

Nosek M.A, Parker, R.M., and Larsen S. 1987. "Psychosocial Independence and Functional Abilities: Their Relationship in Adults with Severe Musculoskeletal Impairments." *Archives of Physical Medicine and Rehabilitation* 68(12): 840-45.

Penrod, J.D. et al. 1995. "Who Cares? The Size, Scope and Composition of the Caregiver Support System." *Gerontologist* 35: 489.

Phillips, CD., Hawes, C., Mor, V., Fries, B.E, and Morris, J.N. 1997-8. "Geriatric Assessment in Nursing Homes in the United States: Impact of a National Program." *Generations* 21(4): 15-24.

Phillips V.L. 1996. "The Role of Case Managers in a United Kingdom Experiment with Self-Directed Care." *Journal of Case Management* 5(4): 142-45.

Phillips, P.D. et al. 1989. "Quality Assurance Strategies for Home-Delivered Long-term Care." *Quality Review Bulletin* 15: 156.

Pita, D.D., Ellison, M.L. and Farkas, M. 2001. "Exploring Personal Assistance Services for People with Psychiatric Disabilities." *Journal of Disability Policy Studies* 12(1): 2-9.

Prince, J., Manley, M. and Whiteneck, G. 1995. "Self-Managed Versus Agency-Provided Personal Assistance Care for Individuals with High Level Tetraplegia." *Archives of Physical Medicine and Rehabilitation* 76(10): 919-923.

Racino, J.A. and Heumann, J.E. 1992. "Independent Living and Community Life: Building Coalitions among Elders, People with Disabilities, and Our Allies." *Generations*, 16: 43-47.

Reid, D., Haas, W. and Hawkings, D. 1977. "Locus of Desired Control and Positive Self-Concept of the Elderly." *Journal of Gerontology* 32(4): 441-50.

Richmond, G.W., Beatty, P.W., Tepper, S. and DeJong, G. 1997. "The Effect of Consumer-Directed Personal Assistance Services on the Productivity Outcomes of People with Disabilities." *Journal of Rehabilitation Outcomes Measurement* 1(4): 48-51.

Rodin, J. 1986. "Aging and Health: Effects of the Sense of Control." *Science* 233: 1271.

Sabatino, C.P. 1999. "The Legal and Functional Status of the Medical Proxy: Suggestions for Statutory Reform." *Law, Medicine and Health Care* 27: 52.

Sabatino, C.P. 1990. Client-Rights Regulations and the Autonomy of Home-Care Consumers. *Generations* 14 (Supplement), 21-24.

Sabatino, C.P. and Litvak, S. 1992. "Consumer-Directed Homecare: What Makes It Possible?" *Generations* 14 (3): 53-58.

Sabatino, C.P. and Litvak, S. 1996. "Liability Issues Affecting Consumer-Directed Personal Assistance Services—Report and Recommendations." *The Elder Law Journal* 4: 247.

Saxton, M., Curry, M.A., Powers, L.E., et al. 2001. "'Bring My Scooter So I Can Leave You'" -A Study of Disabled Women Handling Abuse by Personal Assistance Providers." *Violence Against Women* 7(4): 393-417.

Scala M.A., Mayberry P.S. and Kunkel S.R. 1996. "Consumer-Directed Home Care: Client Profiles and Service Challenges." *Journal of Case Management* 5(3): 91-98.

Scala, M.A. and Nerney, T. 2000. "People First: the Consumers in Consumer Direction." *Generations* 24(3): 55-59.

Seltzer, M.M. 1992. "Training Families to Be Case Managers for Elders with Developmental Disabilities." *Generations* 18: 65-70.

Seltzer, M.M. and Mayer, J.B. 1988. "Families as Case Managers." *Generations* 12: 26-29.

Seltzer, M.M., Ivry, J. and Litchfield, L. 1987. "Family Members as Case Managers: Partnership between the Formal and Informal Support Networks." *Gerontologist* 27: 722-728.

Shaughnessy, P.W., Crisler, K.S., Schlenker, R.E., Arnold, A.G., Kramer, A.M., Powell, M.C., and Hittle, D.F. 1994. "Measuring and Assuring the Quality of Home Health Care." *Health Care Financing Review* 16(1): 35-67.

Shellenbarger, S. 1994. "Home Aide Shortage Upsets Delicate Balance." *Wall Street Journal* June 1, 1994, at B1.

Silverstein, M. and Parrott, T.M. 2001. "Attitudes Toward Government Policies that Assist Informal Caregivers: The Link between Personal Troubles and Public Issues." *Research on Aging* 23(3): 349-374.

Simmons SF and Schnelle JF. 2001. "The Identification of Residents Capable of Accurately Describing Daily Care: Implications for Evaluating Nursing Home Care Quality." *Gerontologist* 41(5): 605-611.

Simon-Rusinowitz, L., Mahoney, K.J., Desmond, S.M., Shoop, D.M., Squillace, M.R., and Fay, R.A. 1997. "Determining Consumer Preferences for a Cash Option: Arkansas Survey Results." *Health Care Financing Review* 19(2): 73-96.

Simon-Rusinowitz, L., Bochniak, A.M.,. Mahoney, K.J. and Marks, L.N. 2000. "Implementation Issues for Consumer-Directed Programs: A Survey of Policy Experts." *Generations* 24(3): 3440.

Simon-Rusinowitz, L. and Hofland, B.F. 1993. "Adopting a Disability Approach to HomeCare Services for Adults." *The Gerontologist* 33(2): 159-167.

Stoddard S. 1980. "Independent Living." *Annual Review of Rehabilitation* 1: 231-78.

Stone, D.A. 1991. "Commentary: Caring Work in a Liberal Polity." *Journal of Health Politics, Policy and Law* 16(3): 547-552.

Stone, R.I. 2001. "Providing Long-Term Care Benefits in Cash: Moving to a Disability Model. The Cause of Patient Autonomy is Well Served by Cash Benefit Programs, Although Challenges Remain" *Health Affairs* 20(6): 96-109.

Stone, R.I. 2000. "Introduction – Consumer direction in Long-Term Care: Opportunities, Challenges, and Limitations of This Increasingly Popular Approach." *Generations*, 24(3): 5-8.

Tanenbaum, S.J. and Hurley, R.E. 1995. "Managed Care, Disability and the 1115 Waiver Frenzy: a Cautionary Note. *Health Affairs* 14 (4): 113-19.

Tennestdt, S.L. Crawford, S.I. and McKinlay, J.B. 1993. "Is Family Care on the

Decline?: A Longitudinal Investigation of the Substitution of Formal Long-term Care Services for Informal Care." *Milbank Quarterly* 71(4): 601-24.

Thomas, D.R., Zdrowski, C.D., Wilson , M.M., et al. 2002. "Malnutrition in Subacute Care." *American Journal of Clinical Nutrition.* 75 (2): 308-313.

Tilly, J., Wiener, J.M., and Cuellar, A.E. 2000. "Consumer-Directed Home-and Community-Based Services Programs in Five Countries: Policy Issues for Older People and Government." *Generations*, 24(3): 74-84.

Ulicny, G.R., White, G.W., Bradford, B. and Mathews, R.M. 1990. "Consumer Exploitation by Attendants: How Often Does It Happen and Can Anything Be Done about It?" *Rehabilitation Counseling Bulletin* 33: 240-46.

Vaidyanathan S., Soni B.M., Mansour, P., et al. 2001. "Community-Care Waiting List for Persons with Spinal Cord Injury." *Spinal Cord* 39 (11): 584-588.

Velgouse, L. and Dize, V. 2000. "A Review of State Initiatives in Consumer-Directed Long-Term Care." *Generations*, 24(3): 28-33.

Verbrugge L.M., Rennert, C. and Madans, J.H. 1997. "The Great Efficacy of Personal and Equipment Assistance in Reducing Disability." *American Journal of Public Health* 87 (3): 384-92.

Verweij M. 2001. "Individual and Collective Considerations in Public Health: Influenza Vaccination in Nursing Homes." *Bioethics* 15 (5-6): 536-546.

Vladeck, B.C., Miller, N.A. and Clauser, S.B. 1993. "The Changing Face of Long-Term Care." *Health Care Financing Review* 14(4): 5-23.

Wagner, D.L. 1999. "Enhancing Consumer Independence through Delegation." *Caring* 18(7): 22-25.

Wall T. 1999. "Long-Term Care at Home." *The New England Journal of Medicine* 341 (13): 1005.

Wehmeyer, M. L. 1993. "Sounding a Certain Trumpet: Case Management as a Catalyst for the Empowerment of People with Developmental Disabilities." *Journal of Case Management* 2: 14-18.

Welch, H.G., Wennberg, D.E. and Welch, W.P. 1996. "The Use of Medicare Home Health Care Services." *The New England Journal of Medicine* 335 (5): 324-29.

Wiener, J.M., Estes, C.L., Goldenson, S.M., and Goldberg, S.C. 2001. "What Happened to Long-Term Care in the Health Reform Debate of 1993-1994? Lessons for the Future." *The Milbank Quarterly* 79 (2): 207-252.

Wiener, J.M.and Cuellar, A.E. 1999. "Public and Private Responsibilities: Home and Community-Based Services in the United Kingdom and Germany." *Journal of Aging and Health* 11: 417.

Wiener, J.M. 1996. "Managed Care and Long-Term Care: The Integration of Financing and Services." *Generations* 20 (2): 47-52.

Williams G.H. and Wood, P.H. 1988. "Coming to Terms with Chronic Illness: The Negotiation of Autonomy in Rheumatoid Arthritis." *International Disability Studies* 10(3): 128-33.

Wilner, M.A. 2000. "Toward a Stable and Experienced Caregiving Workforce." *Generations* 24(3): 60-65.

Wilner, M.A. and Wyatt, A. 1998. "Independent Care System: Managed Care for People with Disabilities." *American Rehabilitation* 24(3): 2-5.

Winick, B.J. 1992. "On Autonomy: Legal and Psychological Perspectives." *Villanova Law Review* 37: 1705-1777.

Woodruff, L. and Applebaum, R.A. 1996. "Assuring the Quality of In-Home Supportive Services: A Consumer Perspective." *Journal of Aging Studies* 10(2), 157-169.

Wong, D. 2000. "Rapid Response: Development of a Home Care Worker Replacement Service." *Generations* 24(3): 88-90.

Yamada Y. 2001. "Profile of Home Care Aides, Nursing Home Aides, and Hospital Aides." *Gerontologist* 41: 395 Sp. Iss. 1.

Young, P.A. 1990. "Home Care Characteristics That Shape the Exercise of Autonomy: A View from the Trenches." *Generations* 14 (Supplement): 17-20.

Zola, I.K. 1982. "Social and Cultural Disincentives to Independent Living." *Archives of Physical Medicine and Rehabilitation* Aug; 63(8): 394-97.

Zimmerman, D.R. 1997-98. "The Power of Information: Using Resident Assessment Data to Assure and Improve Quality of Nursing Home Care." *Generations* 21(4): 52-56.

Index

128
Quality assurance, 160-179
 challenge of, 160-162
 defining and measuring quality,
 166-168
  enabling criteria, 167
  structure, process, and outcomes,
  166
 domains of quality care, 168--170
 twelve quality indicators, 168
 under independent living model,
 168-170
 market vs. regulation, 162-163
  market and medical model, 163-
  165
  market and independent living
  model, 165
 regulation - long-term care, 174-176
  nursing homes, 175
  of home health care, 176
  of institutional care, 175-176
  of personal assistance services,
  176-178
 stakeholders, 170-174
  consumers, 172-174
   satisfaction surveys, 173
  family members, 174
  payors, 172
  providers, 170-171
 total quality management (TQM)
 and continuous quality
 improvement (CQI), 178-179

-R-
Rapid response worker replacement
 system, 97
Recipient, 6
Rehabilitation act of 1973, section
 504, 47
Respite care, 65
Roberts, E.V., 45
Robert Wood Johnson Foundation,
 50

-S-
Security, 120-121
Self-direction, 242

Social security, 242
State institutions, 40
Surrogate, 65, 242

-T-
Terminology, 6
Three models of Long-term care, 70-86
 independent living model, 79-86
  consumers and providers under,
  82-84
  employer-related tasks, 80-81
  future of, 85-86
  payors under, 85
 informal support model, 70-74
  consumers and providers under,
  72-73
  consumers and providers under,76-
  77
  future of, 73-74
   medical model, 75-79
  future of, 78-79
  payers under, 77-78
  violation of medical practice act or
   nurse practice act, 71
 ranges of potential consumer direction and independence, 70
Title I of the Older Americans Act, 49
Total quality management (TQM),
 178-179

-U-
Unionization, 158
University of Illinois, 46
University of California at Berkeley,
 46
 Berkeley center for independent liv-
 ing, 46

-V-
Variations of the independent living
 model, 87-100
 Cash and counseling demonstra-
 tion, 93-97
  Arkansas independentchoices
  Program, 95-97
 Doty, Pamela, 94
 consumer-funded personal assis-

About the Author

Andrew I. Batavia, J.D., M.S., was a Professor at the School of Policy and Management of Florida International University. He formerly served in several key disability policy positions in the federal government, including Associate Director of the White House Domestic Policy Council, Legislative Assistant to U.S. Senator John McCain of Arizona, Special Assistant to U.S. Attorney General Dick Thornburgh, and Executive Director of the National Council on Disability. As a researcher and research administrator, he has served as Research Director for Disability and Rehabilitation Policy at Abt Associates and Associate Director of the National Rehabilitation Hospital Research Center. In 1990, Batavia was appointed a White House Fellow by President Bush, and helped the Department of Justice to promulgate the regulations for the Americans with Disabilities Act (ADA). He has authored two books and over 60 other publications on issues of disability policy. Batavia is a founding Associate Editor of the *Journal of Disability Policy Studies*, the founding President of AUTONOMY , Inc., and a member of the Bar of the U.S. Supreme Court, the State Bars of Florida, California and the District of Columbia, and Georgetown University's Kennedy Institute of Ethics.